EDITION 10

Manter and Gatz's Essentials of Clinical Neuroanatomy and Neurophysiology

EDITION 10

Manter and Gatz's Essentials of Clinical Neuroanatomy and Neurophysiology

Sid Gilman, MD, FRCP
William J. Herdman Professor and Chair
Department of Neurology
University of Michigan Medical School
Ann Arbor, Michigan

Sarah Winans Newman, PhD
Professor Emerita
Department of Anatomy and Cell Biology
University of Michigan Medical School
Courtesy Professor
Psychology Department
Cornell University
Ithaca, New York

Illustrations by Margaret Croup Brudon

F.A. Davis Publishers
Philadelphia

FIRST INDIAN EDITION 2009

As new scientific information becomes available through basic and clinical research, recommended treatments and drug therapies undergo changes. The authors and publisher have done everything possible to make this book accurate, up to date, and in accord with accepted standards at the time of publication. The authors, editors, and publisher are not responsible for errors or omissions or for consequences from application of the book, and make no warranty, expressed or implied, in regard to the contents of the book. Any practice described in this book should be applied by the reader in accordance with professional standards of care used in regard to the unique circumstances that may apply in each situation. The reader is advised always to check product information (package inserts) for changes and new information regarding dose and contraindications before administering any drug. Caution is especially urged when using new or infrequently ordered drugs.

Printed in India

Published by

Jitendar P Vij
Jaypee Brothers Medical Publishers (P) Ltd
B-3 EMCA House, 23/23B Ansari Road, Daryaganj
New Delhi 110 002, India
Phones: +91-11-23272143, +91-11-23272703, +91-11-23282021, +91-11-23245672
Rel: 32558559, Fax: +91-11-23276490, +91-11-23245683
e-mail: jaypee@jaypeebrothers.com
Visit our website: www.jaypeebrothers.com

Branches

- 2/B, Akruti Society, Jodhpur Gam Road Satellite
  Ahmedabad 380 015, Phones: +91-079-26926233 Rel: +91-079-32988717
  Fax: +91-079-26927094 e-mail: ahmedabad@jaypeebrother.com
- 202 Batavia Chambers, 8 Kumara Krupa Road, Kumara Park East,
  Bengaluru 560 001, Phones: +91-80-22285971, +91-80-22382956,
  Rel: +91-80-32714073, Fax: +91-80-22281761 e-mail: bangalore@jaypeebrothers.com
- 282 IIIrd Floor, Khaleel Shirazi Estate, Fountain Plaza, Pantheon Road,
  Chennai 600 008, Phones: +91-44-28193265, +91-44-28194897,
  Rel: +91-44-32972089, Fax: +91-44-28193231 e-mail: chennai@jaypeebrothers.com
- B-2, Sector - 4, Lekhraj Market, Faizabad Road, Indira Nagar
  Lucknow 226 016, Phones: +91-0522-3040553, +91-0522-3040554
  e-mail: lucknow@jaypeebrothers.com
- 4-2-1067/1-3, 1st Floor, Balaji Building, Ramkote Cross Road
  Hyderabad 500 095, Phones: +91-40-66610020, +91-40-24758498
  Rel:+91-40-32940929, Fax:+91-40-24758499 e-mail: hyderabad@jaypeebrother.com
- No. 41/3098, B & B1, Kuruvi Building, St. Vincent Road
  Kochi 682 018, Kerala, Phones: 0484-4036109, +91-0484-2395739, +91-0484-2395740
  e-mail: kochi@jaypeebrothers.com
- 1-A Indian Mirror Street, Wellington Square
  Kolkata 700 013, Phones: +91-33-22451926, +91-33-22276404, +91-33-22276415
  Rel: +91-33-32901926, Fax: +91-33-22456075 e-mail: kolkata@jaypeebrothers.com
- 106 Amit Industrial Estate, 61 Dr SS Rao Road, Near MGM Hospital, Parel
  Mumbai 400 012, Phones: +91-22-24124863, +91-22-24104532, Rel: +91-22-32926896
  Fax: +91-22-24160828 e-mail: mumbai@jaypeebrothers.com
- "KAMALPUSHPA" 38, Reshimbag, Opp. Mohota Science College, Umred Road
  Nagpur 440 009 (MS), Phones: Rel: 3245220, Fax: 0712-2704275
  e-mail: nagpur@jaypeebrothers.com

ISBN 978-81-8448-666-7

Printed by Sanat Printers, Kundli

Preface to the 10th Edition

In the six years since the ninth edition of this book was published, neuroscience has continued to progress at an astonishingly rapid rate. Moreover, the remarkable advances in basic neuroscience of the past three decades have been translated into clinical advances that have begun to change the management of many neurological diseases. We now have means of treating disorders that previously defied even symptomatic benefit. For example, we have an array of medications available for Parkinson's disease, epilepsy, stroke, sleep disorders, multiple sclerosis, migraine headache, and neuromuscular disorders such as myasthenia gravis, myositis, and peripheral neuropathy. We also have symptomatic treatments for Alzheimer's disease, and from the current pace of research in this disorder, it appears that preventive therapies will become available within the next decade. The armamentarium for diagnosis of neurological disorders has also advanced, including an array of imaging studies for examining the structure and function of the nervous system. These approaches have proved invaluable not only in the diagnosis of neurological disorders, but also in understanding some of the most complex functions of the normal brain.

We undertook the present revision to update the book scientifically. To this end, we added considerable new material concerning neuroanatomy, neurophysiology, and neuropharmacology, and yet attempted to keep the book short and succinct. To accomplish this, we shortened and consolidated some of the existing material, including the presentations of the structure and function of the brain stem and thalamus. We have rewritten literally every chapter. We changed many of the illustrations in keeping with the new information presented, and added several new illustrations.

We also added two new features in keeping with our longstanding aim of making the book relevant to clinical practice. We present a clinical case briefly at the beginning of many chapters to illustrate the practical utility of the information contained in that chapter. These real cases pose problems of localization of disease process, type of pathology causing the symptoms, and management of the patient. We present follow-up material on these cases at the end of the chapter. We also added magnetic resonance images taken from neurologically normal adult humans, both to illustrate structural relationships and to give our readers experience in viewing clinical imaging studies. Throughout the current revision we have emphasized physiological concepts within the context of the anatomic organization of the nervous system and pointed out the clinical relevance of the major anatomic structures. We kept the book focused on the student who seeks a brief, clinically oriented overview of neuroanatomy and neurophysiology that summarizes the material in more comprehensive textbooks. We intended the book to be helpful to house officers in neurology, neurosurgery, otolaryngology, psychiatry, and physical medicine and rehabilitation who wish to update their knowledge. We also provided an approach that will be useful to physical therapists, speech pathologists, and nurses.

Sid Gilman, MD, FRCP
Sarah Winans Newman, PhD

Acknowledgments: Consultants for the 10th Edition

We thank the colleagues listed below who graciously gave us their valuable time to review manuscript sections, suggest revisions, and advise us on appropriate references for updating this edition. We do not hold these individuals responsible for any material in the final revision of this book. The authors take full responsibility.

We give special thanks to the Department of Radiology of the University of Michigan and to Dr. Diana Gomez-Hassan, who not only contributed her time and expertise, but also selected the magnetic resonance images of neurologically normal individuals and prepared them for our use.

We also thank Margaret Croup Brudon, who revised some of her previous illustrations and provided new illustrations, all of which are superb.

Harold P. Adams, MD
Department of Neurology
University of Iowa Hospitals

James W. Albers, MD, PhD
Department of Neurology
University of Michigan Medical School

Roger L. Albin, MD
Department of Neurology
University of Michigan Medical School

Robert W. Baloh, MD
Reed Neurological Research Center
University of California, Los Angeles

Louis R. Caplan, MD
Department of Neurology
Beth Israel Deaconess Medical Center

Antonio R. Damasio, MD, PhD
Department of Neurology
University of Iowa

Norman L. Foster, MD
Department of Neurology
University of Michigan Medical School

Diana Gomez-Hassan, MD, PhD
Department of Radiology
University of Michigan Medical School

Susan Hickenbottom, MD
Department of Neurology
University of Michigan Medical School

Jaideep Kapur, MD, PhD
Department of Neurology
University of Virginia HSC

Golda Kevetter Leonard, PhD
Department of Otolaryngology
University of Texas Medical Branch, Galveston

Richard J. Krauzlis, PhD
Salk Institute

Allan I. Levey, MD, PhD
Department of Neurology
Emory University

William Z. Rymer, MD, PhD
Rehabilitation Institute of Chicago

Jeremy D. Schmahmann, MD
Department of Neurology
Massachusetts General Hospital

Steven Telian, MD
Department of Otolaryngology
University of Michigan Medical School

Roy Twyman, MD
R.W. Johnson Pharmaceutical Research Institute

Contents

Section 1 BASIC PRINCIPLES 1

Chapter 1 **Introduction to the Nervous System 1**

- Nerve Cells and Nerve Fibers 1
- Organization of Cells and Fibers in the Nervous System 3
- Functionally Defined Fiber Groups in the Peripheral Nerves 3
- Overview of the Gross Anatomy of the Nervous System 4
- Internal Anatomy of the Spinal Cord 9
- Development of the Nervous System 11

Chapter 2 **Physiology of Nerve Cells 15**

- Resting Membrane Potential 15
- Ion Channels Control Membrane Potential 16
- Action Potential 16
- Action Current 18
- Afterpotentials and Refractory Periods Follow the Action Potential 18
- Synapses 19
- Neuromuscular Junction 21

Section 2 PERIPHERAL NERVOUS SYSTEM 23

Chapter 3 **Fibers of the Spinal Nerves 23**

- Functional Classification 23
- Physiologic Classification 25

Chapter 4 **Spinal Reflexes and Muscle Tone 27**

- Spinal Reflexes 27
- Muscle Spindles 27
- Alpha, Beta, and Gamma Motoneurons of the Spinal Cord 29
- Stretch Reflex 30
- Golgi Tendon Organs and Their Reflexes 30
- Muscle Tone 31
- Reflexes of Cutaneous Origin 31

Chapter 5 **Autonomic Nervous System 33**

- The Autonomic Nervous System Has Two Divisions 33
- Sympathetic Nervous System 34
- Parasympathetic Nervous System 36
- Autonomic Innervation of the Genitourinary System 36
- Autonomic Reflexes of Other Pelvic Viscera 38

Section 3 ASCENDING AND DESCENDING PATHWAYS 41

Chapter 6 **Pain and Temperature 41**

- Somatic Sensation 41
- Overview of the Pathways for Pain, Thermal Sense, and Touch 42
- Dorsal Roots of the Spinal Nerves Supply Dermatomes 42
- Adjacent Spinal Nerves Form Peripheral Nerves 42
- Pain-Temperature Pathways 42
- Perception of Pain 47
- Temperature Sense 47
- Visceral Pain Pathways and Referred Pain 47
- Effect of Cutting the Spinothalamic Tract 48
- Sensory Effects of Dorsal Root Irritation 48
- Endogenous Analgesia 49
- Central Pain (Thalamic Syndrome) 49

Chapter 7 **Proprioception, Touch, and Tactile Discrimination 51**

- Central Nervous System Pathways 51
- Physiologic Aspects of Tactile Discrimination 57
- Effect of Spinal Cord Lesions on Touch Sensation 58

Chapter 8 **Motor Pathways 60**

- Motor Areas of the Cerebral Cortex 60

Descending Fibers from the Cerebral Cortex and Brain Stem Influence Motor Activity 61
Role of Lateral, Medial, and Propriospinal Pathways in Spinal Cord Function 66

Chapter 9 Lesions of the Peripheral Nerves, Spinal Nerve Roots, and Spinal Cord 68

Degeneration and Regeneration of Nerve Cells and Fibers after Injury 68
Clinical Consequences of Peripheral Nerve Lesions 69
Lower Motoneuron Lesions: Hypotonic Paralysis of Muscles 69
Lesions of Dorsal Roots 69
Upper Motoneuron Lesions: Spastic Paralysis of Muscles 70
Abnormal Reflexes Associated with Lesions of the Motor Pathway 72
Transection of the Spinal Cord 73
Hemisection of the Spinal Cord (Brown-Séquard Syndrome) 73
Lesions of the Central Gray Matter of the Spinal Cord 75
Lesions Involving the Ventral Horns and the Corticospinal Tracts 75
Lesions Involving Dorsal and Lateral Funiculi 75
Thrombosis of the Anterior Spinal Artery 75
Tumors of the Spinal Cord 76

Section 4 BRAIN STEM AND CEREBELLUM 77

Chapter 10 Organization of the Brain Stem and Cranial Nerves 77

Surface Anatomy of the Brain Stem 77
Internal Structures at the Transition from Spinal Cord to Brain Stem 82
Classification of Cranial Nerve Nuclei and Fibers according to their Functions 83
Functionally Distinct Cranial Nerve Cell Columns 84
Reticular Formation 86
Atlas of the Brain Stem: Transverse Sections 88
Blood Supply to the Brain Stem and Cerebellum 95

Chapter 11 Cranial Nerves of the Medulla 97

Hypoglossal Nerve (XII) 97
Accessory Nerve (XI) 97
Vagal System: Nervus Intermedius (VII), Glossopharyngeal (IX), Vagus (X) and Cranial Accessory (XI) Nerves 98

Chapter 12 Cranial Nerves of the Pons and Midbrain 104

Abducens Nerve (VI) 104
Trochlear Nerve (IV) 105
Oculomotor Nerve (III) 105
Facial Nerve (VII) 106
Trigeminal Nerve (V) 107

Chapter 13 Lesions of the Brain Stem 111

Principles of Localization 111
Lesions of the Medulla 112
Lesions of the Pons 114
Lesions of the Midbrain 116
Brain Stem Lesions Causing Coma and ''Locked-in'' Syndrome 118

Chapter 14 Hearing 119

Ear 119
Central Auditory Pathways 122
Diagnosing Hearing Deficits from Nerve Damage and from Conductive Defects 124
Auditory Reflexes 125

Chapter 15 Vestibular System 127

Vestibular Portion of the Inner Ear 127
Vestibular Nerve and Its Central Connections 129
Vestibulocerebellar Connections 130
Vestibulospinal Tracts 130
Vestibulo-ocular Systems 131
Vestibulothalamocortical Pathway 133
Sensory Aspects of Vestibular Stimulation 133

Chapter 16 Cerebellum 135

Overview of Cerebellar Function 135
Cerebellar Anatomy 135
Peduncles 139
Major Circuits 141
Integration of the Cerebellum and Cerebral Cortex in Movement and Cognition 143
Clinical Signs of Cerebellar Dysfunction 144
Diseases 145

Section 5 FOREBRAIN 147

Chapter 17 Basal Ganglia 147

Overview 147

Components 149
Connections of the Dorsal Striatum and Pallidum with the Cerebral Cortex 150
Connections of the Pallidum with the Brain Stem 154
Ventral Striatum and Pallidum 154
Function and Dysfunction 154

Chapter 18 Vision 158
Overview of the Visual Pathways 158
Retina 158
Visual Pathways 161
Information Processing in the Visual Pathways 163
Effects of Lesions Interrupting the Visual Pathway 164

Chapter 19 Optic Reflexes and Eye Movements 167
Light Reflexes 167
Reflexes Associated with the Near-Point Reaction 168
Disorders of Pupillary Function 168
Eye Movements 169

Chapter 20 Cerebral Cortex and Thalamocortical Connections 174
Cerebral Cortex 174
Cortical Cell Layers: The Basis for Structure and Function Relationships within and between Cortical Areas 174
Cortical Networks and Information Processing 177
Thalamus 177
Thalamocortical Connections 180
Functional Cortical Regions 182
Disorders of Cortical Networks 189

Chapter 21 Limbic System 193
Overview 193
Telencephalic Limbic System 193
Hypothalamus 197
Hypothalamic Functions 200
Epithalamus 202

Chapter 22 Olfaction 204
Olfactory Receptors 204
Olfactory Bulbs and Their Projections 204
Olfactory Cortical Areas 206
Damage to Olfactory Structures 206

Chapter 23 Chemical Neuroanatomy 207
Characteristics of Neurotransmitter Molecules 207
Functional Characterization of Neurotransmitter Receptors 207
Acetylcholine 208
Monoamines 209
Neuropeptides 214
Amino Acids 218

Section 6 CIRCULATION OF BLOOD AND CEREBROSPINAL FLUID 221

Chapter 24 Cerebral Arteries Supplying the Forebrain 221
Anterior Circulation 221
Internal Carotid Artery and Its Branches 221
Posterior Cerebral Artery and Its Branches 223
Formation of the Circle of Willis and Its Central Branches 225

Chapter 25 Cerebrospinal Fluid 227
Formation and Circulation 227
Composition and Function 228
Blood-Brain Barrier 229
Pressure 229

Section 7 APPROACHES TO PATIENTS WITH NEUROLOGIC SYMPTOMS 233

Chapter 26 Clinical Evaluation of Neurologic Disorders 233
Patient History 234
Physical Examination 236
Neurologic Examination 236

Chapter 27 Neurologic Diagnostic Tests 241
Cerebrospinal Fluid Analysis 241
Electroencephalography and Evoked-Potential Studies 242
Nerve Conduction Studies, Electromyography, and Muscle and Nerve Biopsy 243
Anatomic Imaging Studies 244
Physiologic Imaging Studies 245

Suggested Readings 247

Index 249

SECTION 1

Basic Principles

1

Introduction to the Nervous System

Nerve Cells and Nerve Fibers

The **neuron** (nerve cell) constitutes the primary functional and anatomic unit of the nervous system. All neurons consist of a **cell body** (perikaryon) containing a nucleus and surrounding cytoplasm. From the cell body extend one to several dozen processes (fibers) of varying lengths (Fig. 1–1A, B).

Dendrites consist of **afferent** neuronal processes with branches that **receive signals.** Usually, the signals consist of chemicals acting as **neurotransmitters** that interact with specific molecular receptors in the membrane of the dendrite at chemical **synapses** with other neurons (Fig. 1–1C). These signals transiently alter the electrochemical gradient across the membrane of the dendritic process, and this transient change moves along the dendrites.

The **axon (axis cylinder)** of a nerve cell consists of a single fiber extending to other parts of the nervous system or to a muscle or gland. The term **axon** applies to a fiber that **conducts impulses** (actively propagated electrochemical changes called **action potentials**) away from the dendrites; thus, an axon is an **efferent** fiber or process. At its end, branches of the axon make synaptic contact with other neurons (Fig. 1–1C) or with muscle fibers (Fig. 1–1D).

Most neurons in the mammalian nervous system have a **multipolar** configuration (i.e., have many processes, like neurons A and B in Fig. 1–1). In these neurons, the cell body lies between the dendrites and the axon. In some specialized neurons, however, the dendritic branches attach directly to the axon, and the cell body sits on a process (or **stalk**) near the end of the axon. These are **pseudounipolar** cells (e.g., the dorsal root ganglion cells described in Chapter 3).

Myelinated and Unmyelinated Fibers

Many nerve fibers in the brain, spinal cord, and peripheral nerves have a **myelin sheath,** but only peripheral nerve fibers have, in addition, a **neurolemma (sheath of Schwann)** outside the

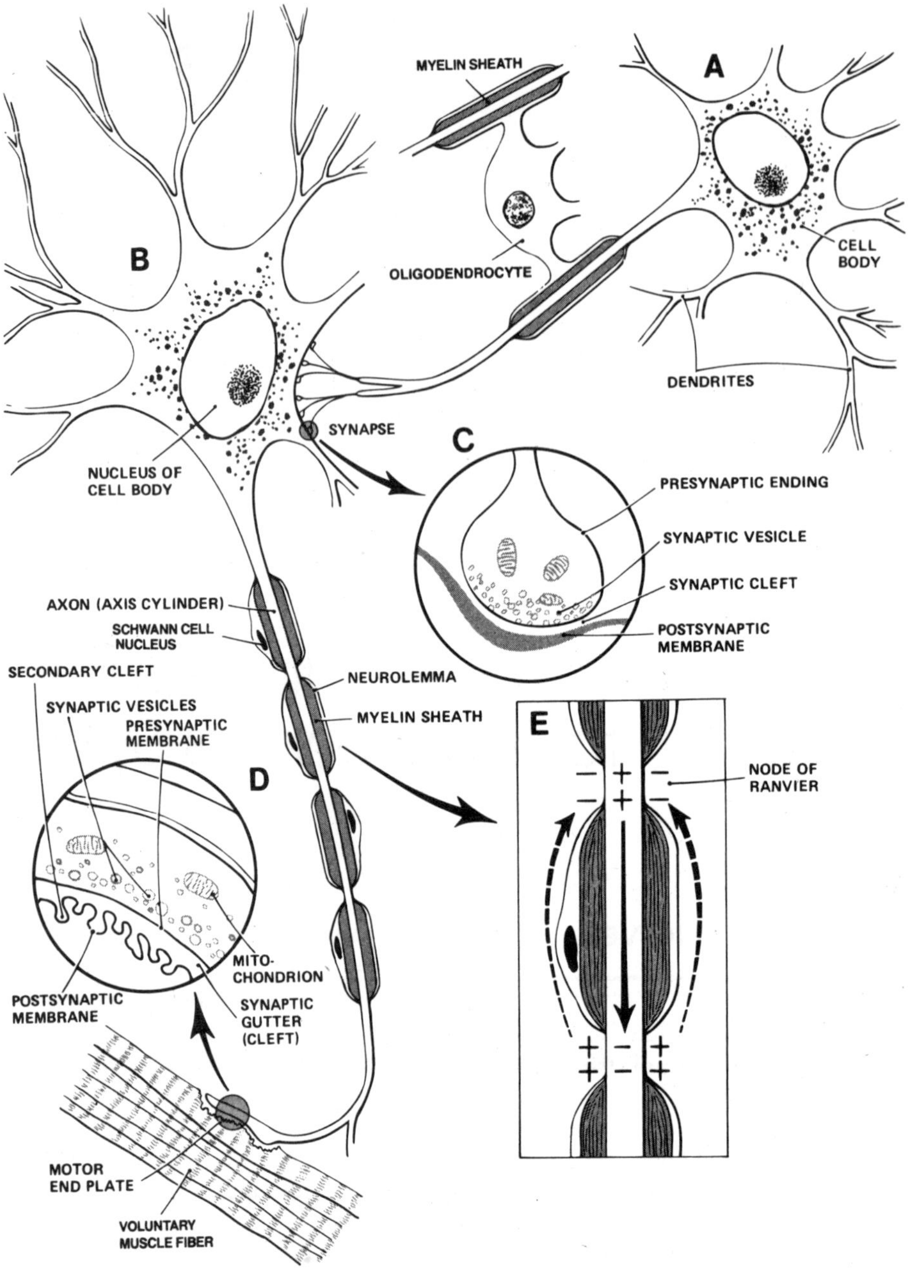

■ **FIGURE 1-1.** **(A** to **E)** Neurons with cell bodies in the central nervous system (CNS). Neuron **A** is confined to the CNS and terminates on neuron **B** at a typical chemical synapse **(C).** Neuron **B** is a motor neuron; its axon extends to a peripheral nerve and innervates a striated (voluntary) muscle at the neuromuscular junction (motor end plate, **D**). In **E,** the action potential is moving in the direction of the *solid arrow* inside the axon; the *dashed arrows* indicate the direction of flow of the action current.

myelin. The myelin of peripheral neurons consists of a spiral wrapping of many layers of cell membranes from the same **Schwann cell** that forms the neurolemma on the outside. The neurolemma constitutes the cell body (nucleus and cytoplasm) of the Schwann cell (see neuron B in Fig. 1–1). Each Schwann cell contributes myelin to one segment (or internode) of a myelinated axon. Between two adjacent myelinated segments lies a small gap called the **node of Ranvier** (Fig. 1–1E). **Unmyelinated fibers** are enfolded into simple cytoplasmic processes of nearby Schwann cells. No layering of cell membranes occurs around unmyelinated fibers. The myelinated fibers in the white matter of the brain and spinal cord possess a myelin sheath but have no neurolemma because their myelin sheaths consist of the cytoplasmic extensions of **oligodendrocytes.** These cytoplasmic extensions radiate away from the cell body of the oligodendrocyte, and each extension contributes myelin to a nearby axon (Fig. 1–1A).

Organization of Cells and Fibers in the Nervous System

Groups of Nerve Cell Bodies Form Ganglia, Nuclei, and Cortical Areas

Nerve cell bodies usually cluster together in groups. Outside the brain and spinal cord, these groups are called the **ganglia** of the **peripheral nervous system** (PNS). Within the brain and spinal cord, which make up the **central nervous system** (CNS), neurons form groups of various sizes and shapes known as nuclei. In this instance, the term **nucleus** has a meaning different from that of the nucleus of an individual cell. The layers (or **laminae**) of nerve cell bodies on the surface of the cerebrum and cerebellum comprise the cerebral **cortex** and cerebellar cortex.

Gray Matter and White Matter of the Central Nervous System

Regions of the brain and spinal cord that contain aggregations of nerve cell bodies (nuclei and cortex) constitute the **gray matter,** so called for its color in the fresh state. In gray matter, the ramifications of the dendrites and the terminal branches of axons that make synapses with the dendrites surround the neuron cell bodies. This delicate network surrounding the neuron cell bodies is known as **neuropil.** Areas of the brain and spinal cord that consist primarily of myelinated axons compose the **white matter.**

Fiber Bundles in the Central and Peripheral Nervous Systems

In the CNS, groups of axons that have a common origin (i.e., cell bodies in the same nucleus) and a common destination (axonal endings in the same area of gray matter) constitute a **tract.** Although a tract occupies a definable position, it does not always form a segregated bundle because some intermingling occurs with fibers of neighboring tracts. Anatomically distinct bundles of fibers in the brain have been given names such as **fasciculus, brachium, peduncle, column,** or **lemniscus.** These structures may contain only a single tract, or they may consist of several tracts running together in the same bundle. Outside the brain and spinal cord, in the PNS, the terms **nerve, nerve root, nerve trunk, nerve cord,** and **ramus** refer to specific bundles of nerve fibers.

Glial Cells

The CNS contains three types of nonneuronal cells called neuroglia or **glial cells:** oligodendrocytes, astrocytes, and microglia. **Oligodendrocytes** form and maintain the myelin sheaths of axons in the CNS (Fig. 1–1A). **Astrocytes** contribute in a variety of important ways to the metabolism of the CNS. They cannot develop action potentials, but they are highly permeable to potassium ions (K^+) and become depolarized if the extracellular concentration of K^+ increases. Astrocytes take up extracellular K^+ during intense neuronal activity and thereby buffer K^+ concentration in the extracellular space. They also take up and store neurotransmitters and thus may regulate extracellular concentrations of neurotransmitters. In addition, they transfer metabolites from capillaries to the extracellular space. Astrocytes are sensitive to many different insults to CNS tissue. Depending on the noxious agent, astrocytes may respond to injury with cytoplasmic swelling, accumulation of glycogen, fibrillar proliferation within the cytoplasm, cell multiplication, or a combination of these reactions. They frequently form a permanent scar or plaque after destruction of neuronal elements has occurred. **Microglia** are phagocytic cells that form part of the nervous system's defense against infection and injury. The glia of the PNS are the myelin-producing **Schwann cells** (Fig. 1–1B) and the **satellite cells** that are found in ganglia associated with the peripheral nerves.

Functionally Defined Fiber Groups in the Peripheral Nerves

The 12 pairs of **cranial nerves** and 31 pairs of **spinal nerves,** with their associated ganglia, compose the human PNS. The two types of motor (or **efferent**) fibers of peripheral nerves are **somatic motor fibers,** which terminate in **skeletal muscle,** and **visceral motor (or autonomic) fibers,** which innervate **cardiac muscle, smooth muscle, glands,** and **adipose tissue (fat).** The termination of a somatic motor fiber on a skeletal muscle fiber occurs at the **motor end plate** or **neuromuscular junction,** which resembles a synapse (Fig. 1–1D). The transmitter released by the vesicles at the motor end plate is acetylcholine.

The sensory (or **afferent**) nerve fibers of the PNS transmit signals from sensory receptors of various types. Each afferent fiber conducts impulses toward the spinal cord or brain from the particular sensory receptors (e.g., touch, pain, auditory, taste) with which it is connected. **Somatic sensory fibers** arise in sensory receptors of the body wall (skin, muscle, and bone), whereas **visceral sensory fibers** arise in the internal organs and in the walls of blood vessels throughout the body.

Overview of the Gross Anatomy of the Nervous System

The CNS consists of the brain and the spinal cord. The brain of a young man averages 1380 g in weight, and the brain of a young woman averages 100 g less. The adult brain is divided into three gross parts: the **cerebrum,** the **cerebellum,** and the **brain stem.**

Cerebral Hemispheres Are Divided into Six Lobes

A deep medial longitudinal fissure separates the left and right cerebral hemispheres. The surface of each hemisphere is wrinkled by the presence of eminences, known as **gyri,** and furrows, which are called **sulci** or **fissures.** The **cerebral cortex** consists of a layer of gray matter that varies from 1.3 to 4.5 mm in thickness and covers the expansive surface of the cerebral hemisphere. This cortex is estimated to contain 14 billion nerve cells.

Two major grooves are found on the lateral surface of the brain (Fig. 1–2). The **lateral fissure (of Sylvius)** begins as a deep cleft on the basal surface of the brain and extends laterally, posteriorly, and upward. The **central sulcus (of Rolando)** runs from the dorsal border of the hemisphere near its midpoint obliquely downward and forward until it nearly meets the lateral fissure. For descriptive purposes, the lateral surface of the hemisphere is divided into four lobes, and each of these lobes is composed of numerous gyri (Fig. 1–2). The **frontal lobe** (approximately the anterior one-third of the hemisphere) is the portion that is rostral (anterior) to the central sulcus and above the lateral fissure. The **occipital lobe** is that part lying behind, or caudal to, an arbitrary line drawn from the **parieto-occipital fissure** to the **preoccipital notch.** This lobe occupies a small area of the lateral surface but has more extensive territory on the medial aspect of the hemisphere (Fig. 1–3), where it includes all cortex posterior to the parieto-occipital fissure. The **parietal lobe** extends from the central sulcus to the parieto-occipital fissure and, on the lateral surface, is separated from the **temporal lobe** below by an imaginary line projecting from the horizontal portion of the lateral fissure to the middle of the line demarcating the occipital lobe. The gyri within each lobe are named, as illustrated in Figures 1–2, 1–3, and 1–6, but their patterns show considerable individual variation. Figure 1–3 depicts the structures that are located on the medial (midsagittal) surface of the brain. This surface is exposed by cutting the brain in half on a plane through the medial longitudinal fissure. This cut severs the **corpus callosum, diencephalon, brain stem,** and **cerebellum,** and it exposes a portion of the ventricular system within the brain (Fig. 1–4). On the medial surface of the cerebral cortex, the gyri and sulci of the frontal, parietal, occipital, and temporal lobes are continuous with those seen on the lateral surface. The central sulcus sometimes extends a short distance over the dorsal crest of the hemisphere onto the medial side and thus marks the boundary between the frontal and parietal lobes. The parieto-occipital fissure, as its name implies, separates the parietal and occipital lobes. Only the temporal pole region of the temporal lobe can be seen on this medial section through the whole brain. Gyri on the ventral surface of the temporal lobe and the frontal lobe are shown on Figure 1–6.

With the brain cut in the midsagittal plane (Fig 1–3) and on the corresponding magnetic resonance image (Fig. 1–5), part of the fifth lobe can be seen on the cerebral cortex. This is the **limbic lobe,** a ring (or limbus) of cortical tissue consist-

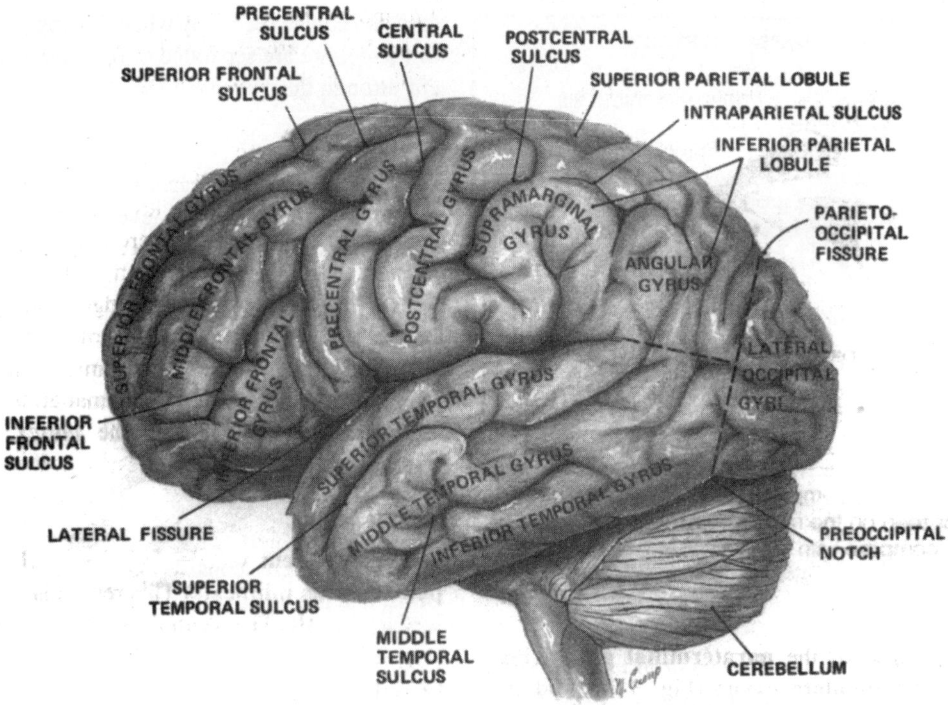

■ **FIGURE 1–2.** Lateral view of the left cerebral hemisphere, cerebellum, and brain stem.

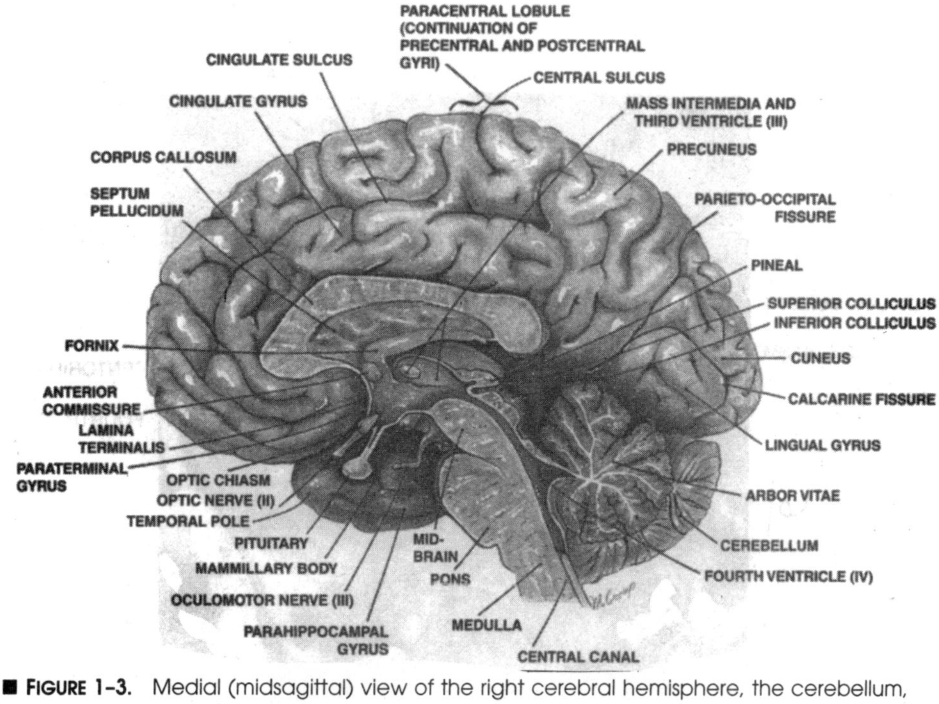

■ **FIGURE 1–3.** Medial (midsagittal) view of the right cerebral hemisphere, the cerebellum, and the brain stem of a hemisected brain.

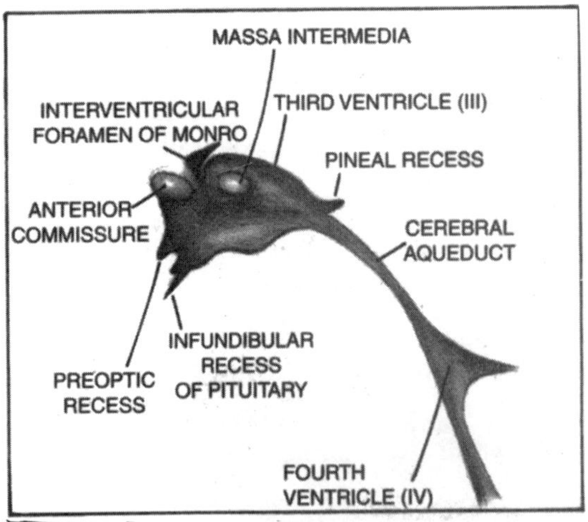

■ **FIGURE 1–4.** Components of the ventricular system as seen on the midsagittal section of the brain (compare with Fig. 1–3).

ing primarily of the **paraterminal gyrus** (Fig. 1–3), the **cingulate gyrus** (Fig. 1–3), and the **parahippocampal gyrus** (Fig. 1–6), which is partially hidden by the cerebellum and brain stem. The full limbic lobe can been seen in Figure 20–3.

A sixth lobe, the **insular lobe,** cannot be seen in any of these figures. It consists of the cortical tissue that forms the floor of the deep lateral fissure and can be seen only when the lips (opercula) of this fissure are separated or on coronal sections cut through the brain (see Fig. 17–1).

Cerebellum

The **cerebellum** is attached to the dorsal surface of the brain stem at the level of the pons. Its surface, like that of the cerebral hemispheres, consists of a layer of gray matter, the **cerebellar cortex,** which is arranged in ridges and grooves. In the cerebellum, the ridges of cortical gray matter are called **folia.** On the midsagittally cut brain (Fig. 1–3), a core of white matter, the **arbor vitae,** can be seen under the cortex of the cerebellar folia.

Brain Stem

The **brain stem** consists of the **medulla,** the **pons,** and the **midbrain.** This region is described in Chapter 10. The ventral surface of the brain (Fig. 1–6) shows the 12 pairs of cranial nerves (I to XII) exiting from the brain. All but pairs I (olfactory) and II (optic) attach to the brain stem.

Ventricles, Meninges, and Cerebrospinal Fluid

Cavities within the brain, called the **ventricles,** are filled with **cerebrospinal fluid** (CSF) (Figs.

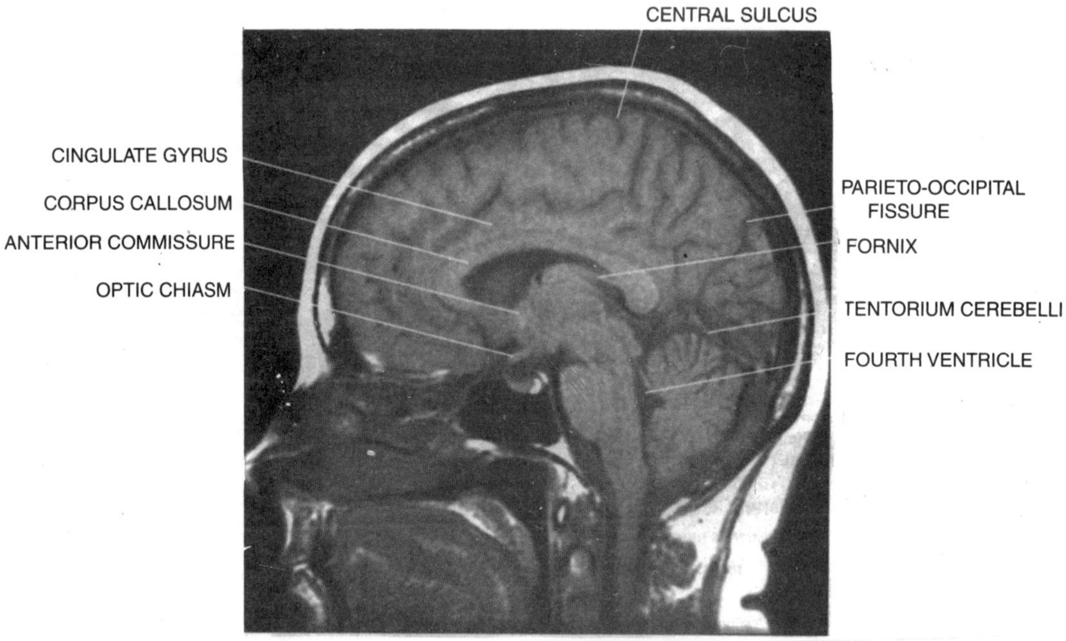

■ **FIGURE 1–5.** Magnetic resonance image (T1-weighted sequence) of a normal brain in the midsagittal plane (compare with Figs. 1–3 and 25–1).

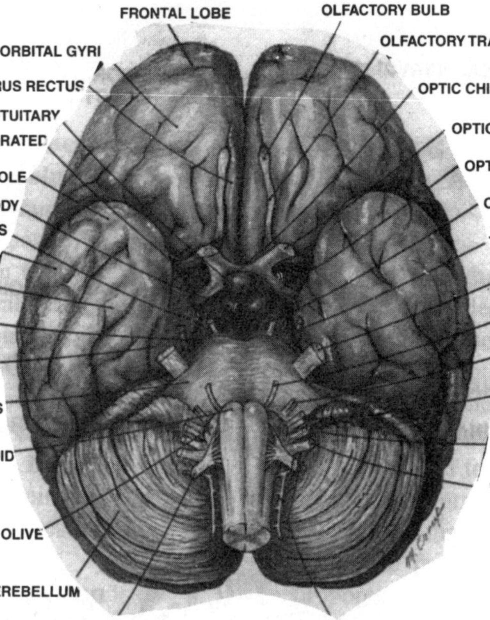

■ **FIGURE 1–6.** Ventral surface of the brain.

1–3 to 1–5; also see Fig. 25–1). Specialized tissue inside the ventricles called the **choroid plexus** produces the CSF. The ventricular system opens to the space outside of the brain at three sites in the medulla. Through these three openings, CSF flows from the ventricles into the **subarachnoid space,** which surrounds the brain and spinal cord. This space is located between the pia mater and the arachnoid, two layers of the three connective-tissue membranes that enclose the **CNS.** The **pia mater** is intimately attached to the surface of the brain and spinal cord. Fine strands of connective tissue, the trabeculae, stretch across the subarachnoid space between the pia mater and the **arachnoid.** Outside the arachnoid, the tough **dura mater** lines the bony cranial cavity around the brain and the vertebral canal around the spinal cord. Together, the pia mater, arachnoid, and dura mater constitute the meninges. Additional details on the meninges and CSF can be found in Chapter 25.

Spinal Cord

The human **spinal cord** consists of a slender cylinder less than 2 cm in diameter. It is closely surrounded by the pia mater and is anchored through the arachnoid to the dura mater by paired lateral septa of pia. These septa are called the **denticulate ligaments.** From its rostral junction with the medulla to its caudal end, the spinal cord is divided arbitrarily into five regions: **cervical, thoracic, lumbar, sacral,** and **coccygeal.** Enlargements in the lower cervical region and in the lumbosacral region contain the cell bodies of nerve fibers supplying the upper and lower limbs.

Spinal Nerve Roots and Spinal Nerves

Spinal nerves are attached to the spinal cord in pairs: 8 cervical pairs, 12 thoracic pairs, 5 lumbar pairs, 5 sacral pairs, and 1 coccygeal pair (Fig. 1–7). The union of a **dorsal root,** composed of sensory or afferent fibers, and a **ventral root,** composed mostly of motor or efferent fibers, forms each nerve. The sensory fibers of the dorsal roots are processes of sensory neuron cell bodies in the **dorsal root ganglia.** The motor fibers in the ventral root are axons of neuron cell bodies in the spinal cord (see Fig. 3–1). The spinal cord does not extend to the lowest level of the bony vertebral canal, but rather ends at the level of the lower border of the first lumbar vertebra. Its tapered end is called the **conus medullaris.** The pia mater continues caudally as a connective-tissue filament, the **filum terminale,** which passes through the subarachnoid space to the end of the dural sac at the level of vertebra S1 (Fig. 1–7), where it receives a covering of dura and continues to its attachment to the coccyx. Because the spinal cord is about 25 cm shorter than the vertebral column, the lower segments of the

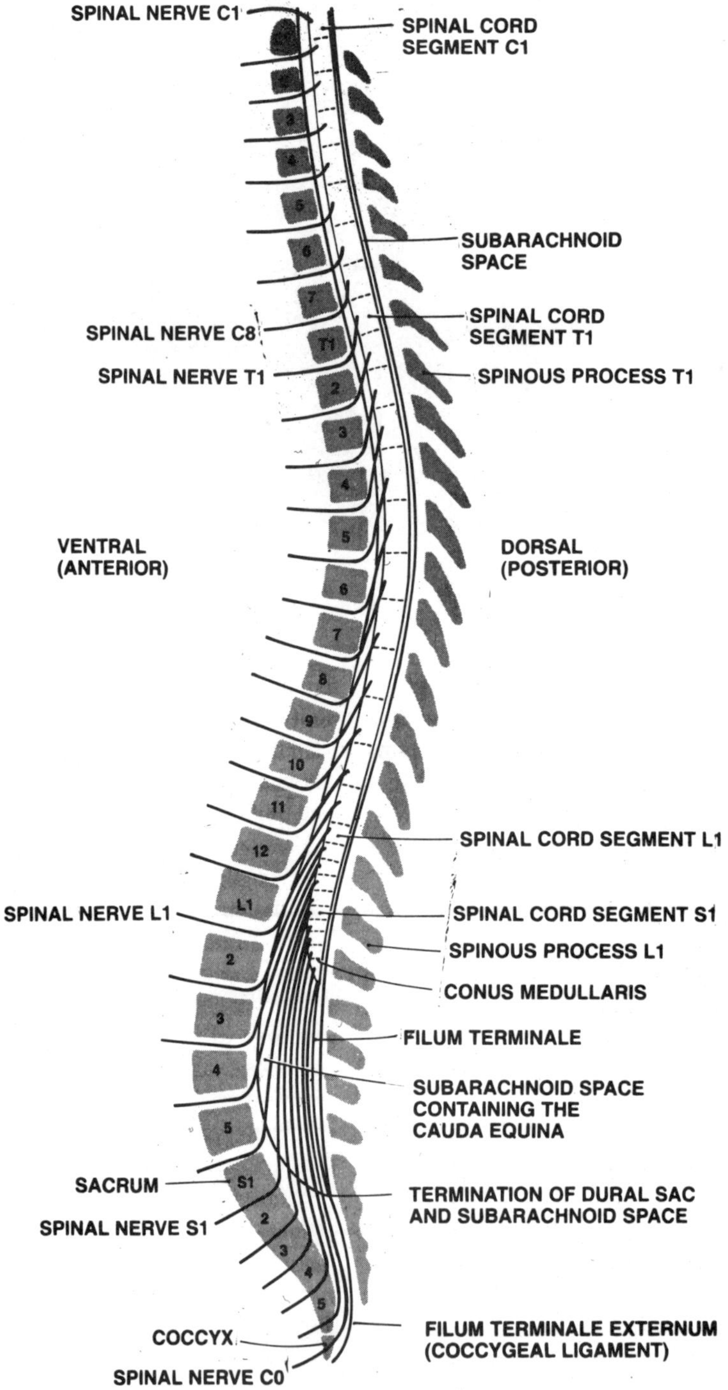

■ **FIGURE 1-7.** Diagram of the relation of the spinal cord segments and spinal nerve roots to the dural sac and vertebrae of the spinal column. The bodies of the individual vertebrae on the ventral side of the spinal cord are numbered. The spinous processes of the vertebrae are dorsal to the spinal cord. The dural sac, filum terminale, and filum terminale externum (coccygeal ligament), which are all connective-tissue structures, are shown in color.

spinal cord are not aligned opposite corresponding vertebrae. Thus, the lumbar and sacral spinal nerves have very long roots, extending from their respective segments in the spinal cord to the lumbar and sacral **intervertebral foramina,** which are openings in the bony vertebral canal. At each intervertebral foramen, a dorsal root and a ventral root join to form a **spinal nerve.** The spinal nerve roots descending in a bundle from the conus resemble the tail of a horse, and thus this formation is known as the **cauda equina.**

Internal Anatomy of the Spinal Cord

In describing the spinal cord, the terms **posterior** and **dorsal** are used interchangeably. Similarly, the terms **anterior** and **ventral** are interchangeable. Sections of the spinal cord cut perpendicular (i.e., transverse) to the length of the cord reveal a butterfly-shaped area of gray matter surrounded by white matter (Fig. 1–8).

The White Matter Is Divided into Funiculi

The white matter consists mainly of nerve fibers that run longitudinally through the spinal cord and therefore are cut in cross section in a transverse section of the cord. Midline grooves on the dorsal and ventral surfaces are known as the **dorsal median sulcus** and the **ventral median fissure.** The lateral surface shows a **dorsolateral sulcus** and a **ventrolateral sulcus,** which correspond to the dorsal root zone and the ventral root zone, respectively. These markings divide the white matter of the spinal cord into **dorsal, lateral,** and **ventral funiculi.** The dorsal root zone is interposed between the dorsal and lateral funiculi, and the ventral root zone lies between the lateral and ventral funiculi.

The ratio of white matter to gray matter in the spinal cord varies systematically from its rostral end to its caudal end. This ratio is much greater at cervical levels than in the lumbosacral region (Fig. 1–8). This is because the white matter in the cervical region contains fibers connecting the entire spinal cord with the brain (i.e., fibers passing through that region to and from lower levels, as well as fibers arising or terminating in the cervical region). In contrast, the white matter of the lumbosacral cord contains only fibers serving the caudal end of the spinal cord.

The Gray Matter Is Divided into Horns

The gray matter of the spinal cord contains dorsal and ventral areas known as the **dorsal horns** and the **ventral horns.** Small **lateral horns** also are found in the thoracic and upper lumbar segments of the spinal cord (see segment T5 in Fig. 1–8). The ventral horns are larger in the cervical and lumbosacral enlargements of the spinal cord than in the thoracic segments. This is because the muscle mass of the limbs is greater than that of the trunk, and these horns are made up largely of cell bodies of neurons that innervate skeletal muscles. Accordingly, the ventral horn of the lumbosacral enlargement is more massive than that of the cervical enlargement because of the greater muscle mass in the lower limbs.

Nuclei, Cell Columns, and Laminae within the Horns of the Spinal Cord

In a transverse section of the spinal cord, the gray matter can be subdivided into groups of neuronal cell bodies that are called **nuclei** (left side of Fig. 1–9). When the spinal cord is cut along its length, these nuclei are seen to be longitudinal **cell columns.** They can also be viewed as distinctive layers or laminae, arranged from dorsal to ventral within the gray matter. Rexed divided the cord into 10 laminae (Fig. 1–9, right side). Each **lamina** extends the length of the cord. Lamina I is the most dorsal part of the dorsal horn, lamina IX is the most ventral part of the ventral horn, and lamina X surrounds the central canal.

Laminae I through VI are confined to the dorsal horn. Cells in these laminae receive and transmit information concerning sensory input from the spinal nerve afferents. Fiber pathways from other spinal cord levels and the brain also synapse on cells in these laminae. Within laminae I to VI are found several classically defined nuclei or cell columns of the spinal cord. For example, lamina II corresponds to the **substantia gelatinosa,** which receives information from pain and temperature afferents. Functions and connections of the cells of laminae I through VI are described in Chapters 6 and 7.

Lamina VII is located in the intermediate gray area and extends into the anterior horn. It contains

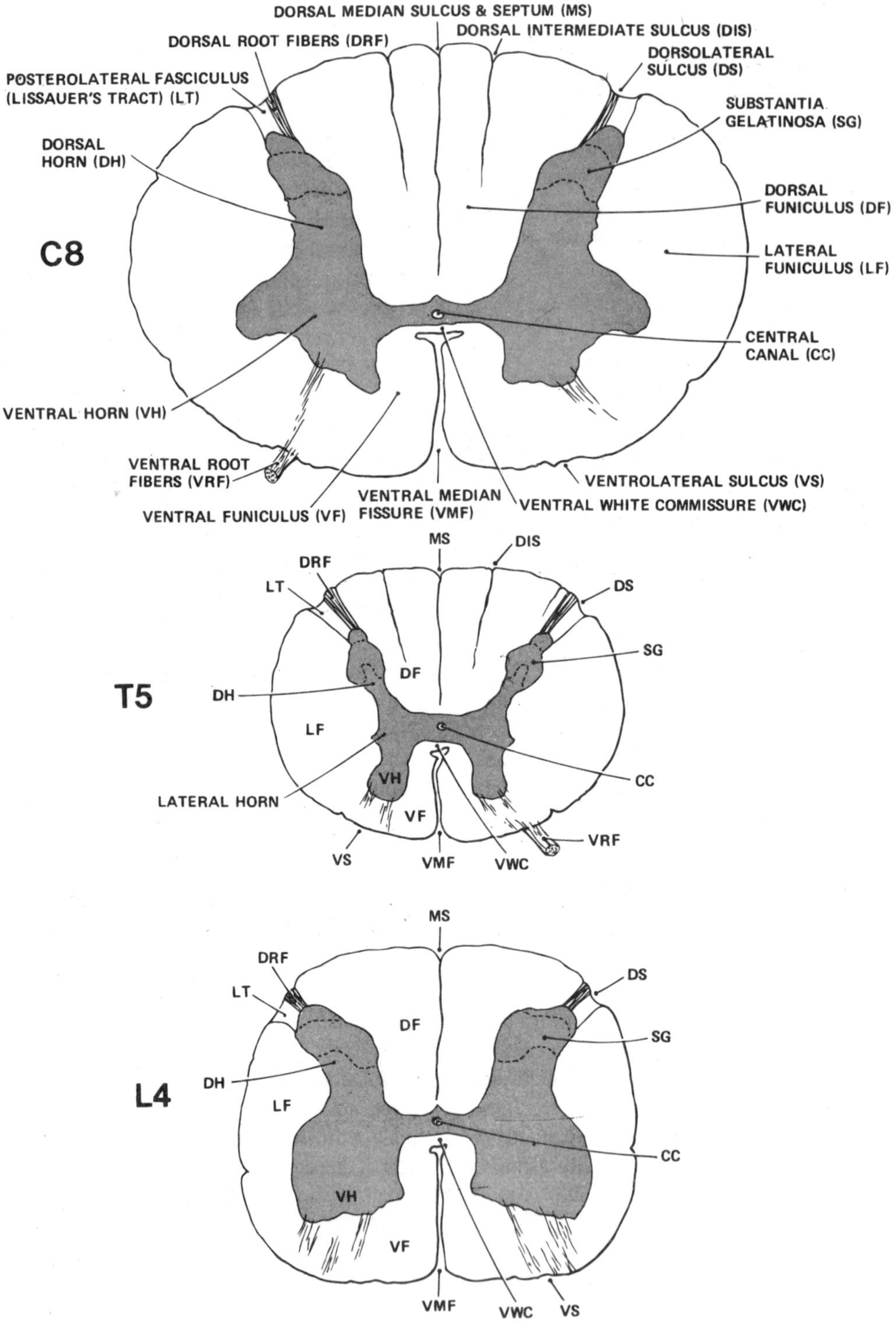

■ **FIGURE 1-8.** Transverse sections of the human spinal cord at approximately the eighth cervical (C8), fifth thoracic (T5), and fourth lumbar (L4) segmental levels.

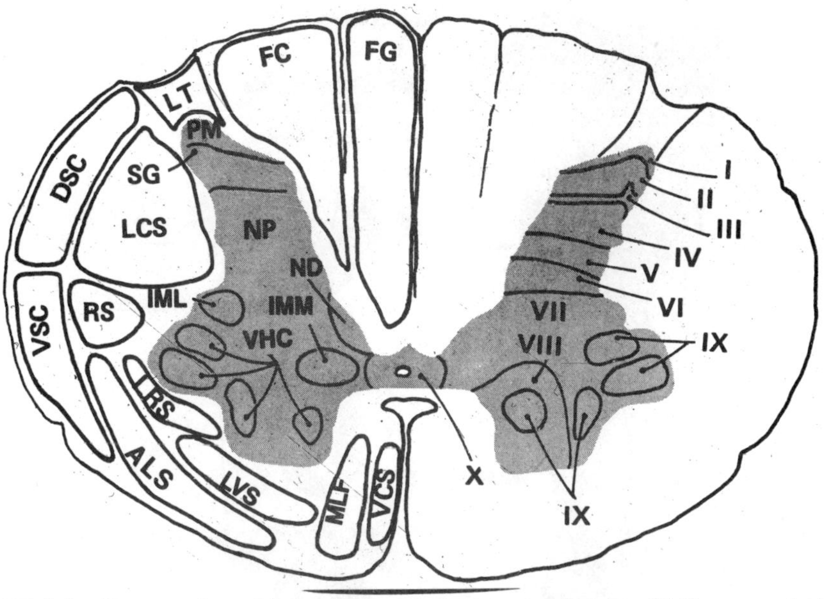

■ **FIGURE 1-9.** Cross section of the spinal cord at approximately the C8-T1 segmental level. Tracts and nuclei of the spinal cord are illustrated on the *left;* Rexed's laminar organization of the gray matter is illustrated on the *right.* ALS = anterolateral system; DSC = dorsal spinocerebellar tract; FC = fasciculus cuneatus; FG = fasciculus gracilis; IML = intermediolateral cell column; IMM = intermediomedial cell column; LCS = lateral corticospinal tract; LRS = lateral reticulospinal tract; LT = Lissauer's tract; LVS = lateral vestibulospinal tract; MLF = medial longitudinal fasciculus; ND = nucleus dorsalis; NP = nucleus proprius; PM = posteromarginal nucleus; RS = rubrospinal tract; SG = substantia gelatinosa; VCS = ventral corticospinal tract; VHC = ventral horn cell columns; VSC = ventral spinocerebellar tract.

the **nucleus dorsalis** and the **intermediolateral** and **intermediomedial cell columns.** The connections and functions of the nucleus dorsalis are described in Chapter 7, and those of the other two cell groups are described in Chapter 5. Lamina VIII is located in the ventral horn and contains many neurons that send **commissural axons** to the opposite side of the spinal cord. Lamina IX is restricted to the ventral horn and consists of several different columns of cells. Each of these cell columns contains **alpha, beta,** and **gamma motoneurons,** which send their axons into the ventral roots of the spinal nerves and innervate skeletal muscles.

Development of the Nervous System

Neural Tube

The adult human nervous system originates in the ectoderm of the embryo. Initially, a rostrocaudal groove appears in the midline of the embryonic ectoderm. This **neural groove** is flanked by **neural folds,** which then close to form a **neural tube** (Fig. 1–10). The rostral end of this tube develops into the brain, and the remainder differentiates into the spinal cord. The tube closes first at the level destined to become the upper cervical region of the spinal cord. From this point, closure proceeds both rostrally and caudally. The final closure at the ends of the tube, at the **anterior and posterior neuropores,** normally occurs during the fourth week of embryonic life. Thus, the final form of the early CNS consists of a hollow tube that is closed at both ends. Partial or complete failure of closure of the posterior neuropore results in **spina bifida,** a common developmental abnormality.

The tissue comprising the neural tube contains several different types of cells. **Neuroblasts,** the primordial neurons, and **glioblasts,** the primordial astrocytes and oligodendrocytes, compose most of this structure. The single layer of cells lining the tube later becomes the **ependyma,** which lines the ventricles of the adult brain.

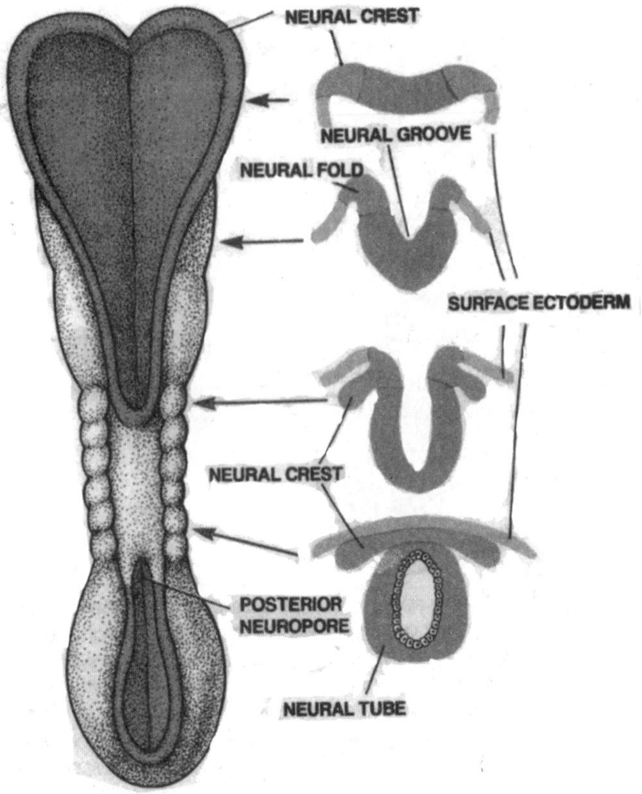

■ **FIGURE 1–10.** (*Left*) A dorsal view of the central nervous system (CNS) in a human embryo at the end of the third week of development. (*Right*) Histologic sections through the CNS at the levels of the *arrows*.

Neural Crest and Ectodermal Placodes

Ectodermal tissue lateral to the neural tube constitutes the **neural crest** (Fig. 1–10). It is a collection of cells that differentiate into the neurons and glia of the PNS, as well as a variety of nonneural structures including melanocytes, chromaffin cells of the adrenal medulla, and mesenchymal derivatives in the head. Elements derived from the neural crest ultimately give rise to autonomic ganglia and most of the sensory ganglia of the body and head (Fig. 1–11C; also see Fig. 3–1), as well as glial cells of the PNS.

Other sources of neural structures in the embryo are the **epidermal (sensory) placodes.** Along with the neural crest, these paired placodes contribute to the developing sense organs and sensory ganglia of the head. For example, the nasal placodes and otic placodes are precursors of the olfactory epithelium and the auditory and vestibular receptors and ganglia, respectively.

Development of the Brain and Spinal Cord from the Neural Tube

External Development from Tube to Three-Vesicle and Five-Vesicle Brain

Development of the brain begins with differentiation of three swellings, or **vesicles,** at the rostral end of the neural tube: the **prosencephalon,** the **mesencephalon,** and the **rhombencephalon** (Fig. 1–11A, B). This stage quickly proceeds to a five-vesicle stage of development in which the brain consists of the embryonic **telencephalon, diencephalon, mesencephalon, metencephalon,** and **myelencephalon** (Fig. 1–11C, D). The first three of these vesicles eventually differentiate into the cerebral hemispheres, the diencephalon (including the thalamus and hypothalamus), and the midbrain, respectively. The metencephalon becomes the cerebellum and pons, whereas the embryonic myelencephalon becomes the medulla oblongata. This basic arrangement of five vesicles

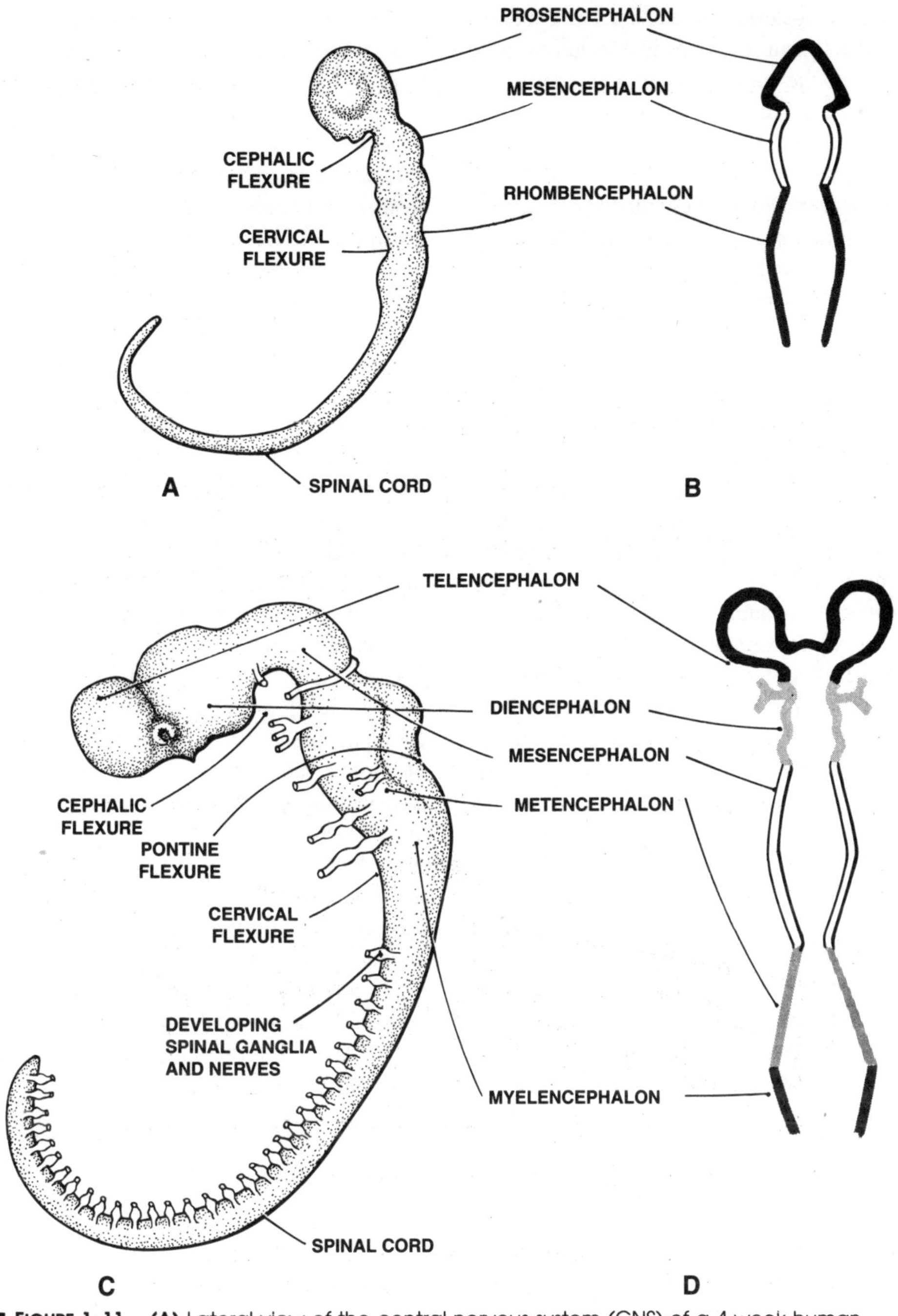

■ **FIGURE 1-11.** **(A)** Lateral view of the central nervous system (CNS) of a 4-week human embryo. **(B)** Dorsal view of a section through the three-vesicle brain in **A.** **(C)** Lateral view of the CNS and sensory ganglia in a 6-week human embryo. **(D)** Dorsal view of a section through the five-vesicle brain in **C.**

is established by the time the embryo is 6 weeks of age. Thereafter, the major change in form that produces the adult human brain consists of a tremendous growth of the cerebral hemispheres and cerebellum relative to other parts of the brain.

Internal Development of Functionally Defined Cell Groups

The internal development of the embryonic neural tube proceeds with differentiation of cell groups both in the medial-lateral dimension and in the anterior-posterior dimension. The development of medial neuron groups is directed by gene expression in the underlying mesendoderm: by the notochord posteriorly (in the region of the future spinal cord and brain stem) and by the prechordal plate anteriorly (the future diencephalon and telencephalon). These medial cell groups form the ventral neurons, or **basal plate,** which is a **motor** cell column, such as the ventral horn of the spinal cord. The development of the lateral neuron cell groups, which become **alar plate** structures, is influenced by gene expression in adjacent nonneural ectoderm. These lateral neuron groups will assume largely **sensory and integrative** functions, as in the dorsal horn of the spinal cord.

The simple anatomic and functional organization of motor and sensory cell columns described previously remains preserved in the ventral and dorsal horns of the adult spinal cord. In the brain stem, however, the organization changes because of shifts in the course of the long tracts connecting the brain and spinal cord and because of the migration of cell groups from the alar plate to form unique relay nuclei. (This is discussed further in Chapter 10.)

Mechanisms Underlying Histogenesis of the Nervous System

The development of the nervous system into a specific pattern of functionally related cell groups and fiber bundles results from complicated processes including the migration of nerve cells, the growth of their axons and dendrites, and the establishment of synaptic connections. The mechanisms controlling these processes are critical for the establishment of appropriate contacts among the various parts of the system; that is, the development of functional systems such as the visual, auditory, or motor systems.

Although the mechanisms that determine **cell migration, neuritic outgrowth,** and **synaptogenesis** remain only partially understood, **chemical guidance** is clearly of great importance. Both neuron cell bodies and fibers migrate along chemically marked pathways and in response to chemical gradients. In some instances, however, the **physical scaffolding** on which this migration occurs is also important. For example, in the developing cerebral cortex and other laminated structures, the migrating neuron cell bodies follow the processes of radial glial cells to their place in the appropriate cell layer. Similarly, a neuroglial bridge of tissue between the developing cerebral hemispheres provides a necessary substrate for the migration of fibers forming the corpus callosum.

Contacts between neurons are essential for normal development of the nervous system and for its maintenance in the adult. Synaptic contacts provide a mechanism for exchange of **trophic and regulatory influences** for both presynaptic and postsynaptic cells. In most cases, exchange of these factors prevents cell death of the presynaptic and postsynaptic neuron, but in some cases, this contact through active synapses actually appears to enhance cell death. Thus, cell contacts play a role in the control of **cell death,** which, like cell migration, is a fundamental process through which the adult form of the nervous system can be achieved.

2

Physiology of Nerve Cells

Resting Membrane Potential

Neurons rely on both electrical (ionic) and chemical signals to communicate. In general, electrical signals provide intraneuronal communication, and chemical compounds provide signals between neurons. In some cases, however, interneuronal signals result from ionic shifts.

Nerve cell membranes consist of bilayers of lipoproteins. These cellular membranes maintain an electrical charge across the external and internal surfaces of the cell. At rest, nerve cells contain positive charges on the outside and negative charges on the inside. This electrical charge is termed the **resting membrane potential.** Arbitrarily, the outside of the cell is designated as zero, and because the inside of the cell is negative in relation to the outside, the resting membrane potential is a negative number. From direct measurements with microelectrodes, the resting membrane potential of various nerve cells has been found to be between –40 and –75 millivolts (mV) (a millivolt is one-thousandth of a volt). An increase in resting membrane potential, which makes it more negative, is termed **hyperpolarization.** A decrease in membrane potential, which makes it more positive, is called **depolarization.**

The ions principally responsible for membrane potential include sodium (Na^+) and chloride (Cl^-), which are concentrated outside the cell, and potassium (K^+) and organic anions (A^-), which are concentrated inside the cell. Organic anions are negatively charged amino acids and proteins. Nerve cells are variably permeable to Na^+, Cl^-, and K^+, but they are impermeable to A^-.

Obeying simple chemical diffusion principles, ions such as K^+ tend to diffuse down their concentration gradients. The electrical force of repulsion of like charges opposes the chemical force of diffusion and sets up movement in the opposite direction. The membrane potential at which the electrical force of repulsion of an ion balances the chemical force of concentration gradient of the ion is called the **equilibrium potential.** The **Nernst equation** describes this equilibrium state mathematically:

$$E = RT/ZF \ln C_2/C_1$$

Where: E = the difference in electrical potential between the inside and the outside of the cell (i.e., the resting membrane potential)

R = the universal gas constant

T = absolute temperature

Z = the valence of the ions under consideration

F = Faraday's constant (the electric charge per gram equivalent of univalent ions)

ln = the natural logarithm (this term can be replaced by $2.3 \times \log_{10}$)

C_2 = the concentration of ion outside the membrane

C_1 = the concentration of ion inside the membrane

At resting membrane potential, neuronal membranes are much more permeable to K^+ than to Na^+. As a consequence, the resting membrane potential (–40 to –75 mV) is much closer to the K^+ equilibrium potential (–80 mV) than to the Na^+ equilibrium potential (+50 mV).

For cells to maintain a steady resting membrane potential, the separation of charges across the membrane must be constant; that is, the efflux of charge must exactly balance the influx of charge. Because of constantly open channels in the membrane and the differences in ion concentrations between the inside and outside of the cell, Na^+ constantly leaks into the cell and K^+ constantly leaks out of the cell. Opposing this migration is a **sodium-potassium pump,** which moves Na^+ out of the cell and K^+ into the cell and requires adenosine triphosphate as its energy source. Thus, metabolic energy must be expended to maintain the ionic gradients across the membrane. In contrast to Na^+ and K^+, Cl^- is free to diffuse into or out of the cell, and, in most cells, chloride is not pumped actively. Thus, Cl^- is described as being **passively distributed** across the membrane, whereas Na^+ and K^+ are pumped and therefore are actively distributed.

Ion Channels Control Membrane Potential

As described in the previous section, the membrane potential of a neuron depends on the relative permeability of the membrane to various ions. Changes in membrane ion permeability result from the opening and closing of **ion channels,** which are selectively permeable, multiple-subunit proteins that span the cell membrane. These channels fall into two broad classes, those that open or close (i.e., they are "gated") in response to the presence or absence of neurotransmitters **(ligand-gated channels)** and those that open or close in response to changes in voltage across the membrane **(voltage-gated or voltage-sensitive channels).** Some types of channels have been named by their characteristic physiologic behavior, such as ion selectivity or responses to various pharmacologic agents. These characteristics, in turn, depend on the assembled subunits that comprise the channel protein. Voltage-gated channels have strict ion selectivity. Second messenger systems within neurons influence the activity of many of these channels. The processes by which neurotransmitters induce changes in neuronal activity through changes in ion channel activity are termed **signal transduction.**

Neurons can be modeled as electrical circuits. The electrical potential described previously as a resting potential can be viewed as the sum of different **electromotive forces** (i.e., batteries). The electromotive force components of nerve cells result from the concentration gradient of the ions distributed along the inside and outside of the nerve cell membranes. The channels spanning the membrane have the property of **(variable) conductance.** Conductance is the inverse of **resistance,** which is the opposition to current flow. The conductance properties of a nerve cell result from the characteristics of individual ion channels. The lipid bilayer in the nerve cell membrane results in **capacitance,** which is the ability to store charges of opposite sign on two opposing surfaces. Capacitance is important in shaping the temporal profile of currents flowing across nerve membranes.

Action Potential

Nerve cells use an electrical signal called the **action potential** for intraneuronal signaling. The action potential, also known as the **spike** or **nerve impulse,** consists of a regenerative, stereotyped, all-or-none, transient sequence of rapid membrane depolarization followed by repolarization. When a nerve cell becomes depolarized, voltage-sensitive Na^+ channels open and allow the influx of Na^+ ions. The greater the depolarization, the greater is the fraction of open channels; the results are greater permeability to Na^+ and a net increase in positive charge flowing through the membrane. Positive charges thus accumulate inside the membrane and cause further depolarization (Fig. 2–1A). The increasing depolarization results in the opening of more voltage-gated Na^+ channels and leads to a greater influx of positive charge, thereby increasing depolarization still further. Thus, a positive feedback cycle occurs that drives the membrane potential toward the equilibrium potential of sodium, about +90 mV.

Depolarization of a nerve cell membrane also results in the opening of voltage-sensitive K^+ channels (Fig. 2–1B), but this lags behind the opening of Na^+ channels (Fig. 2–1D). Once they are open, however, these K^+ channels increase the efflux of K^+. The sodium channels rapidly close and become inactivated. Depolarization continues with the increased K^+ flux, and the result is a net efflux of positive charge from the cell. The process continues until the cell repolarizes to its resting value (Fig. 2–1B). The events described previously, influx of Na^+ followed by efflux of K^+, result in the development of an action

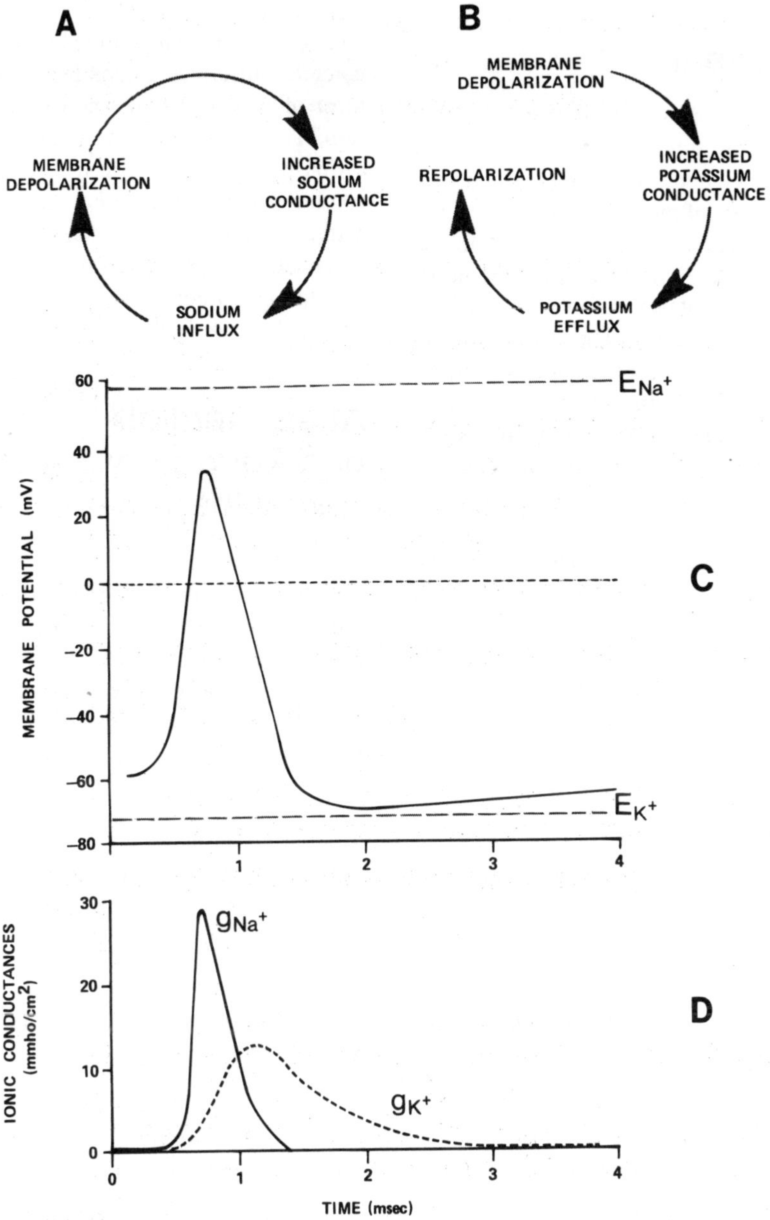

■ **FIGURE 2-1.** Events that occur during the action potential. **(A)** The depolarization phase of the nerve impulse has a regenerative aspect resulting from the positive feedback of membrane potential, sodium conductance, and sodium influx. **(B)** Membrane repolarization occurs when potassium efflux restores the internal negativity of the membrane. **(C and D)** Theoretical solution of the Nernst equation for changes in membrane potential **(C)** and sodium and potassium conductances **(D)** as a function of time.

potential (Fig. 2–1C). The action potential has characteristics determined only by the properties of the cell, independent of the characteristics of the exciting stimuli.

Action Current

The flow of current during the action potential, termed the **action current** (see Fig. 1–1E), depolarizes the neighboring membrane and provides for movement of the action potential along the membrane. The action potential can be propagated a very long distance along the nerve cell body or axon without variation of waveform and at a constant velocity. The action current meets far less electrical resistance in larger-diameter axons than in smaller-diameter axons, and, as a consequence, nerves with larger-diameter axons have greater conduction velocities than nerves with smaller-diameter axons. Conduction velocity is also substantially greater in **myelinated axons** than in **unmyelinated axons.** In myelinated axons, during the propagation of the action potential, the action current does not flow across the myelin sheath, but it flows only across the cell membrane at the nodes of Ranvier (see Fig. 1–1E). The unmyelinated membrane at the nodes contains large numbers of voltage-dependent Na^+ and K^+ channels, whereas the intervening myelinated membrane has few channels. Thus, the action current can efficiently depolarize the node of Ranvier without leakage through the intervening membrane, and the action potential, in effect, jumps from node to node, a form of propagation termed **saltatory conduction.** This is an efficient method of transmitting action potentials because it results in maximum conduction velocities with a minimum amount of active-membrane and metabolic activity. In unmyelinated fibers, nerve impulses are propagated by the continuous progression of the action potential along the length of the fiber.

Afterpotentials and Refractory Periods Follow the Action Potential

In most nerve cells, a brief period of hyperpolarization, termed the **hyperpolarizing afterpotential,** follows the action potential. This brief increase in the negativity of the membrane potential occurs because the voltage-sensitive K^+ channels that open during the late phase of the

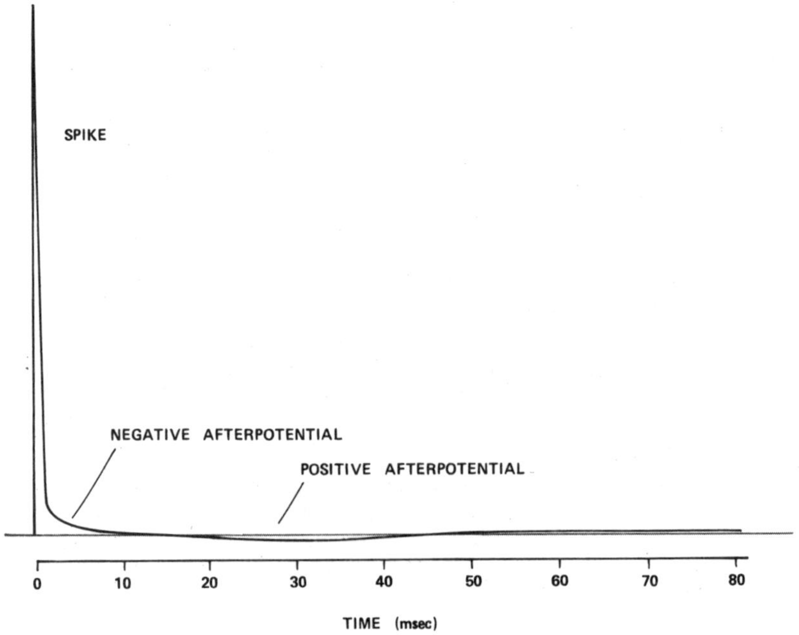

■ **FIGURE 2–2.** Scale drawing of an action potential and related afterpotentials resulting from electrical stimulation, recorded extracellularly from the saphenous nerve of the cat. (Adapted from Erlanger, J, and Gaser, HS: Electrical Signs and Nervous Activity. University of Pennsylvania Press, Philadelphia, 1938.)

action potential do not all close immediately. It takes a few milliseconds for all of them to return to the closed state. A brief period of **refractoriness,** consisting of the **absolute and relative refractory periods,** also follows the action potential. The absolute refractory period comes immediately after the action potential, and, during this interval, the cell cannot be excited to produce another action potential no matter how large a stimulating current it receives. The relative refractory period follows the absolute refractory period and consists of an interval during which an action potential can be evoked by a stimulus that is stronger than the usual threshold stimulus necessary to evoke an action potential. Both periods of refractoriness result from the residual opening of K^+ channels and the residual inactivation of Na^+ channels.

The previous description pertains to events that follow activation of single nerve cells. Activation by electrical stimulation of a whole nerve consisting of large myelinated fibers produces in extracellular recordings a **spike potential,** followed by a **negative afterpotential,** and then a **positive afterpotential** (Fig. 2–2). The negative afterpotential results from residual depolarization of the nerve fiber membrane, and the positive afterpotential reflects hyperpolarization of the membrane.

Synapses

Communication between neurons occurs at the **synapse,** which is the specialized contact zone where neurons communicate with each other. Two distinct types of synapses have been described: **electrical synapses** and **chemical synapses.** Electrical synapses have bridges interconnecting the cytoplasm of the presynaptic and postsynaptic cells. These synapses are called **bridged junctions** or **gap junctions.** Ionic current mediates transmission at electrical synapses, so little synaptic delay occurs. Only the speed of electrical transmission across the short distance separating the presynaptic and postsynaptic elements limits transmission. Electrical synapses can conduct equally well in forward or backward directions (i.e., from presynaptic to postsynaptic cell or from postsynaptic to presynaptic cell). In addition, channels between the two neurons at an electrical synapse allow for the direct exchange of molecules between the cells. Neurons of the human central nervous system (CNS) contain chiefly chemical synapses, although some electrical synapses have been described. Glial cells frequently contain gap junctions, which allow for electrical coupling and the potential for widespread communication between these cells.

Chemical Synapses

Chemical synapses consist of presynaptic and postsynaptic neurons completely separated by a specialized synaptic cleft (see Fig. 1–1C). The presynaptic terminal usually contains synaptic vesicles, which contain a chemical neurotransmitter. The postsynaptic membrane active zone contains specialized receptors, which are ligand-gated channels, complex proteins that mediate the effect of the neurotransmitter. Neurotransmitters such as acetylcholine and norepinephrine must be released, must diffuse across the synaptic cleft, and must bind to postsynaptic receptors; thus, transmission is associated with a substantial synaptic delay, usually at least 0.3 ms (one-thousandth of a second) and sometimes up to 1 millisecond or even longer. This transmission can occur only in a single direction, from presynaptic cell to postsynaptic cell, but it can have either excitatory or inhibitory effects on the postsynaptic membrane. Many single neurons of the CNS receive thousands of synaptic connections from other neurons; thus, the level of depolarization or hyperpolarization of the cell results from the summation of activity at many thousands of receptors.

Neurotransmitters

Many chemical substances presumed to be **excitatory neurotransmitters** have been identified. The most widely distributed of these is **glutamate,** which is found in all parts of the CNS. Fewer chemical substances thought to be **inhibitory neurotransmitters** have been identified. **Gamma-aminobutyric acid** (GABA) and **glycine** are the best characterized. In the adult, GABA is distributed throughout the brain, whereas glycine is found chiefly in the spinal cord. Glycine is also found in small amounts within the cerebral cortex, where it has excitatory effects on glutamatergic synapses. Many other chemicals have been identified as putative neurotransmitters, including the following: acetylcholine; monoamines such as dopamine, norepinephrine, and serotonin; and numerous peptides, including substance P, vasopressin, cholecystokinin, endorphin, and enkephalins. Only some of these have met the rigorous experimental criteria that establish them as neurotransmitters.

Events of Synaptic Transmission

When an action potential moves down an axon and enters the axon terminal on the presynaptic side of the synapse, the opening of voltage-dependent **calcium (Ca^{2+}) channels** allows the influx of Ca^{2+} ions, which initiate neurotransmitter release. As may be expected, Ca^{2+} channels occur more abundantly at presynaptic terminals than along the axons of nerve cells. Increasing extracellular Ca^{2+} concentration enhances transmitter release; decreasing Ca^{2+} concentration decreases release; and increasing magnesium (Mg^{2+}) concentration blocks release. Several Ca^{2+} channel subtypes are recognized, with different physiologic and pharmacologic properties; only some of these are coupled to transmitter release. After the transmitter is released, it diffuses across the synapse and binds to postsynaptic receptors.

Stimulation of a single presynaptic excitatory neuron evokes in the postsynaptic neuron an **excitatory postsynaptic potential (EPSP),** which is a small, nonpropagated depolarization. The EPSP results from the opening of excitatory ligand-gated channels, usually cholinergic or glutamatergic channels. If increasing numbers of presynaptic neurons making connections with the same postsynaptic neuron become activated simultaneously, the EPSP will progressively increase in amplitude until it brings the neuronal membrane to the threshold needed to generate an action potential. At this point, the postsynaptic neuron becomes depolarized, Na^+ channels have opened, and an all-or-nothing action potential travels along the cell's axon.

Electrical stimulation of a single inhibitory presynaptic neuron contacting a single postsynaptic neuron results in the development of an **inhibitory postsynaptic potential (IPSP),** which consists of a transient hyperpolarization of the postsynaptic membrane. The IPSP results from transient opening of transmitter-gated Cl^- or G-protein–associated K^+ channels (see later). Opening of Cl^- channels leads to movement of Cl^- into the cell; this hyperpolarizes the cell because it increases the negative charge intracellularly. Opening K^+ channels results in movement of K^+ out of the cell and thus decreases the amount of positive charge within the cell and augments the hyperpolarization.

Neurotransmitters are released from presynaptic terminals in small packets termed **quanta.** A quantum of transmitter, probably released from a single vesicle, evokes a small potential of fixed size in the postsynaptic neuron. This is known as a **unit potential** or **miniature end-plate potential.** Usually, a **synaptic potential** consists of many unit potentials. The amount of Ca^{2+} that enters the presynaptic neuron affects the number of quanta of transmitter that are released.

Synaptic Transmission Is Affected by Drugs and Toxins

The processes of transmitter release, receptor activation, and the subsequent reuptake or chemical inactivation of the transmitter molecules are susceptible to the actions of chemicals at the synapses. Drugs and toxins, as well as endogenous compounds, can interfere with presynaptic events, including the action potential, the synthesis of transmitter molecules, and the release of transmitters from vesicles. These compounds can also affect the fate of the transmitter within the cleft and its influence on the postsynaptic membrane. All these substances influence ion channel activity (and thus neuronal activity) indirectly, but some drugs, such as Ca^{2+} channel blockers, also can influence ion channels directly.

Neurotransmitter Receptors

All neurotransmitter **receptors** consist of proteins concentrated in the cell membranes of either postsynaptic neurons or presynaptic terminals **(autoreceptors).** Receptors act through two general mechanisms. In the first, the receptor is an integral part of a ligand-gated channel. Binding of a transmitter to its recognition site induces a conformational change in the channel, an associated ion flux, and either depolarization or hyperpolarization. This mechanism operates rapidly and underlies physiologic processes that require speed. Receptors of this type are called **ionotropic receptors.** The second mechanism involves a neurotransmitter-receptor interaction that leads to a signal inside the cell mediated by second messengers. These receptors are called **metabotropic** or **G-protein–coupled receptors.** They are linked to other membrane-bound proteins called G proteins, which, when activated, influence ion channel activity directly or indirectly by numerous different biochemical pathways.

Neuromuscular Junction

Communication from neuron to voluntary muscle occurs at the **motor end plate,** or **neuromuscular junction** (see Fig. 1–1D). Here, the synaptic vesicles contain acetylcholine, which, on release, activates the receptor channels in the postsynaptic membrane. The physiologic and molecular processes at the motor end plate are essentially identical to those at chemical synapses between neurons, and, as at these neural junctions, drugs and toxins can affect function. For example, botulinum toxin inhibits the release of acetylcholine and thereby leads to loss of muscle activation. Clinically in botulism, this effect is seen as muscle weakness. If large amounts of the toxin have been ingested in inadequately processed food, weakness leads to a widespread paralysis that can be fatal. Tiny amounts of botulinum toxin can be injected into muscles to weaken them. This is used in the treatment of certain neurologic disorders such as severe dystonia, a disorder consisting of abnormal postures resulting from constant focal muscle contractions.

The physiologic contact between neuron and muscle has long been recognized as a trophic and regulatory contact as well as a point of activation. Denervation of striated muscles leads to death of the muscle fibers and atrophy of the muscle. Research has demonstrated that this trophic function is also characteristic of contact between neurons in the CNS. If a neuron is deprived of its synaptic contacts as a result of injury or disease, rapid changes in metabolism, transmitter receptor production, and even morphology (e.g., dendritic structure) of the postsynaptic cell can occur.

Section 2

Peripheral Nervous System

3

Fibers of the Spinal Nerves

In peripheral nerves, the fibers that innervate the muscles, joints, and skin of the body wall are termed **somatic;** those that innervate the internal organs of the body cavities and blood vessels throughout the body are termed **visceral.** Sensory fibers are designated **afferent,** and motor fibers are designated **efferent.** In addition, nerve fibers designated **general** innervate skin, muscles, bones, and viscera throughout the body, whereas the term **special** is reserved for sensory organs and muscles found only in unique regions in the head (e.g., retina, inner ear). Thus, all nerve fibers in spinal nerves are general, but the cranial nerves as a group contain both general and special fibers.

Functional Classification

General Afferent Fibers

General afferent fibers of the spinal nerves are sensory fibers with cells of origin in the **dorsal root ganglia.** These cells differ in shape from the neurons shown in Figure 1–1. Dorsal root ganglion cells are round and have only one process leaving the cell body. This process splits into a peripheral branch, which enters the nerve, and a central branch, which passes through the dorsal root to the spinal cord (Fig. 3–1).

- **General somatic afferent (GSA)** fibers (Fig. 3–1A) carry **exteroceptive** and **proprioceptive** information. An organism receives **exteroceptive** information from receptors in the skin that mediate pain, temperature, and touch and **proprioceptive** information from sensory endings in muscles, tendons, and joints that mediate position sense, muscle length, rate of change of muscle length, and muscle contraction.
- **General visceral afferent (GVA)** fibers (Fig. 3–1B) carry **interoceptive** information from receptors in visceral structures. They mediate data concerning distension and contraction of these structures.

General Efferent Fibers

General efferent fibers are motor fibers with cells of origin in the spinal cord (in the case of general somatic efferent and general visceral efferent preganglionic fibers) or in autonomic

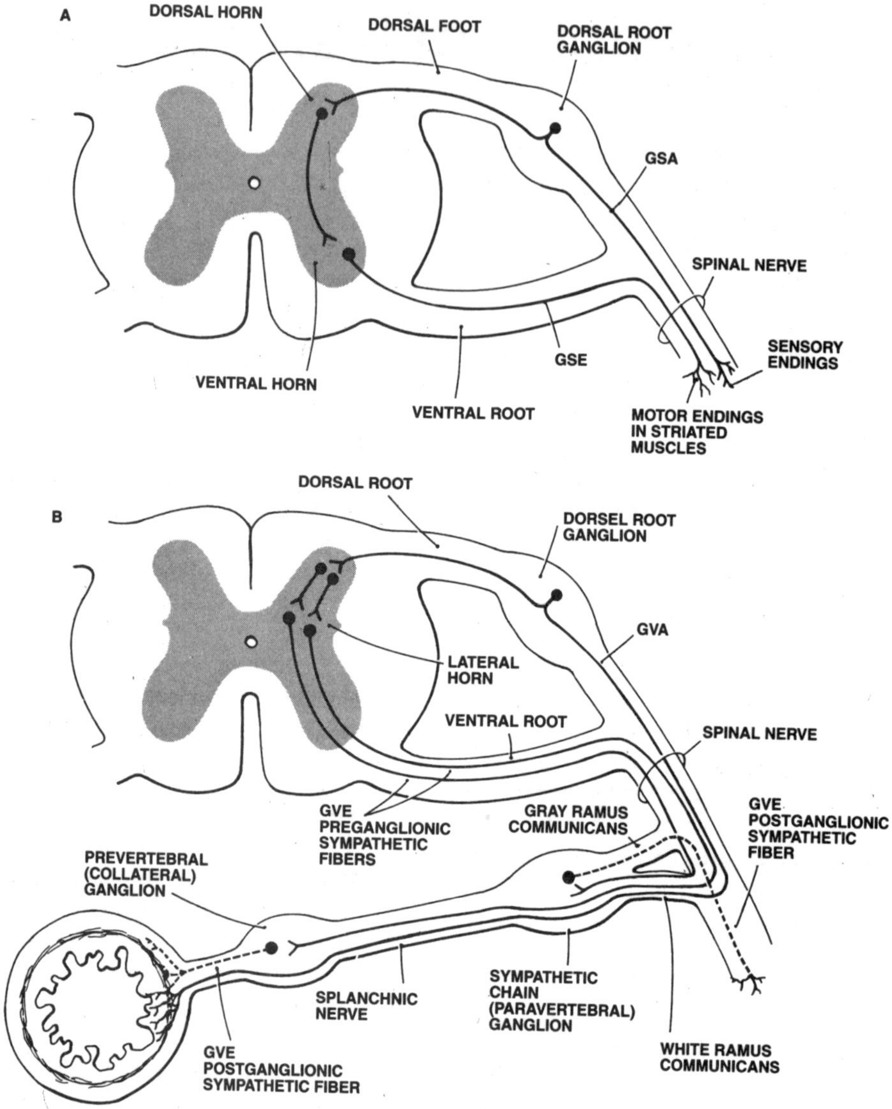

■ **FIGURE 3–1.** Functional components of a spinal nerve. Afferent neurons (and interneurons) are shown in *black*. Efferent neurons are shown in *color*. **(A)** General somatic afferent (GSA) and general somatic efferent (GSE) components of a polysynaptic somatic reflex arc illustrated on a transverse section through the spinal cord and spinal nerve roots. **(B)** General visceral afferent (GVA) and general visceral efferent (GVE) components of visceral reflex arcs through the spinal cord. In **(B)**, presynaptic GVE fibers are shown in *solid color lines;* postsynaptic GVE fibers are indicated with *dashed color lines.*

ganglia (in the case of general visceral efferent postganglionic fibers).

- **General somatic efferent (GSE)** fibers (Fig. 3–1A) consist of motor fibers originating from the cell bodies of alpha, beta, and gamma motoneurons in lamina IX. These fibers innervate striated skeletal muscles.
- **General visceral efferent (GVE)** fibers (Fig. 3–1B) consist of preganglionic and postganglionic autonomic fibers that innervate smooth muscle and cardiac muscle and regulate glandular secretion. **Preganglionic sympathetic** cell bodies are located in the intermediolateral cell column within lamina VII, which forms the lateral horn and extends only from segment T1 to segment L2 or L3 of the spinal cord. **Preganglionic parasympathetic** cell bodies are located in lamina VII of the sacral spinal cord (S2 to S4). In sympathetic ganglia throughout the body and in parasympathetic ganglia in the pelvis, preganglionic fibers from the spinal cord synapse on the cell bodies of postganglionic autonomic neurons (see paravertebral and prevertebral ganglia, Fig. 3–1B).

Physiologic Classification

Nerve fibers can be categorized according to fiber diameter and conduction velocity of the nerve impulse. As mentioned in Chapter 2, in general, the larger the diameter of the fiber, the thicker is the myelin sheath and the greater is the action potential conduction velocity. Two classifications of nerve fibers are in use (Table 3–1).

An electrophysiologic classification is based on the **conduction velocities of different types of motor and sensory nerve fibers.** With electrical stimulation of an entire compound nerve (i.e., a nerve containing many motor and sensory fibers) and extracellular recording, peaks in the compound action potential reveal these velocities. The compound action potential consists of the sum of the action potentials of individual fibers within the nerve. In this classification, fibers fall into **three groups: A, B, and C** (Fig. 3–2). A and B fibers are myelinated, and C fibers are unmyelinated. A fibers are further subdivided on the basis of mean conduction velocity, and hence fiber size, into several subgroups: alpha (α), beta (ß), gamma (γ), and delta (δ). The A fiber group includes separate motor components that inner-

■ TABLE 3-1. CLASSIFICATION OF NERVE FIBERS

Sensory and Motor Fibers	Sensory Fibers	Largest Fiber Diameter (μm)	Fastest Conduction Velocity (m/s)	General Comments	
Aα		22	120	Motor	Axons of alpha motoneurons of lamina IX, innervating extrafusal muscle fibers
Aα	Ia	22	120	Sensory	Primary afferents of muscle spindles
Aα	Ib	22	120	Sensory	Afferents of Golgi tendon organs, touch and pressure receptors
Aβ		13	70	Motor	Motor axons innervating both extrafusal and intrafusal (muscle spindle) muscle fibers
Aβ	II	13	70	Sensory	Secondary afferents of muscle spindles, touch and pressure receptors, and Pacinian corpuscles (vibratory sensors)
Aγ		8	40	Motor	Axons of gamma motoneurons of lamina IX, innervating intrafusal fibers (muscle spindles)
Aδ	III	5	15	Sensory	Small, lightly myelinated fibers; touch, pressure, pain, and temperature receptors
B		3	14	Motor	Small, lightly myelinated preganglionic autonomic fibers
C		1	2	Motor	Postganglionic autonomic fibers (all are unmyelinated)
C	IV	1	2	Sensory	Unmyelinated pain and temperature fibers

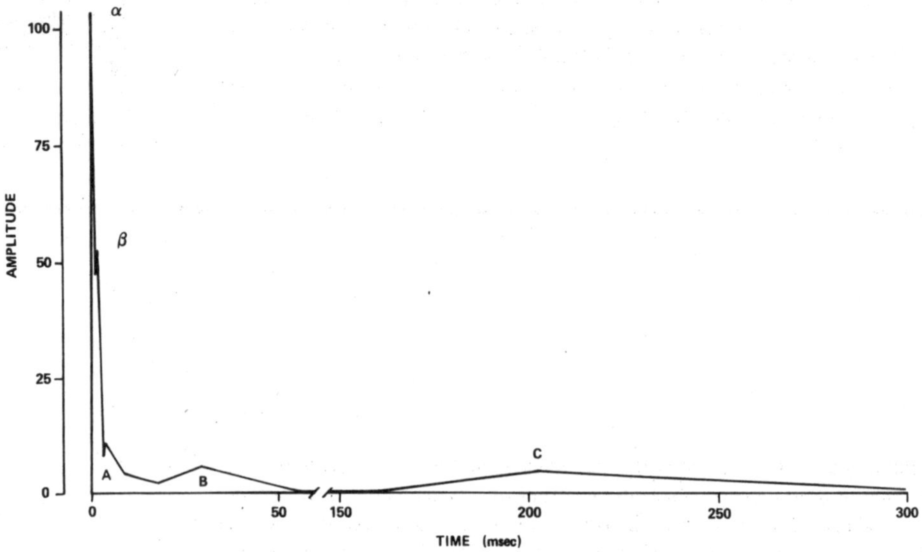

■ **FIGURE 3–2.** A complete compound action potential resulting from electrical stimulation of the sciatic nerve of a frog. Subcomponents of the A group of fibers cannot be distinguished because the time scale was chosen to illustrate the B and C fiber peaks. The amplitude of the action potential is plotted relative to the A peak. (Adapted from Erlanger, J, and Gaser, HS: Electrical Signs and Nervous Activity. University of Pennsylvania Press, Philadelphia, 1938.)

vate two types of muscle fiber. **Extrafusal muscle** consists of striated skeletal muscle outside the muscle spindles, and large-diameter **Aα fibers** innervate these muscle fibers. **Intrafusal muscle** fibers are located within muscle spindles, and small-diameter **Aγ fibers** innervate these muscle fibers. The intermediate-sized **Aß** group includes fibers that innervate both types of muscle. C fibers are subdivided into two classes: sC fibers (postganglionic efferent sympathetic C fibers) and drC fibers (afferent dorsal root C fibers).

A second classification system for peripheral nerve pertains to sensory fibers. In this system, fibers are divided into four groups (I to IV) that are differentiated chiefly on the basis of diameter (and thus speed of conduction). Because this system pertains specifically to sensory fibers, the categories also divide fibers into groups according to the sensory receptors they innervate (Table 3–1).

4

Spinal Reflexes and Muscle Tone

Case Study

A 23-year-old male medical student is carrying six large books between his hands, with the books leaning against his chest, as he descends a stairway. His foot misses a stair and he falls backward, landing hard on his gluteal region. He experiences a severe pain in his low back that radiates into his right leg posteriorly and extends down to the ankle. On arising, he finds that his back is stiff and sore, and he has difficulty in walking, owing to weakness in lifting the right foot. Examination reveals mild weakness of dorsiflexion (upward movement) and eversion (upward and outward rotation) of the right foot at the ankle, moderate weakness of dorsiflexion of the great toe, and mild weakness of the small muscles of the right foot (with difficulty in flexing and inverting the foot). The deep tendon reflexes at the knees are equal, but the right ankle reflex is absent whereas the left is present. Sensation, as tested with pinprick and light touch, is decreased along the lateral dorsal and ventral border of the right foot and along the lateral aspect of the right leg below the knee.

Where is the injury that caused the pain, muscle weakness, reflex change, and sensory disturbance? What can be done to help this man?

Spinal Reflexes

A reflex action consists of a **specific, stereotyped response to an adequate stimulus.** The adequate stimuli for somatic spinal reflexes involve input to the spinal cord from sensory receptors in muscles, skin, and joints. (Visceral reflexes are discussed in Chapters 5 and 11.) The response involves contraction of striated skeletal muscle fibers. A reflex response may be mediated by as few as two neurons, one afferent and one efferent, and in this case it is termed a **monosynaptic reflex.** The stretch reflex, or deep tendon reflex, which is important in clinical neurology, is a monosynaptic reflex. Most reflexes involve several **interneurons** in addition to the afferent and efferent neurons. A reflex mediated by more than two neurons is termed **polysynaptic.** The flexor reflex and crossed extensor reflex described at the end of this chapter are examples of polysynaptic reflexes.

A reflex may involve the following: (1) neurons in just one or a few spinal cord levels, as in the case of segmental reflexes (those restricted to a single spinal cord segment); (2) neurons in several to many spinal cord levels, as in the case of intersegmental reflexes; or (3) neurons in structures of the brain that influence the spinal cord, as in the case of supraspinal reflexes.

Muscle Spindles

Function, Size, and Distribution of Muscle Spindles

Muscle spindles are receptor organs within striated muscles that provide the central nervous system with information about the length and the rate of change in length of muscles. They also provide afferent input for stretch reflexes. Muscle spindles contain a motor nerve supply that can alter the sensitivity of the receptor to muscle stretch. They are encapsulated structures, found in most skeletal muscles of the body, varying in length from 1 to 3 mm in small muscles, such as the lumbricals, to 7 to 10 mm in large muscles. Muscle spindles also vary in number, or density, in different muscles of the body and are particularly numerous in the small, delicate muscles of the hand.

Anatomy of Muscle Spindles

Each spindle contains 2 to 12 thin muscle fibers of modified striated muscle. Because the fibers are enclosed within the capsule of the spindle-shaped, or fusiform, bag, they are termed **intrafusal** muscle fibers, to differentiate them from the large **extrafusal** fibers (Fig. 4–1). Muscle spindles are attached to the connective tissue septa that run between extrafusal fibers. Consequently, the entire muscle spindle structure is connected to the muscle's tendons in parallel with the extrafusal fibers, a feature that is important in muscle spindle function. This parallel arrangement means that increases in force during muscle contraction

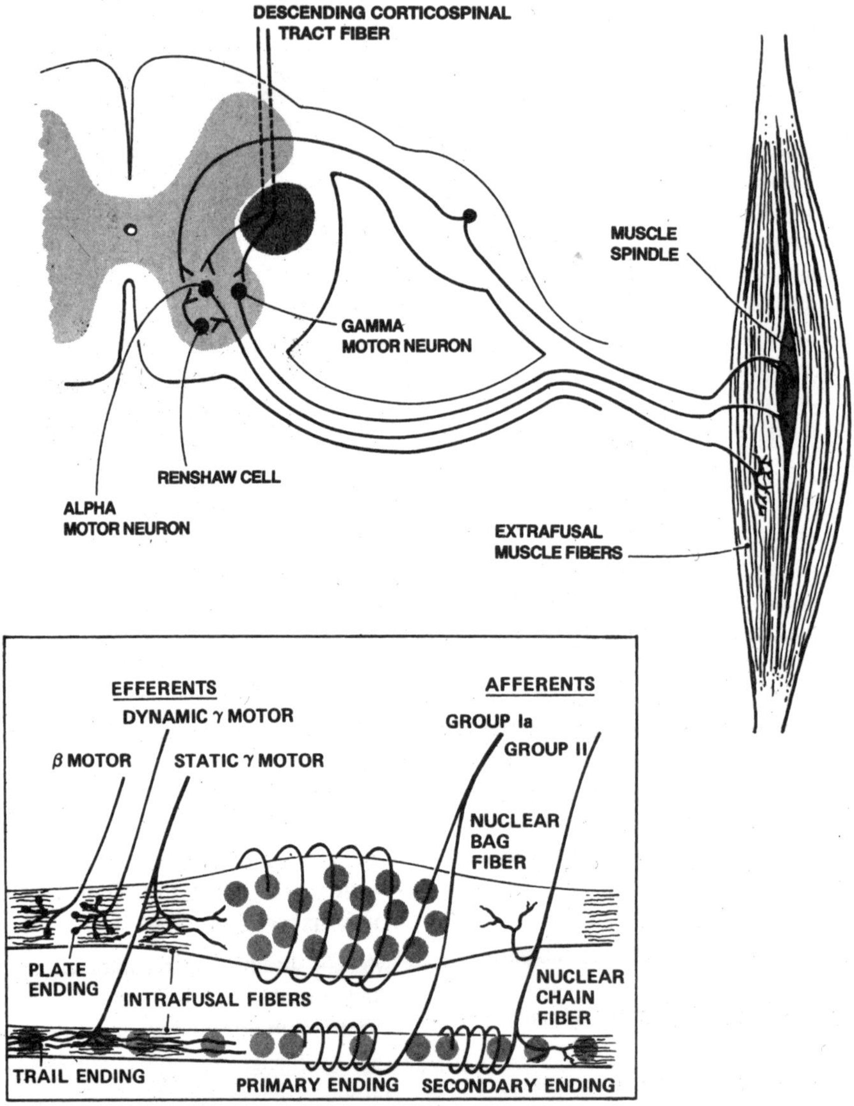

■ **FIGURE 4–1.** A cross section of the spinal cord shows a Ia afferent fiber originating in a muscle spindle, passing through a peripheral nerve, entering a dorsal root, and making synaptic connection with an alpha motoneuron. The axon of the alpha motoneuron emerges through the ventral root, passes through the peripheral nerve, and terminates on extrafusal muscle fibers. The axon of the gamma motoneuron terminates on intrafusal fibers within the muscle spindle. The *inset* shows an enlarged view of one nuclear bag and one nuclear chain **intrafusal fiber** within the muscle spindle and the principal nerve endings on these fibers.

induce modest lengthening of the tendon, accompanied by a relative reduction of spindle fiber length and a decline in spindle afferent firing.

There are two distinct types of intrafusal fibers and a third, intermediate type. The longest and largest type of fiber contains numerous large nuclei closely packed in a central bag and hence is called a **nuclear bag** fiber (Fig. 4–1). Shorter and thinner, the other main type contains a single row, or chain, of central nuclei and is termed a **nuclear chain** fiber (Fig. 4–1). A third type of intrafusal fiber is intermediary in structure and is termed bag_2 to differentiate it from the larger type of bag fiber, which is termed bag_1.

Innervation of the Muscle Spindle

Gamma or beta motoneurons innervate the contractile ends of both bag and chain fibers, terminating in two types of endings, **plates** and **trails** (Fig. 4–1). Plate endings occur chiefly on nuclear bag fibers and rarely on nuclear chain fibers. Trail endings occur mostly on nuclear chain fibers but are frequently found on bag fibers as well.

Muscle spindles contain abundant sensory nerve endings that generate action potentials with stretching of the intrafusal fibers. The types of endings are primary endings, derived from group Ia nerve fibers, and secondary endings, derived from group II fibers. **Primary** afferents arise in the central region of both bag and chain fibers. The Ia fibers from these endings make monosynaptic contact with alpha motoneurons innervating the same (homonymous) muscle (Fig. 4–1) and synergistic (heteronymous) muscles. **Secondary** endings arise predominantly on nuclear chain fibers and lie to either side of the primary endings. Their group II fibers excite homonymous alpha motoneurons monosynaptically.

Alpha, Beta, and Gamma Motoneurons of the Spinal Cord

Alpha, beta, and gamma motoneurons of lamina IX in the spinal cord regulate skeletal muscle activity. **Alpha motoneurons** are the largest of the anterior horn cells. They can be stimulated monosynaptically by (1) the Ia (primary) afferents and group II (secondary) afferents of the muscle spindles, (2) corticospinal tract fibers in primates (Fig. 4–1), (3) lateral vestibulospinal tract fibers, and (4) reticulospinal and raphe spinal tract fibers. Although these pathways can stimulate alpha motoneurons monosynaptically, interneurons in the spinal cord gray matter primarily influence ongoing alpha motoneuron activity. These interneurons mediate polysynaptic segmental, intersegmental, and supraspinal reflexes as well as the activity from additional descending tracts.

Alpha Motor Neurons Innervate Extrafusal Muscle Fibers

Each alpha motoneuron innervates a group of extrafusal muscle fibers within a specific muscle. The functional unit defined by this neuron and its muscle fibers is called a **motor unit.** Motor units in proximal muscles, which are used for postural control, are much larger (i.e., many muscle fibers are controlled by a single motoneuron) than motor units in distal limb muscles, which are used for finely controlled movements. In the muscles of the shoulder, for example, there may be hundreds of muscle fibers in each motor unit, whereas in an intrinsic muscle of the hand, each alpha motoneuron may innervate fewer than 10 muscle cells.

Special interneurons in the ventral horn, called **Renshaw cells,** also influence alpha motoneurons. Collateral fibers emerging from the axons of the alpha motoneurons excite Renshaw cells (Fig. 4–1). Renshaw cells, in turn, inhibit alpha motoneurons and can thereby modify the probability of firing of these neurons.

Gamma and Beta Motor Neurons Innervate Intrafusal Muscle Fibers

Gamma motoneurons, which are also termed **fusimotor neurons,** innervate intrafusal muscle fibers. Gamma motoneurons differ from alpha motoneurons in several important ways. Gamma motoneurons (1) do not innervate extrafusal muscle fibers; (2) are regulated primarily by intersegmental and supraspinal pathways and little by segmental sensory inputs; (3) do not receive inhibitory feedback through Renshaw cells; and (4) tend to discharge spontaneously, often at high frequencies. Despite these differences, when they do respond to the same sensory stimulus or descending pathway, gamma and alpha motoneurons respond similarly (i.e., with excitation or inhibition). The reticular formation, vestibular nuclei, cerebellum, and basal ganglia exert particularly strong control over the gamma motoneurons through descending pathways, as described in Chapter 8. The axons of **beta motoneurons** are comparable in diameter to those of alpha motoneurons. Beta motoneurons innervate both extrafusal and intrafusal muscle fibers, and they provide a significant fraction of the innervation of muscle spindles.

The sensory function of the spindle receptors is to inform the nervous system of the **length and rate of change in length** of the extrafusal fibers. The primary afferents respond to both the length of muscle and the rate of change in length of muscle. In contrast, the secondary endings respond chiefly to muscle length. Because muscle spindles are located in parallel with extrafusal fibers, muscle contraction can decrease the effective stretch on the spindles and thereby can decrease the sensitivity of the spindle. Activation of gamma motoneurons makes the intrafusal muscle fibers contract, and this contraction, in turn, can make the sensory portion of the muscle spindles more responsive to stretch and can maintain the sensitivity of the spindle.

In addition to their role in modulating the stretch reflex, gamma motor neurons participate in producing and controlling complex movements. Two types of gamma motoneurons have been described. One type affects the afferent responses to phasic extension more than the responses to static tension. This type of neuron is called the **dynamic gamma motoneuron.** The other type of neuron increases the spindle response to static extension and thus is called the **static gamma motoneuron.** Dynamic gamma motoneurons terminate in plate endings solely on nuclear bag fibers, whereas static gamma fibers terminate in trail endings on both bag and chain fibers. Thus, gamma motoneurons can adjust the length of intrafusal fibers so the spindle receptors can operate on a sensitive portion of their response scale. In addition, during a powerful contraction with considerable shortening, it may be advantageous for the spindle receptors to continue firing to reinforce the power of the contraction in reflex fashion.

Information from muscle spindles reaches higher levels of the nervous system, particularly the cerebellum and cerebral cortex. These areas control the descending pathways that facilitate and inhibit both alpha and gamma motoneuron activity. Most supraspinal and intersegmental systems influence the discharge of both alpha and gamma motoneurons innervating a particular muscle. This phenomenon is known as alpha-gamma **coactivation.** Finally, muscle spindles convey information needed for the conscious perception of limb position and movement.

Stretch Reflex

The **stretch (myotatic) reflex** is a segmental reflex. Stretching a single muscle spindle induces contraction limited to the part of the muscle containing the spindle. Stretching a single muscle or a group of synergistic muscles therefore produces a discrete response, limited to the same muscle or to the group of synergistic muscles. This imposes an orderly relation between muscle length change and the resultant force, and it causes the muscle to act as a compliant spring, an important attribute for posture and gait.

The **deep tendon reflex** is a fractional manifestation of the stretch reflex that can be tested by tapping the tendon of a muscle. For example, tapping the patellar tendon stretches most of the extrafusal fibers of the quadriceps femoris muscle group simultaneously. Because muscle spindles are arranged in parallel with the extrafusal fibers of the quadriceps, the intrafusal fibers in many muscle spindles are also stretched. This stretching stimulates the sensory endings on the intrafusal fibers, particularly the primary afferents (group Ia fibers). The Ia afferents monosynaptically stimulate the alpha motoneurons that innervate the quadriceps muscle and polysynaptically inhibit the alpha motoneurons of the antagonist muscle group (the hamstring muscles). Consequently, the quadriceps suddenly contracts and the hamstrings relax, thereby causing the leg to extend at the knee.

Golgi Tendon Organs and Their Reflexes

Golgi tendon organs consist of encapsulated structures attached in series with the large, collagenous fibers of tendons at the insertions of muscles and along the fascial covering of muscles. Within the capsule, sensory nerve endings (Ib afferents) terminate on small bundles of collagenous fibers of tendons. When muscle contraction occurs, shortening of the contractile part of the muscle stretches the noncontractile region containing the tendon organs. This leads to vigorous firing of the afferent fibers innervating Golgi tendon organs. Thus, these receptors respond primarily to muscle contraction. Their Ib afferent fibers project to the spinal cord, where they polysynaptically inhibit the alpha motoneurons innervating the agonist muscle and facilitate motoneurons of the antagonist muscle. Golgi tendon organs provide continuous and accurate information about **muscle force,** which both segmental and supraspinal pathways use to control movement.

Muscle Tone

The term **muscle tone** indicates the resistance that an examiner perceives when passively manipulating the limbs of a patient. A more precise term for this is **resistance to passive manipulation.** In a relaxed normal person, during manipulation of a limb at one of the joints, the examiner detects a certain amount of resistance in muscle. This resistance is not related to any conscious effort. There are two general abnormalities of muscle tone: hypotonia and hypertonia. **Hypotonia** is a decrease of resistance to passive manipulation of the limbs, and **hypertonia** is an increase of resistance to passive manipulation.

Hypotonia occurs in a muscle immediately if the ventral roots containing the motor nerve fibers to the muscle are cut. It also results from transection of the dorsal roots that contain sensory fibers from the muscle. Thus, reflex activity of the nervous system maintains and regulates muscle tone, and muscle tone is not a property of isolated muscle. Hypotonia also occurs in disease that affects certain parts of the nervous system, particularly the cerebellum.

Hypertonia appears in one of two general forms: spasticity and rigidity. In **spasticity,** which usually results from disease of the corticospinal and corticobulbar pathways, there is an increased resistance to externally imposed stretch, sometimes accompanied by a ''clasp-knife'' inhibition. The clasp-knife phenomenon begins with a marked increase in resistance to passive manipulation (in flexion or extension) during the initial portion of the manipulation. As the manipulation proceeds, the resistance suddenly decreases and disappears. The disappearance of resistance previously was thought to result from activation of Golgi tendon organs, but more recent evidence indicates that group III and IV (Aδ and C) muscle afferents are also responsible. Group III and IV afferents are those that respond to a variety of stimuli, including thermal, chemical, mechanical, and noxious stimuli. In **rigidity,** which usually results from disease of the basal ganglia, there is a plastic or ''cogwheel'' type of resistance to passive manipulation, often without changes in muscle stretch reflexes.

Reflexes of Cutaneous Origin

The sensory receptors in skin and subcutaneous tissues respond to touch, pressure, temperature, and tissue damage. These receptors generate signals that alter the activity of spinal motoneurons through interneurons and produce polysynaptic reflexes (see Fig. 3–1A). The **flexor reflex** and **crossed extensor reflex** are examples of polysynaptic responses to aversive stimuli that cause a limb to be withdrawn from a source of injury and a postural compensation to prevent falling. A noxious stimulus to a limb results in flexion of the ipsilateral limb and extension of the contralateral limb. For example, when a person steps on something hot or sharp, the stimulated extremity withdraws in reflex fashion. This results from the polysynaptic facilitation of alpha motoneurons innervating the ipsilateral flexor muscles and inhibition of motoneurons innervating the extensor muscles of the same leg (the flexor reflex). Simultaneously, the opposite limb extends to support the weight of the body. This extension results from facilitation of motoneurons innervating extensor muscles and inhibition of motoneurons innervating flexor muscles (i.e., the crossed extensor reflex).

Case Follow-up

The patient described at the beginning of this chapter sustained an injury of the L5 and S1 nerve roots on the right from the fall. These nerve roots innervate the dorsiflexors of the foot and great toe, the everters of the foot, and the intrinsic muscles of the foot. These nerve roots are also responsible for the integrity of the deep tendon reflex at the ankle and for sensation along the lateral border of the foot and lower leg. His fall caused herniation of intervertebral discs in his lumbosacral region, and this injured the nerve roots. After treatment with pain medication and bedrest for 1 week, the pain improved greatly, and both the muscle weakness and sensory loss disappeared. The ankle reflex remained absent. The patient was given a course of exercises to strengthen his back, with later resolution of all symptoms.

5

Autonomic Nervous System

Case Study

A 20-year-old woman develops an aching pain in her fingers and toes after walking outside for 15 minutes in an ambient temperature of 10°F during her first winter in a cold climate. Removing her thin gloves, she finds that her fingers initially turn white and then blue. After she returns to a warm room, her fingers turn red and develop a throbbing pain. She consults a physician for these symptoms. Examination in a warm room reveals no abnormalities on general physical or neurologic examination, and exposure to a cold ambient temperature reproduces the symptoms and findings.

What caused this disorder? Can it be treated?

The autonomic nervous system (ANS) is the functional division of the peripheral nervous system that innervates **smooth and cardiac muscle** and the **glands** of the body. Although by its original definition the ANS consists only of motor (general visceral efferent) fibers, the sensory (general visceral afferent) fibers accompanying the motor fibers to the viscera are integrally related, both anatomically and functionally, with the motor fibers and must be considered part of the ANS. Only the efferent system is described here. Description of the visceral afferent fibers that accompany the sympathetic nerves is in Chapter 6 (Visceral Pain Pathways and Referred Pain), and the visceral afferents associated with the cranial parasympathetic system are described in Chapter 11 (Sensory Functions of the Vagal System). Under ordinary circumstances, the ANS functions at the subconscious level. It regulates the ongoing, reflexively driven activity of smooth muscle, cardiac muscle, and glands, and it integrates visceral systems with each other and with somatic motor function. Many of the tissues innervated by the ANS can carry out their most basic functions (e.g., cardiac contractions, peristalsis of the intestinal tract) without external regulation from the autonomic fibers. In situations that require rapidly fluctuating or extreme responses, however, the autonomic nerves are essential for appropriate visceral function.

Visceral motor neurons are controlled by visceral and somatic sensory inputs, as well as by integrative influences through descending pathways from the brain stem and hypothalamus. Unlike the somatic motor system, the peripheral ANS reaches its effector organs by a two-neuron chain.

The cell bodies and fibers of this chain are classified as follows:

1. The **preganglionic neuron,** the presynaptic or primary neuron, is located in the brain stem (cranial nerve nuclei III, VII, IX, X, and XI) or spinal cord (intermediolateral cell column in lamina VII).
2. The **postganglionic neuron,** the postsynaptic or secondary neuron, is located in an outlying ganglion and innervates the end organ. Within these autonomic ganglia, synapses between preganglionic and postganglionic ANS neurons are modulated by a variety of interneurons.

The Autonomic Nervous System Has Two Divisions

Cell bodies of the preganglionic ANS neurons are found in three regions of the brain stem and two regions of the spinal cord. The **thoracolumbar**

outflow consists of the fibers that arise in the **intermediolateral cell column** of the thoracic and the first two lumbar segments of the spinal cord. This is the origin of the **sympathetic division of the ANS.** The **cranial outflow** consists of fibers that arise in the nuclei of cranial nerves III, VII, IX, X, and XI. These fibers follow the cranial nerve branches to their destinations. The **sacral outflow** consists of fibers that arise from cell bodies in the intermediate cell column of sacral segments 2 through 4. These fibers form the pelvic splanchnic nerves (nervi erigentes). The cranial and sacral outflows share many anatomic and functional features and together form the **parasympathetic division of the ANS.**

The sympathetic and parasympathetic divisions of the ANS differ not only in their sites of origin in the central nervous system but also on the basis of the neurotransmitters released at the terminals of their postganglionic fibers. The terminals of the parasympathetic postganglionic fibers liberate acetylcholine and thus are classified as **cholinergic.** The terminals of the sympathetic postganglionic fibers release **norepinephrine and epinephrine** and thus are classified as **adrenergic.** The terminals of sympathetic fibers on sweat glands do not follow this pattern, because they are cholinergic. Although the neurotransmitters released by postganglionic fibers distinguish the sympathetic and parasympathetic divisions, the preganglionic neurons in both systems release acetylcholine.

Many organs receive postganglionic innervation from both the sympathetic and parasympathetic systems. Moreover, the fibers from the two systems frequently have opposing effects. For example, parasympathetic fibers to the stomach increase peristalsis and relax the sphincters, whereas sympathetic fibers decrease peristalsis and tighten the sphincters.

Sympathetic Nervous System

The preganglionic neurons of the sympathetic nervous system are located in the intermediolateral cell column of the thoracolumbar spinal cord. Their axons, the myelinated preganglionic fibers (B fibers; see Table 3–1) of the sympathetic system, leave the spinal cord with the motor fibers of ventral roots T1 to L2. The axons then separate from the spinal nerves to form the **white rami communicantes,** which enter the **chain ganglia** of the **sympathetic trunks** (see Fig. 3–1B). The trunks consist of paired, ganglionated chains of nerve fibers that extend along either side of the vertebral column from the base of the skull to the coccyx. Some of the fibers of the white rami synapse with postganglionic neurons in the chain ganglion (also called **paravertebral ganglion**) nearest their point of entrance (see Fig. 3–1B). Other preganglionic fibers pass up or down the chain to end in paravertebral ganglia at higher or lower levels than the point of entrance (not shown in Fig. 3–1). A third group of preganglionic fibers passes through the paravertebral ganglion into the **splanchnic nerves** and terminates in the **prevertebral ganglia** of the abdomen and pelvis (see Fig. 3–1B).

Sympathetic Innervation of the Body Wall

Some of the nonmyelinated postganglionic fibers (C fibers) originating from the neurons in the sympathetic chain ganglia form the **gray rami communicantes** (see Fig. 3–1B). Each spinal nerve receives a gray ramus that delivers postganglionic fibers to be distributed to the blood vessels in the muscles and the blood vessels, erector pili muscles, and sweat glands of the skin throughout the **dermatome** (see Figs. 6–1 and 6–2) innervated by that nerve. In regions of the body that do not have separate chain ganglia for each segment, more than one gray ramus arises from each ganglion. For example, the large superior cervical ganglion provides postganglionic fibers in gray rami to cervical nerves 1 through 4 in addition to its postganglionic supply to the head. Thus, there are 31 gray rami on each side of the body, one for each spinal nerve, but only 14 white rami. As mentioned previously, the white rami carry the preganglionic fibers from the 12 thoracic and 2 upper lumbar segments to the sympathetic chain (trunk). Therefore, the cervical, lower lumbar, and sacral ganglia of the chain receive preganglionic fibers that have traveled up or down the trunk from the thoracolumbar levels.

Sympathetic Innervation of the Head and Neck

The **cervical part** of the sympathetic trunk consists of ascending preganglionic fibers from the first four or five thoracic segments of the spinal cord. There are three ganglia: **superior cervical,**

middle cervical, and **cervicothoracic** (stellate). The last is formed by fusion of the inferior cervical and first thoracic ganglia. The superior cervical ganglion cells give rise to the **carotid plexus,** a network of postganglionic fibers that follow the ramifications of the carotid arteries and furnish the sympathetic innervation of the entire head. Some fibers end in blood vessels and sweat glands of the head and face; others supply the lacrimal and salivary glands. The eye receives sympathetic fibers that innervate the dilator muscles of the pupil and the smooth muscle fibers in the muscle that raises the eyelid, the levator palpebrae superioris. In addition, the three cervical chain ganglia give rise to postganglionic fibers that form the **cardiac nerves** to the cardiac plexus.

Sympathetic Innervation of the Thoracic Viscera

The cardiac nerves from the cervical chain ganglia and postganglionic fibers from the upper five thoracic chain ganglia supply the viscera of the thorax. All these fibers enter the plexuses of the heart and lungs.

Sympathetic Innervation of the Abdominal and Pelvic Viscera

The pattern of sympathetic innervation of the viscera of the abdominal and pelvic cavities differs from that of the thorax. Preganglionic neurons in spinal cord segments T5 to T12 regulate the abdominal viscera. Their fibers pass through the sympathetic trunk without synapsing and enter the **thoracic splanchnic nerves.** The greater, lesser, and least thoracic splanchnic nerves carry these fibers to the **prevertebral (collateral) ganglia** (see Fig. 3–1B) of the abdomen. The prevertebral ganglia include the **celiac, superior mesenteric, and aorticorenal ganglia,** which are located at the roots of the arteries for which they are named. Neurons in these ganglia give rise to postganglionic axons that travel along the arterial walls to reach most of the abdominal viscera. Sympathetic innervation of the lower abdomen and pelvis arises from preganglionic neurons in the upper lumbar spinal cord. Their axons pass through the sympathetic trunk into the **lumbar splanchnic nerves,** which terminate in the **inferior mesenteric and hypogastric ganglia.** The postganglionic fibers from these prevertebral ganglia follow the ramifications of the visceral arteries to the organs.

Sympathetic Innervation of the Adrenal Gland

Stimulation of the sympathetic nervous system can, under certain circumstances, produce generalized physiologic responses rather than discrete localized effects. This results in part from the wide dispersion of sympathetic fibers, but the release of epinephrine from the adrenal glands into the bloodstream augments these effects. Preganglionic fibers from the lesser and least splanchnic nerves supply the medulla of the adrenal gland and end directly on the adrenal medullary cells without synapsing in an interposed ganglion. The chromaffin cells in the adrenal medulla are derivatives of the neural crest, as are the autonomic ganglia. Thus, in effect, the adrenal medulla constitutes a modified sympathetic ganglion. Pain, exposure to cold, and strong emotions such as anxiety, anger, and fear evoke sympathetic activity that mobilizes the body's resources for action. This mobilization suspends the functions of the gastrointestinal tract and shunts blood away from the splanchnic area. Heart rate and blood pressure increase, the coronary arteries dilate, and the bronchioles of the lungs widen. The spleen releases extra red cells to the blood. This activity has been described as the **fight or flight phenomenon** and results primarily from activation of the sympathetic nervous system and the adrenal medulla.

Clinical Aspects of Sympathetic Function

Injury to the sympathetic innervation of the orbit causes **Horner's syndrome.** Constriction of the **pupil** of the eye on the injured side results from paralysis of its dilator muscle. This is called **miosis.** Partial ptosis of the eyelid results from denervation of the smooth muscle fibers in the levator palpebrae superioris muscle, but the eyelid can still be raised voluntarily through the action of the general somatic efferent fibers in cranial nerve III on the skeletal muscle fibers in the same muscle. An apparent enophthalmos (the eye appears to be sunken into its socket) may be noted as well. **Absence of sweating (anhidrosis)** and **vasodilatation** on the affected side cause the skin of the face and neck to appear reddened and to feel warmer and drier than the normal side. Horner's syndrome results from lesions that interrupt the central or peripheral sympathetic pathways to the face, including the pathways from the hypothalamus and reticular formation descending ipsilaterally through the brain stem to the spinal cord. It can also occur when a lesion of the spinal cord destroys the preganglionic neurons in the upper thoracic segments or their axons in the cervical sympathetic trunk or after injury to the postganglionic cells in the superior cervical ganglion or to its postganglionic fibers in the carotid plexus.

Parasympathetic Nervous System

The preganglionic fibers of the parasympathetic system extend to the **terminal ganglia** located within, or very close to, the organs they supply. As a result, the postganglionic fibers are short.

The **cranial division** of the parasympathetic system originates in cranial nerves III, VII, IX, X, and XI. Parasympathetic fibers to the eye, which innervate the ciliary muscle and sphincter muscle of the pupil, pass through the oculomotor nerve (III) to the **ciliary ganglion,** which supplies postganglionic fibers to the eye. Secretory preganglionic fibers from the nervus intermedius of cranial nerve VII synapse in the **pterygopalatine** and **submandibular ganglia.** Postganglionic fibers from the pterygopalatine ganglion innervate glands in the mucous membrane of the nasal chamber, the air sinuses, the palate and pharynx, and the lacrimal gland, whereas fibers of the submandibular ganglion supply the sublingual and submandibular salivary glands. The **otic ganglion,** which receives preganglionic fibers through cranial nerve IX, sends postganglionic fibers to the parotid gland. The vagus nerve (X) supplies the preganglionic fibers to the heart, lungs, and abdominal viscera. Postganglionic neuron cell bodies in plexuses adjacent to or within the walls of the viscera innervate these organs. The cranial, or bulbar, part of cranial nerve XI also contributes to the preganglionic parasympathetic innervation of the heart.

The **sacral division** arises from parasympathetic preganglionic neurons in the intermediate gray column of lamina VII in spinal cord segments S2, S3, and S4. Axons of these cells form the **pelvic splanchnic nerves** and supply fibers to ganglia in the muscular coats of the urinary and reproductive tracts, the descending and sigmoid colon, and the rectum. In the pelvic region, the parasympathetic system is primarily concerned with mechanisms for emptying the bladder and rectum. In highly emotional circumstances, these fibers may discharge along with a generalized sympathetic response and may empty these organs involuntarily.

Autonomic Innervation of the Genitourinary System

Role in Sexual Function

Sexual activity requires both the parasympathetic and sympathetic divisions of the ANS. In women, the parasympathetic fibers cause increased vaginal secretions, erection of the clitoris, and engorgement of the labia minora. In men, the parasympathetic fibers induce penile erection, but stimulation by sympathetic fibers initiates the contractions of the ductus deferens and seminal vesicles to start the processes of emission and ejaculation. Final ejaculation through the urethral canal results from parasympathetic activity. Disease of the parasympathetic fibers, as in diabetic neuropathy, causes impotence, with failure of erection and ejaculation. Disease of the sympathetic fibers or drug treatment with adrenergic blocking agents can impair ejaculation. Sympathetic hyperactivity, often related to emotions, can cause weakness of erection and premature ejaculation. Loss of both libido and potency can be caused by cerebral lesions or by the use of various drugs, including antihypertensives, diuretics, antidepressants, antipsychotics, and sedatives.

Motor Innervation of the Urinary Bladder

Motor control of the urinary bladder results primarily from **parasympathetic function** that is purely reflex in infants but comes under voluntary regulation in neurologically normal adults. The preganglionic fibers of the parasympathetic nerves to the bladder have their cell bodies in the intermediate region of the gray matter of spinal cord segments S2, S3, and S4. They enter the pelvic splanchnic nerves, pass through the vesical plexus, and terminate on ganglia located in the wall of the bladder (Fig. 5–1). Short postganglionic fibers innervate the detrusor muscle, which

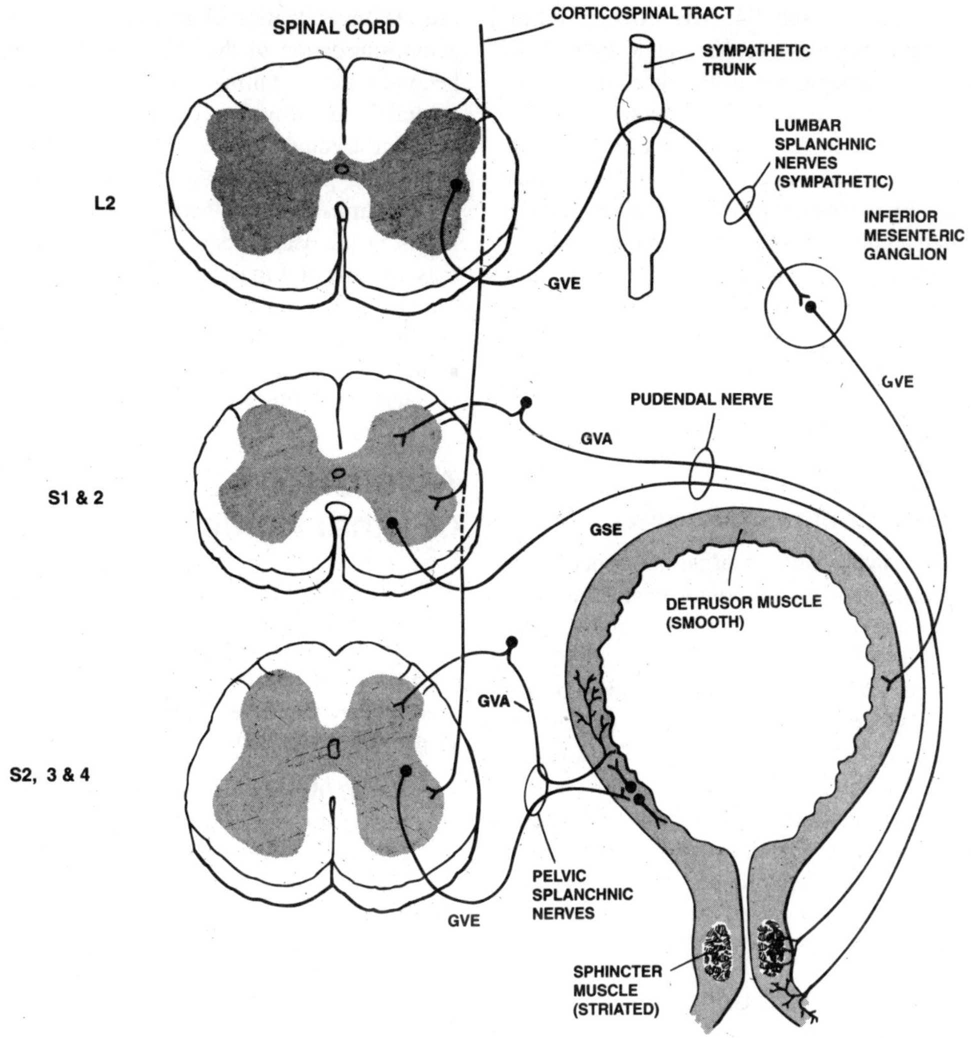

■ **FIGURE 5-1.** Autonomic innervation of the urinary bladder and associated somatic innervation of the sphincter. GSE = general somatic efferent; GVA = general visceral afferent; GVE = general visceral efferent.

forms the wall of the bladder. Stimulation of the parasympathetic nerves of the bladder contracts the detrusor muscle, opens the neck of the bladder into the urethra, and empties the bladder.

The **sympathetic supply** to the bladder originates in upper lumbar spinal cord segments from cells of the intermediolateral gray column whose axons pass through the sympathetic trunk and reach the inferior mesenteric ganglion through the lumbar splanchnic nerves. Postganglionic fibers continue through the hypogastric and vesical plexuses to the wall of the bladder. The functions of the sympathetic nerves are uncertain. They may assist the filling of the bladder by relaxing the detrusor muscle, but they have little influence on emptying mechanisms. Cutting the sympathetic nerves to the bladder does not seriously affect its function.

The external sphincter of the urethra consists of striated muscle and, along with other muscles of the perineum, receives innervation from **somatic motor fibers** of the pudendal nerve. The external sphincter may be closed voluntarily, but it relaxes by reflex action as soon as urine enters the urethra at the beginning of micturition.

Vesical Reflex

The smooth muscle of the bladder responds to a stretch reflex operated by **proprioceptors** in its wall that send afferent signals to spinal cord segments S2, S3, and S4. The efferent reflex fibers return impulses over the pelvic splanchnic nerves to maintain tonus in the detrusor muscle while the bladder fills. Reflex contraction of the detrusor muscle in response to bladder filling is called the **vesical reflex.** It can be evaluated clinically by **cystometry,** which involves placing measured amounts of sterile fluid into the bladder and measuring the resulting pressure. Ultrasound instruments can be used clinically to determine whether the vesical reflex results in complete bladder emptying. In infants, the uninhibited bladder fills to nearly its normal capacity, then a strong reflex response takes place, and the bladder empties automatically.

Voluntary Control of Urination

Voluntary suppression of urination depends on fibers that descend in the corticospinal tracts from the paracentral lobules of the cerebral cortex. This system is described in Chapter 8. These fibers can inhibit the vesical reflex. The sensation of increased bladder tension and the desire to void are conveyed by sensory impulses in the afferent fibers of the pelvic nerves and visceral afferent pathways (spinoreticular tracts) deep to the lateral spinothalamic tracts in the lateral funiculus of the spinal cord. The dorsal columns, however, may mediate the sensations of urethral touch and pressure. (See Chapters 6 and 7.)

Lesions That Affect Urinary Bladder Function

Lesions of the dorsal roots of the sacral segments interrupt afferent reflex fibers and produce an **atonic bladder.** The bladder wall becomes flaccid, and its capacity greatly increases. The sensation of fullness of the bladder is entirely lost. As the bladder becomes distended, incontinence and dribbling occur. Voluntary emptying remains possible, but emptying becomes incomplete, leaving residual urine in the bladder. Lesions of the conus medullaris of the spinal cord interrupt the central connections of the same reflex arc. Lesions of the cauda equina that destroy the second and third sacral roots interrupt both the afferent and efferent pathways of the reflex. Thus, all three of these lesions can cause an atonic bladder.

Injuries of the spinal cord above the level of the conus medullaris derange bladder reflexes and usually result initially in contraction of sphincter muscles and retention of urine. In the patient with acute transection of the spinal cord, the bladder becomes atonic, failing to empty when full. It is essential to provide constant or intermittent drainage through a catheter inserted through the urethra to prevent abnormal stretching of the bladder musculature. After several weeks, reflexes in the sacral segments of the spinal cord may recover and may begin to function, thereby establishing an automatic bladder. In this condition, the bladder fills and empties, either spontaneously or after scratching the skin over the sacral cutaneous area for stimulation.

Autonomic Reflexes of Other Pelvic Viscera

Several important reflexes, including pupillary, lacrimal, salivary, coughing, vomiting, and carotid sinus, are described in Chapter 11 with the account of the vagal system. Some of the reflexes mediated by the ANS in the pelvis are described in the following list.

- **Rectal (defecation) reflex:** Distension of the rectum or stimulation of rectal mucosa results in contraction of the rectal musculature. Sacral segments S2, S3, and S4 mediate this reflex.
- **Internal anal sphincter reflex:** Contraction of the internal anal sphincter can be detected on introduction of the examiner's gloved finger into the anus. Postganglionic sympathetic fibers through the hypogastric plexus mediate the reflex.
- **Bulbocavernosus reflex:** Pinching the dorsum of the glans penis causes contraction of the bulbocavernosus muscle and the urethral constrictor. The contraction can be palpated by placing a finger on the perineum behind the scrotum, with pressure on the bulbous or membranous portion of the urethra. An accompanying contraction of the external anal sphincter can be detected with a gloved finger placed in the anus. The third and fourth sacral nerves mediate this reflex.

Case Follow-up

The patient described at the beginning of this chapter has Raynaud's phenomenon, which consists of an episodic decrease of blood supply to the digits, manifested clinically by the sequential development of digital blanching (pallor) and cyanosis (blueness) after cold exposure, and rubor (redness) after rewarming. A thorough evaluation of the patient failed to disclose evidence of a disease that could cause Raynaud's phenomenon, and the patient was advised to wear thick gloves and socks before exposure to cold. These measures successfully minimized or prevented her symptoms. Vasospasm of the digital arteries causes Raynaud's phenomenon, and the vasospasm probably results from excessive activation of sympathetic nerve fibers innervating the digital arteries after exposure to cold. During the ischemic phase, capillaries and venules dilate, and cyanosis results from the deoxygenated blood in these vessels. Sensations of pain, numbness, and paresthesias of the digits result from stimulation of sensory nerves in the digits. With rewarming, the digital vasospasm resolves, and blood flow into the dilated arterioles and capillaries increases, with a reactive hyperemia imparting a bright red color to the digits. About 50% of people with Raynaud's phenomenon have Raynaud's disease, and the remaining 50% have the phenomenon as a consequence of another disease such as systemic lupus erythematosus, dermatomyositis, or arteriosclerosis.

SECTION 3

Ascending and Descending Pathways

6

Pain and Temperature

Case Study

A 60-year old woman develops numbness, tingling, and then a continuous severe, sharp, and burning pain on the right front and side of her chest wall that extends around the right side onto her back. After about 4 days, the skin in the area of the pain becomes red, and 1 to 2 days later, an eruption of clear, fluid-containing vesicles replaces the redness. Her pain continues and intensifies. After a few days, a crust covers the vesicles, and after another 2 weeks, the crust clears away, leaving a pigmented scar.

What disorder did this patient develop? What accounts for her severe pain? Is a treatment available for this?

Somatic Sensation

Our contact with the external world occurs through specialized structures termed **sensory receptors.** There are three general types: (1) **exteroceptive receptors** respond to stimuli from the external environment, including visual, auditory, and tactile stimuli; (2) **proprioceptive receptors** receive information about the relative positions of the body segments and of the body in space; and (3) **interoceptive receptors** detect internal events such as changes in blood pressure.

The somatic system receives information primarily from exteroceptive and proprioceptive receptors. There are four major subclasses of **somatic sensation:** (1) **pain sensation** results from noxious stimulation of the body surface; (2) **thermal sensation** consists of the separate senses of cold and warmth and occurs with exposure to temperatures colder or warmer than the body surface; (3) **position sense** results from mechanical changes in the muscles and joints, but it includes the sensations of static limb position and limb movement (kinesthesia); and (4) **touch-pressure sensation** occurs with mechanical stimulation of the body surface.

Overview of the Pathways for Pain, Thermal Sense, and Touch

The **anterolateral system** mediates the sensations of pain, itching, temperature, and simple touch. Itching sensation is related to pain. Simple touch is a form of touch-pressure sensation that includes a feeling of light contact with the skin associated with light pressure and a crude sense of tactile localization. Touch sensation is discussed further in Chapter 7. The anterolateral system originates from neurons located in several layers of the dorsal horn of the spinal cord. Most of the axons projecting from these neurons cross the midline through the ventral white commissure and ascend the spinal cord, to give rise to a diffuse bundle of fibers projecting through the anterior and lateral funiculi (see Fig. 1–9). The cells of origin are activated by small-diameter, lightly myelinated and unmyelinated dorsal root afferents, including Aδ (III) and C (IV) fibers, as well as larger myelinated cutaneous afferents. This system includes the **spinothalamic tracts** and the **spinoreticular tracts,** which do not reach the thalamus and thus cannot be termed spinothalamic.

Dorsal Roots of the Spinal Nerves Supply Dermatomes

The dorsal roots convey to the spinal cord essentially all sensations from receptors below the face. The area of skin supplied by one dorsal root is a **dermatome,** or skin segment. The approximate boundaries of human dermatomes are shown on the left side of Figures 6–1 and 6–2. A few sensory fibers have been discovered in the ventral roots. Many of these ventral root afferents respond to painful stimuli from superficial or deep tissues. The cell bodies of the dorsal root fibers are located in the spinal, or dorsal root, ganglia. Each pseudounipolar ganglion cell possesses a single nerve process that divides in the form of a T, with a central branch running to the spinal cord and a peripheral branch coming from a receptor organ or organs (Fig. 6–3). There are no synapses in a dorsal root ganglion. Dorsal root fibers enter the spinal cord through the **dorsal root entry zone,** which is in the region of the dorsolateral sulcus. The largest and most heavily myelinated fibers (Aα and Aβ) generally occupy the most medial position in this zone, and the small myelinated and unmyelinated fibers (Aδ and C) occupy the most lateral position.

Adjacent Spinal Nerves Form Peripheral Nerves

The dorsal and ventral roots converge to form the **spinal nerves** (see Fig. 3–1). Peripheral to this union, a mixture of sensory and motor fibers from individual spinal nerves separates into bundles or fascicles that join those of adjacent spinal nerves to form **peripheral nerves.** The cutaneous branches of each peripheral nerve therefore carry fibers from more than one spinal nerve, and the skin territory of each of these peripheral nerves covers portions of several dermatomes (Figs. 6–1 and 6–2, right side).

Pain-Temperature Pathways

Receptors for Pain

The naked terminals of small (Aδ and C) nerve fibers constitute the peripheral receptors for pain. Many of these may be specialized chemoreceptors that are excited by tissue substances released in response to noxious and inflammatory stimuli. Many substances have been implicated, including histamine, bradykinin, serotonin, acetylcholine, substance P, high concentrations of potassium, and substances involved in the arachidonic acid cascade, including products related to the cyclooxygenases. The concentration of hydrogen ion in these substances is critical in the activation of pain receptors. The stimulus that evokes pain is usually intense and may cause damage or destruction of tissue.

Dorsal Root Afferents Convey Pain Stimuli to the Dorsal Horn

The cell bodies of Aδ and C axons mediating noxious stimuli are in the dorsal root ganglia. The axons enter the spinal cord through the lateral part of the dorsal root zone and immediately divide into short ascending and descending branches that run longitudinally in the **posterolateral fasciculus** (**Lissauer's tract;** see Figs. 1–9 and 6–3). Within one segment or two, these fibers leave Lissauer's tract to connect synaptically with neurons in the dorsal horn, including those in **lami-**

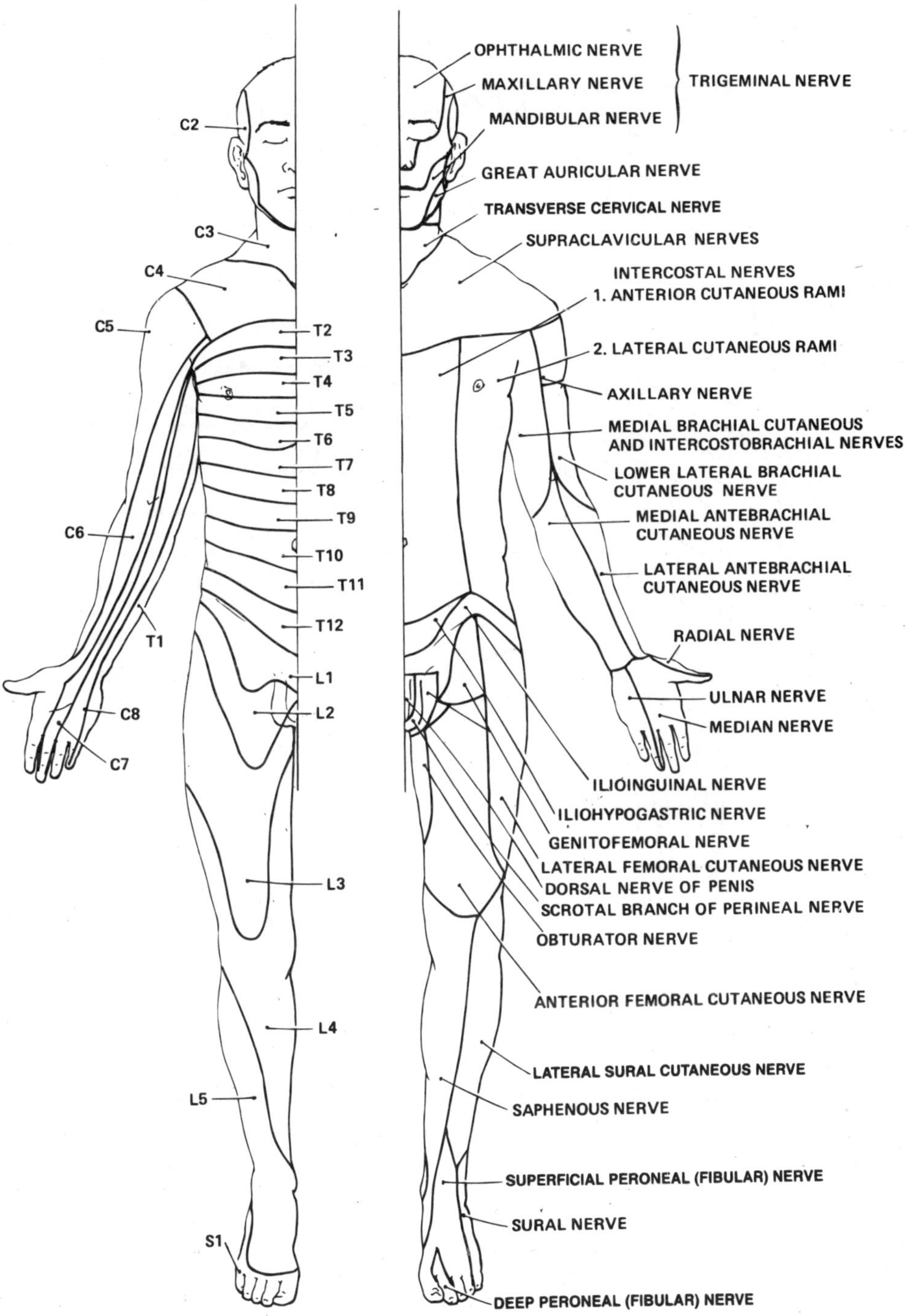

■ **FIGURE 6–1.** The pattern of innervation of the anterior surface of the body by dorsal roots (*left*) and peripheral nerves (*right*).

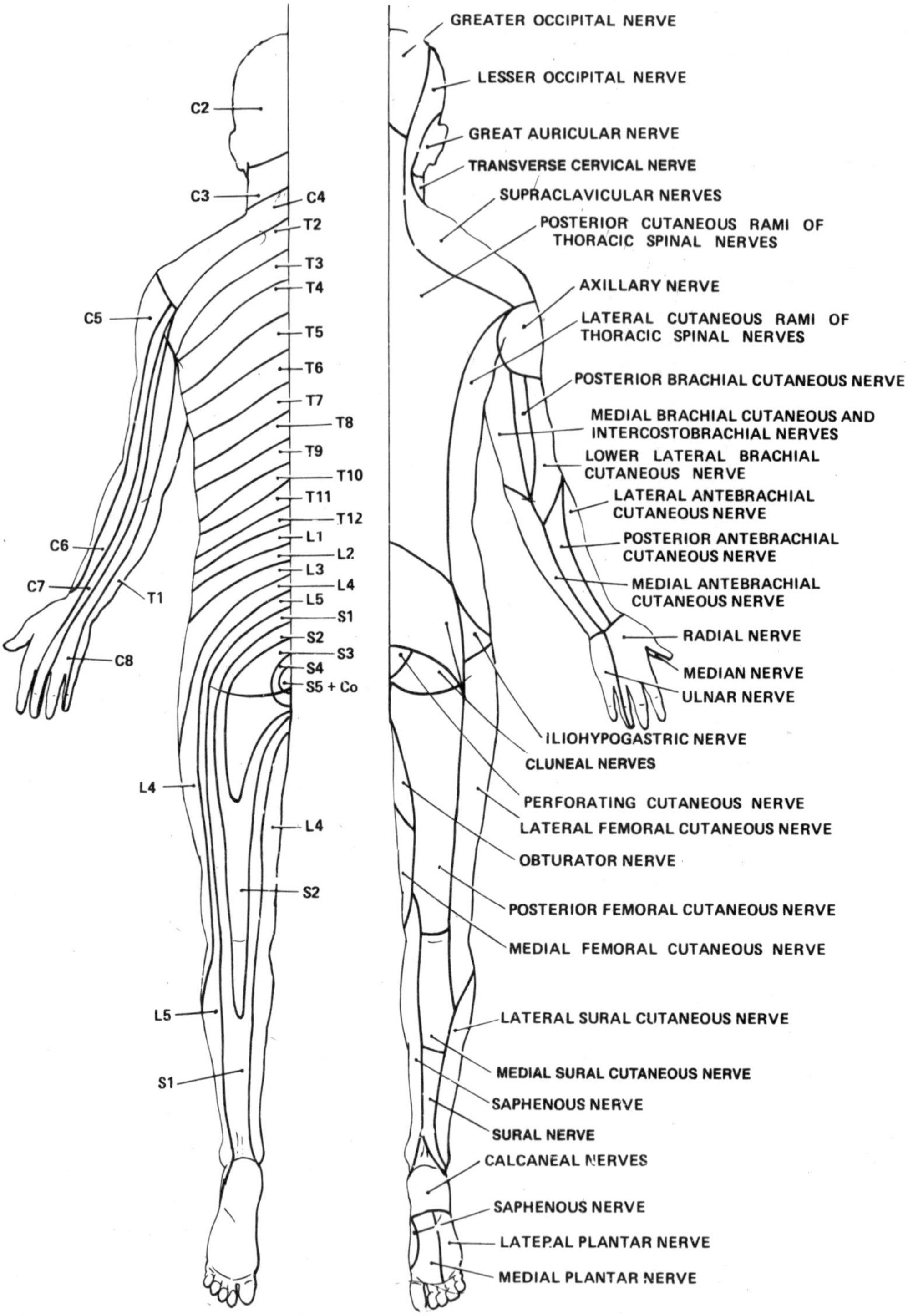

■ **FIGURE 6-2.** The pattern of innervation of the posterior surface of the body by dorsal roots (*left*) and peripheral nerves (*right*).

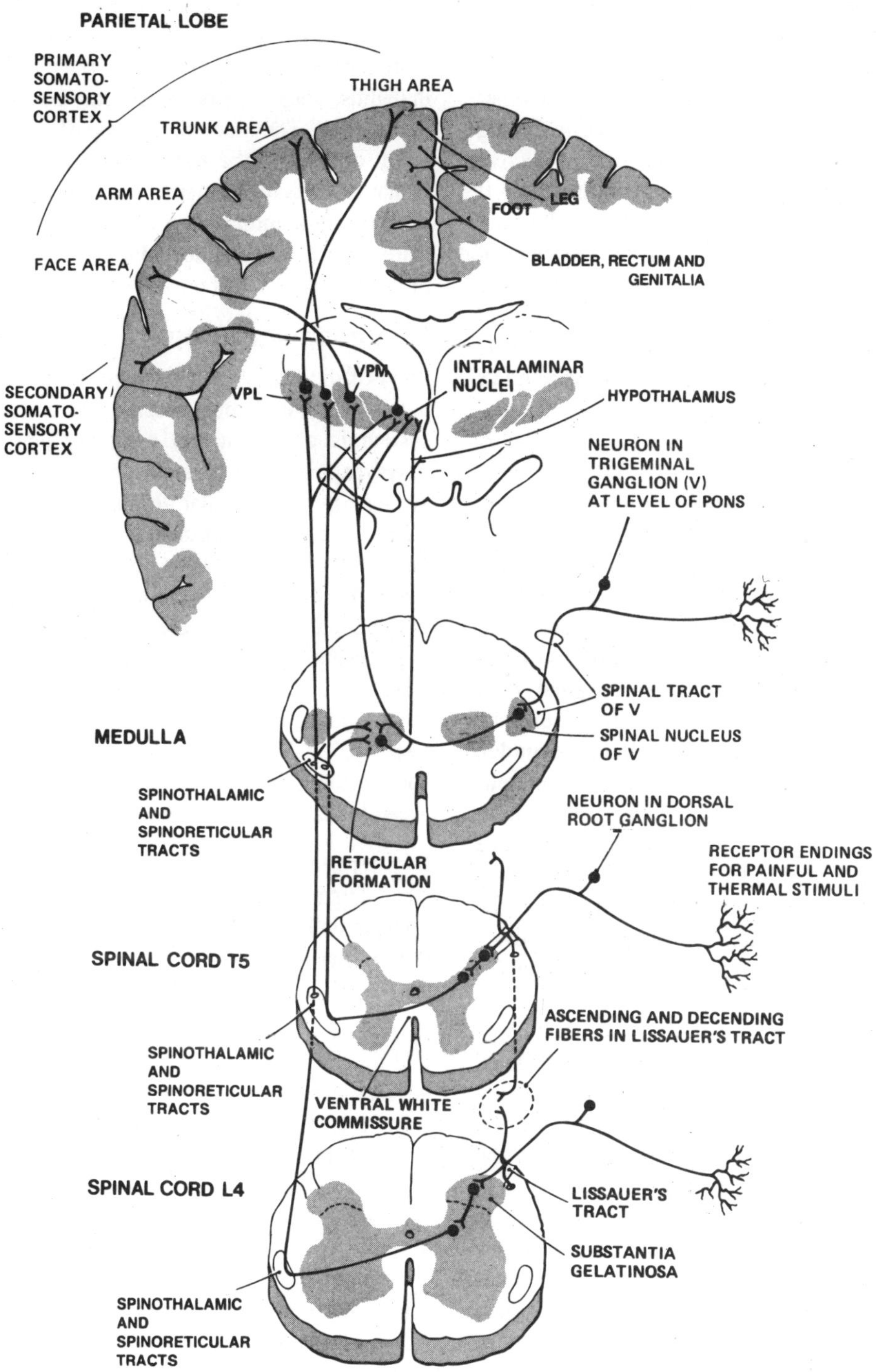

■ **FIGURE 6–3.** The central nervous system pathways that mediate the sensations of pain and temperature. VPL = ventral posterolateral nucleus; VPM = ventral posteromedial nucleus.

nae I (posteromarginal nucleus), II (substantia gelatinosa), III, IV, and V. These neurons contain receptors for numerous neurotransmitters, including excitatory amino acids and neuropeptides. At their connections with these neurons, Aδ and C fibers release glutamate and substance P and other substances that have been implicated, including calcitonin gene–related peptide and vasoactive intestinal peptide. Interneurons in laminae II through IV project to neurons in laminae V and there make synaptic connection on the cells of origin of the anterolateral system, including the spinothalamic tracts and the spinoreticular projections. Neurons in lamina I also give rise to fibers that contribute directly to the spinothalamic tracts (not shown in Fig. 6–3).

Spinothalamic Tracts

The axons of **spinothalamic tract** cells in laminae I and in laminae V cross anterior to the central canal in the **ventral white commissure** and then course rostrally in the **anterolateral funiculus.** The spinothalamic and spinoreticular tracts ascend through the spinal cord and brain stem and supply inputs to other spinal cord segments and to the **reticular formation,** the **superior colliculus,** and several **thalamic nuclei,** including the **intralaminar nuclei** and the **ventral posterolateral nucleus (VPL)**. These areas are discussed in greater detail in Chapter 20. The VPL is considered to be part of the **ventrobasal complex,** in which activity mediated by the spinothalamic projections converges with activity carried by the lemniscal system. (See Chapter 7.) Projections of the anterolateral system to the VPL are organized somatotopically, so the fibers carrying input from the upper body are located medial to those with input from the lower body (Fig. 6–3). This somatotopic organization is maintained in the projections of fibers from the VPL conveying painful and thermal sensations to the **primary somatosensory cortex:** Brodmann's areas 3, 1, and 2 of the **postcentral gyrus** (see Figs. 6–3, 20–1, and 20–2). The primary somatosensory cortex is organized by body parts (i.e., somatotopically), like the adjacent primary motor cortex. The fibers from the upper parts of the body project to cortical areas near the lateral fissure, and those from the lower limb and perineum terminate on the medial surface of the hemisphere in the **paracentral lobule** (see Figs. 1–3 and 20–2). The postcentral gyrus is interconnected with the posterior portions of the parietal lobe. Together, these areas are responsible for localizing pain stimuli and for integrating the pain modality with other types of sensory stimuli.

In humans, only a few fibers in the anterolateral system project directly from the spinal cord to the thalamus; these fibers constitute the spinothalamic tracts. They include a group of phylogenetically old fibers, the **paleospinothalamic tract,** which projects to the medial portions of the thalamus (the intralaminar nuclei), and the phylogenetically newer **neospinothalamic tract,** which projects to the ventral posterolateral region.

Spinoreticular Tracts

Most of the fibers in the anterolateral system do not reach the thalamus directly. The anterolateral system is predominantly a slowly conducting, polysynaptic system, and most of the fibers synapse in the reticular formation of the brain stem. These are the **spinoreticular tracts.** From the cells of the reticular formation, ascending fibers relay pain information to the medial and intralaminar nuclei of the thalamus and to the hypothalamus and limbic system (Fig. 6–3). (See Chapter 21.) Although most fibers of the anterolateral system cross the midline before ascending, some, particularly those conveying visceral sensory information in the spinoreticular tracts, ascend ipsilaterally (not shown in Fig. 6–3).

Trigeminothalamic and Trigeminoreticular Tracts Transmit Pain Sensations from the Head

Pain fibers from the face, the cornea of the eye, the sinuses, and the mucosa of the lips, cheeks, and tongue travel in the **trigeminal nerve** to its sensory ganglion, which is known as the **semilunar, trigeminal,** or **gasserian ganglion.** On entering the brain stem in the pontine region, the central processes of the trigeminal ganglion neurons form an ipsilateral descending tract, the **spinal tract of V,** which courses to the level of the upper cervical segments of the spinal cord. Along the course of this tract, terminals of its fibers form synapses in an adjacent nucleus, the **spinal nucleus of V.** Axons of cells in the spinal nucleus of V cross to the opposite side and ascend to the **ventral posteromedial nucleus (VPM)** of the thalamus (see Figs. 6–3 and 12–1).

The ascending trigeminal pathway also projects to the reticular formation and the medial and intralaminar thalamic nuclei, which receive projections from the anterolateral system of the spinal cord. The cortical projections of the VPM are to the part of the somatosensory cortex closest to the lateral fissure. The areas of the body most sensitive to somatosensory stimuli (e.g., lips and fingers) have disproportionately large areas of neuronal representation in the somatosensory cortex. Thalamocortical fibers from neurons in the intralaminar thalamic nuclei and parts of the VPL-VPM complex relay pain information to the **secondary somatic sensory area** of the cerebral cortex (Fig. 6–3).

Perception of Pain

Although physicians continually manage pain in their patients, they do so despite wide gaps in their knowledge concerning the structure and function of the receptors and central pathways involved. Pain has several aspects including a distinctive sensation, the individual's reaction to this sensation (including accompanying emotional overtones), activity in both somatic and autonomic systems, and both reflex and volitional efforts of avoidance or escape. Three types of pain sensation occur after acute noxious events. The first, **fast pain,** consists of a sharp, pricking sensation that can be localized accurately and results from activation of Aδ fibers, which are myelinated. The second is **slow pain,** a burning sensation that has a slower onset, greater persistence, and a less clear location. Slow pain results from the activation of C fibers, which are unmyelinated. The third type is **deep** or **visceral pain,** which is described either as aching, sometimes with a burning quality, or as cramping. Visceral pain results from stimulation of visceral and deep somatic receptors such as those in joints and muscles. The cramping type of visceral pain may signify the obstruction of a hollow viscus. Visceral receptors are innervated by both unmyelinated C fibers and Aδ myelinated fibers that pass through the sympathetic nerves (see Fig. 3–1B). There is no convincing evidence that separate central nervous system pathways mediate fast pain and slow pain. Good evidence indicates that the neospinothalamic pathway, projecting to the VPL of the thalamus and from there to the primary somatosensory cortex, is essential for the spatial and temporal discrimination of painful sensations. The paleospinothalamic pathway and the spinoreticular pathways, with their connections to the secondary somatosensory cortex, hypothalamus, and limbic system, mediate systemic autonomic responses to pain and probably the emotional and affective responses as well. Cortical activation patterns revealed using positron emission tomography indicate that the cingulate cortex is one of these limbic areas activated by pain.

In patients with complete destruction of the somatosensory areas of cerebral cortex on one side of the brain, painful stimuli can be detected on the contralateral side of the body, provided the thalamus and lower structures remain intact. Destruction of the posterior and intralaminar nuclei of the thalamus can relieve intractable pain. Such lesions may be effective only briefly, however, and pain may return. Lesions of the dorsomedial and anterior nuclei of the thalamus, or transection of the fibers linking these nuclei to the frontal lobe and anterior cingulate cortex (i.e., **prefrontal leukotomy**), can diminish the anguish of constant pain by changing the psychologic response to painful stimuli. Unfortunately, marked negative changes in personality and intellectual capacities occur after creation of these lesions. However, bilateral section of the cingulum bundle (i.e., **cingulotomy**) has proved to be effective in relieving patients' reaction to pain without causing the drastic personality changes that occur with prefrontal leukotomy.

Temperature Sense

The receptors in the skin for the sensations of cold and warmth consist of naked nerve endings. The peripheral nerve fibers mediating these sensations are thinly myelinated Aδ and some C fibers. Other types of C fibers mediate only the painful components of the extremes of hot and cold stimuli. The central nervous system pathway for thermal sensation appears to follow the same course as the pain pathway. The two systems are so closely associated in the central nervous system that they cannot be distinguished anatomically, and injury to one usually affects the other to a similar degree.

Visceral Pain Pathways and Referred Pain

The parenchyma of internal organs, including the brain itself, contains no pain receptors. Pain receptors are located within the walls of arteries, all peritoneal surfaces, pleural membranes, and the dura mater covering the brain. These structures can be sources of severe pain, especially with inflammation or mechanical deformation. Abnormal contraction or dilatation of the walls of hollow viscera, including blood vessels, also causes pain. Pain fibers from viscera project to the spinal cord as components of the sympathetic nerves. In contrast, fibers conveying primarily nonpainful visceral sensations project to the central nervous system as components of parasympathetic nerves, principally the vagus and the parasympathetic nerves of the pelvis. Parasympathetic afferents are discussed in Chapter 11.

General visceral afferents from pain receptors in the viscera follow the peripheral sympathetic nerves (e.g., splanchnic nerves) from the viscera to the sympathetic trunk. They reach the spinal cord by passing from the trunk to the thoracic and lumbar spinal nerves over the white rami (see Fig. 3–1B). Their cell bodies are in the dorsal root ganglia of segments T1 to L2, and their axons terminate at synapses in the dorsal horn and intermediate gray matter, including the **intermediomedial nucleus** of lamina VII (see Fig. 1–9). These nuclei, in turn, project axons bilaterally through the anterolateral system to the brain stem reticular formation, intralaminar thalamic nuclei, and hypothalamus. In addition, evidence suggests that some visceral pain is mediated by neurons with cell bodies in the deep central spinal gray matter, whose axons ascend in the dorsal midline with the dorsal columns. These fibers terminate on neurons in the nuclei of the dorsal columns, which project to the ventral posterior thalamus.

Pain of visceral origin is apt to be vaguely localized. It may be perceived in a surface area of the body far removed from its actual source, a phenomenon known as **referred pain.** For example, the pain of coronary heart disease may be felt in the chest wall, the left axilla, or down the inside of the left arm. In addition, inflammation of the peritoneum covering the diaphragm may be felt over the shoulder. In each of these cases, the peripheral afferents that supply the skin area of the referred pain enter the same segment of the spinal cord as visceral afferents conducting pain from the affected visceral organ. Referring to the pain of coronary artery disease mentioned earlier, spinal cord segments T1 and T2 receive sensory fibers from skin areas of the left upper extremity and from the heart. Moreover, segments C3, C4, and C5 supply the skin of the shoulder area and also receive sensory fibers from the diaphragm. One of the many theoretical explanations of referred pain is that visceral sensory fibers discharge into the same pool of neurons in the spinal cord as fibers from the skin, and an "overflow" of impulses results in misinterpretation of the true origin of the pain.

Referred pain can result from noxious stimuli affecting deep somatic as well as visceral structures. For example, injury of ligaments and muscles associated with the vertebral column can lead to pain affecting a segmental distribution different from the level of origin of the painful stimuli.

Effect of Cutting the Spinothalamic Tract

The lateral spinothalamic tracts can be sectioned in the human spinal cord to relieve intractable pain, a procedure known as **tractotomy.** The neurosurgeon makes a cut in the anterior part of the lateral funiculus. There is usually some damage to the ventral spinocerebellar tract, and perhaps to certain extrapyramidal motor fibers, but no permanent symptoms develop, except a loss of pain sensibility on the contralateral side beginning one or two segments below the cut (see Fig. 7–4B). In some patients, pain relief occurs only temporarily, a finding suggesting that other routes may be available or that both crossed and uncrossed tracts mediate nociceptive sensations in the spinal cord. Visceral pain, in particular, often persists after spinothalamic tractotomy.

Sensory Effects of Dorsal Root Irritation

Mechanical compression or local inflammation of dorsal nerve roots irritates pain fibers and commonly produces pain along the distribution of the affected roots. Pain distributed over an area that is consistent with the boundaries of one dermatome or more than one adjacent dermatome is known as **radicular pain.** Sensory changes other than pain may be associated with dorsal root irritation. There may be localized areas of **paresthesias,** which are spontaneous sensations of prickling, tingling, or numbness. Zones of **hyperesthesia,** in which tactile stimuli appear to be grossly exaggerated, may be present. If the pathologic process progresses and gradually destroys fibers, the dorsal roots will eventually lose their ability to conduct sensory impulses. There will then be **hypesthesia** (i.e., diminished sensitivity) and eventually **anesthesia** (i.e., complete absence of all forms of sensibility) in the affected dermatomes. Essentially all areas of skin receive fibers from more than a single dorsal root; consequently, damage to a single dorsal root may cause little or no sensory loss.

Endogenous Analgesia

Studies in animals have shown that analgesia results from electrical stimulation of peripheral nerve fibers or of discretely distributed loci in the brain, particularly in an irregular series of sites along the medial periventricular and periaqueductal axis, including the **midline raphe nuclei** of the brain stem. The raphe nuclei are found throughout the brain stem. These nuclei are densely populated with neurons that produce the neurotransmitter **serotonin.** The axons of the caudal raphe nuclei descend to the spinal cord through the dorsolateral fasciculus. (See Chapter 8.) These axons terminate in the dorsal horn, where they attenuate the responses of spinothalamic and other dorsal horn cells to spinal nerve afferents mediating noxious stimuli.

The analgesia produced by electrical stimulation of the central nervous system probably results primarily from the release of **opioid peptides,** although other nonopioid neurotransmitters such as serotonin, dopamine, and norepinephrine also mediate analgesia. Enkephalin, beta-endorphin, and dynorphin represent the three families of the opioid peptides, which are naturally occurring substances that bind to the same receptors in the central nervous system as opiate drugs. Opioid peptide neurotransmitters and their opioid-binding receptors are found in the brain structures involved in the modulation of pain transmission. (See Chapter 23.) Enkephalin interneurons are found in laminae I through III of the dorsal horn of the spinal cord. Inputs from the descending serotonergic and noradrenergic fibers activate these interneurons, and, in turn, they inhibit the transmission of painful sensations at the first synaptic connection in the pain pathway. This is one of several ways in which pain may be suppressed through intrinsic, endogenous central nervous system mechanisms.

Central Pain (Thalamic Syndrome)

Injury of the central nervous system, usually affecting the spinothalamic or trigeminothalamic tracts, can result in severe, spontaneous pain in portions of the body represented in the damaged tracts. This is called **central pain.** Often, cutaneous stimulation of the affected region of the body triggers or worsens central pain, although the pain can also occur without provocation. Commonly, the affected portions of the body have an elevated threshold to the perception of pain and temperature. Lesions of many portions of the central nervous system can lead to central pain, including the cerebral cortex, thalamus, brain stem, and spinal cord.

A frequently encountered form of central pain occurs after injury to the thalamus, which often results from vascular disease (stroke). The VPL and VPM are usually involved, and, correspondingly, the patient develops a marked decrease of all modalities of sensation on the contralateral side of the body. Usually, the affected limbs are also paralyzed because of damage to the corticospinal tract, which is located in the internal capsule adjacent to the thalamus. After a brief interval, generally several weeks, the patient develops an agonizing burning pain in the affected parts of the body, worsened by any sort of sensory stimulation of the painful areas. The combination of hemianesthesia with spontaneous pain and hemiparesis is called the **thalamic syndrome.** Fortunately, medical therapy can sometimes relieve the pain that occurs with this syndrome. The thalamic syndrome results in one of the more severe forms of pain that follows damage to the central nervous system.

Case Follow-up

The patient presented at the beginning of this chapter developed herpes zoster, a viral disease causing inflammation of the dorsal root ganglia along with severe pain and a cutaneous eruption in the skin area, or dermatome, to which the ganglion cells distribute peripheral nerve endings. The disease is caused by the varicella virus, which causes chickenpox. Herpes zoster affects only people who have had chickenpox earlier in life, and it occurs when the latent virus becomes reactivated, often in people with immunologic disorders. The pain results from inflammation of neurons in the dorsal root ganglia that convey pain sensations. Currently available medications can reduce the inflammation and the severity of the pain resulting from herpes zoster.

7

Proprioception, Touch, and Tactile Discrimination

Case Study

A boy begins developing an irregular, staggering gait at about 7 years of age. This problem progresses and leads to frequent falls, and his speech becomes difficult to understand because of "slurring." His arm and hand coordination becomes affected at age 10 years, and about 5 years later, he develops leg weakness. By age 25 years, he is confined to a wheelchair. Examination at that time reveals abnormalities in eye movements, a speech disorder, and marked weakness of the legs. Coordinated movements with the arms and legs are slow and clumsy, and he develops a lateral tremor of the arm or leg he uses with reaching movements. He has markedly impaired cutaneous sensation of all four limbs, worse in the legs than the arms, with impairment of pain and tactile discrimination as well as position sense and vibration sense. Deep tendon reflexes are absent in his arms and legs.

Which pathways and structures are involved in this disorder? What disorder does he have? Is treatment available for him?

Tactile sensations are complex because they involve a blending of light cutaneous contact (touch) and variable degrees of pressure, depending on the intensity of the stimuli. In addition, tactile stimuli can be either static or dynamic with respect to space and time. Tactile sensation is divided into **light touch** and **tactile discrimination.** Light touch involves detection of contact with the skin. Tactile discrimination involves perception of the size and shape of objects. In neurologically normal persons, even light tactile stimuli that reach threshold can be localized with precision. Tickling and itching sensations are related to pain and not to tactile sense.

Contacting the skin with a wisp of cotton wool can test light touch. Von Frey hairs are used for experimental work. These are fine hairs of graduated stiffness used to apply stimuli at calibrated intensities to the skin. Several methods can be used to test tactile discrimination. The first is to ask the subject, with eyes closed, to identify common small objects placed in one hand **(stereognosis).** The second is to determine whether one touch stimulus or two simultaneous stimuli have been applied to the skin **(two-point discrimination).** The third is to ask the subject to identify numbers or letters written on the surface of the skin with a blunt object **(complex tactile discrimination).**

The sense of flutter-vibration is also an important component of tactile sensation. The sense of **flutter** is a feeling of repetitive movement, and the sense of **vibration** is a more diffuse and penetrating feeling of "humming" when the base of a vibrating tuning fork contacts a bony prominence of the body.

Proprioceptive sensation includes both **static limb position** and **kinesthesia** (i.e., the sense of movement). Proprioception can be tested by asking the patient to determine whether a distal joint is moving up or down as the examiner moves the joint while the patient's vision is occluded.

Central Nervous System Pathways

Two different sets of sensory pathways in the spinal cord provide essential information to the brain about muscle action, joint position, and the objects with which a person is in contact. The pathways in one of these groups project to the cerebellum, which uses the information for the coordination of movement but not for conscious perception. This group includes four named pathways: the dorsal and ventral spinocerebellar tracts, the cuneocerebellar tract, and the rostral spinocerebellar tract. The second set of pathways includes three tracts that project to the cerebral cortex by way of the thalamus. Information carried by these pathways is perceived consciously. They are the spinal lemniscus, the spinothalamic tract, and the lateral cervical system. Both sets of sensory pathways use mechanoreceptors.

Mechanoreceptors

Mechanoreceptors in the muscles, joints, and skin mediate the various separate and integrated sensations of proprioception, touch, and tactile discrimination. Mechanoreceptors include muscle spindles, Golgi tendon organs, Pacinian corpuscles, Meissner's corpuscles, and other encapsulated receptors, as well as free nerve endings, in muscles, tendons, ligaments, joint capsules, and skin. Information about static limb position comes chiefly from **muscle spindle** afferents. Kinesthetic (joint movement) sensation is not mediated solely by the **joint receptor** afferents, which appear to play a minor role, but by a combination of receptors in the skin, muscles, and joints. **Pacinian corpuscles,** which are found in the skin and connective tissues surrounding bones and joints, detect vibration. **Meissner's corpuscles** mediate superficial phasic touch sensation. In addition, the movement of hairs, detected by **free nerve endings** in hair follicles, conveys a sense of touch. Large-diameter myelinated fibers innervate most of the mechanoreceptors, with the exception of free nerve endings. The cell bodies of these peripheral nerve fibers are in the dorsal root ganglia, and their central processes enter the medial side of the dorsal root zone.

After entering the spinal cord, afferent fibers from mechanoreceptors distribute to three different sites. These are (1) interneurons and motoneurons in the ventral horn of the spinal cord, (2) neurons in the dorsal and intermediate gray areas of the spinal cord that are the origin of the ascending pathways, and (3) neurons of the dorsal column nuclei in the medulla.

Mechanoreceptor Reflexes

Afferent fibers from muscle spindles (Aα Ia and Aβ II fibers) make excitatory monosynaptic connections on alpha motoneurons innervating the muscles of origin of the respective spindle afferents. These connections form the basis of the stretch (deep tendon) reflex (see Fig. 4–1). Afferent fibers from muscle spindles also make inhibitory polysynaptic connections with motoneurons innervating the physiologic antagonists of the muscles of origin of the spindles.

Golgi tendon organ afferents (Aα Ib fibers) synapse on interneurons that inhibit motoneurons innervating the muscle in which the tendon organ is located. They also make excitatory polysynaptic connections with motoneurons of antagonist muscles.

Pathways to the Cerebellum from the Lower Limb

Two pathways carry proprioceptive and other somatosensory stimuli from the lower limbs to the cerebellum. These are the ventral and dorsal spinocerebellar tracts. Some proprioceptive fiber collaterals, especially from Golgi tendon organs, as well as fibers conveying other sensory modalities such as pressure and pain, synapse with neurons in the intermediate gray area and the base of the posterior horn of the spinal cord (Fig. 7–1). At lumbar and, to a lesser extent, sacral levels of the spinal cord (but not at more rostral levels), these neurons give rise to the primarily crossed **ventral spinocerebellar tract,** the most peripheral tract in the ventral margin of the lateral funiculus.

The **nucleus dorsalis,** or Clarke's nucleus, is located at the base of the posterior horn in spinal segments T1 through L2. This column of neurons receives afferents from muscle spindles, cutaneous touch receptors, and joint receptors. Axons of these neurons ascend rostrally on the ipsilateral side in the **dorsal spinocerebellar tract,** which is located just posterior to the ventral spinocerebellar tract in the lateral funiculus (Fig. 7–1). Whereas the proprioceptive afferents from dorsal roots T1 to L2 synapse in the nucleus dorsalis at the level where they enter the spinal cord, the corresponding afferents from dorsal roots L3 to S5 ascend in the fasciculus gracilis of the dorsal funiculus to reach the nucleus dorsalis. There they synapse in the lowest part of the nucleus at segmental levels L1 and L2. Thus, the dorsal

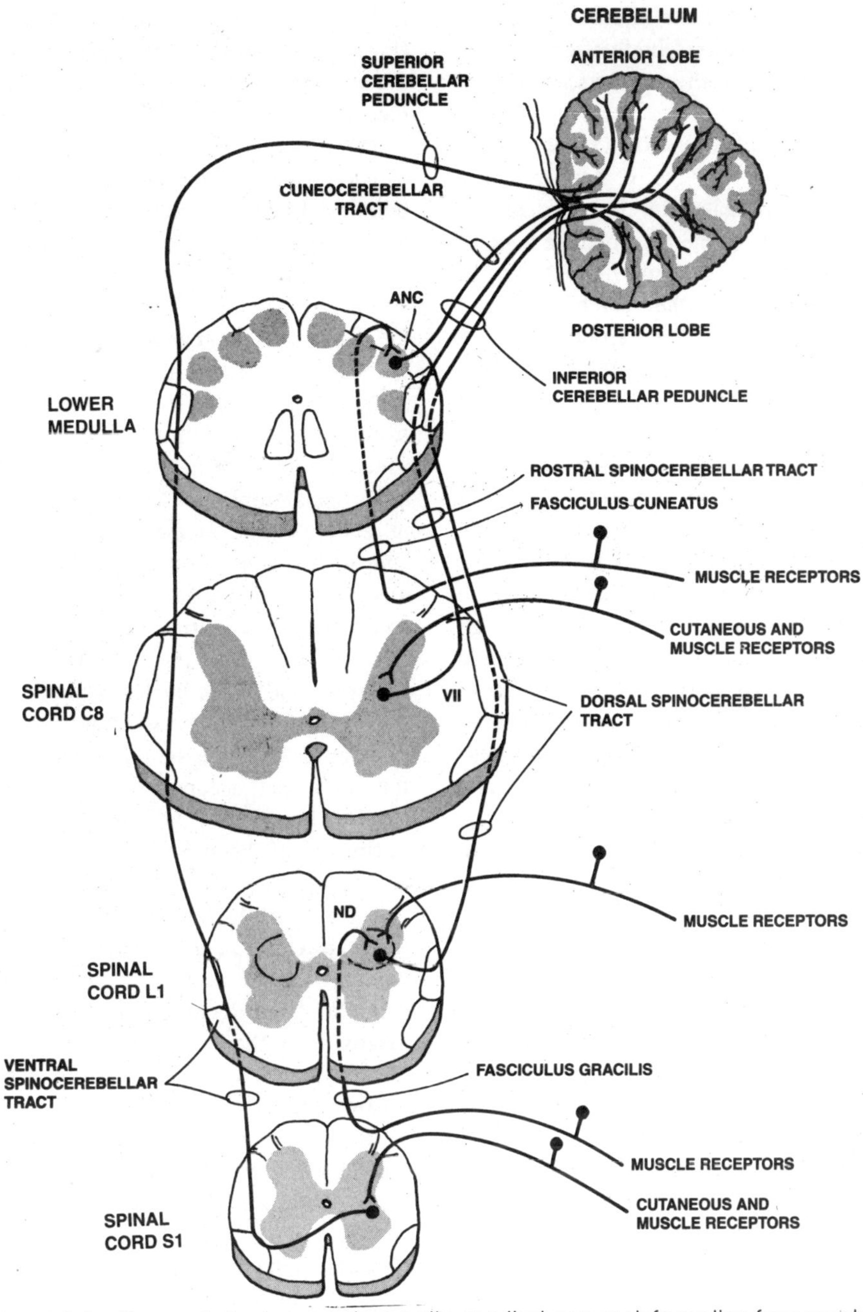

■ **FIGURE 7-1.** The central nervous system pathways that convey information from mechanoreceptors in the muscles, joints, and skin to the cerebellum. ACN = accessory cuneate nucleus; ND = nucleus dorsalis; VII = lamina VII.

spinocerebellar tract, as a fascicle of fibers on the surface of the lateral funiculus, begins at the L2 segment of the spinal cord.

Pathways to the Cerebellum from the Upper Limbs

Mechanoreceptor information from the upper limbs reaches the cerebellum through two additional pathways: the cuneocerebellar tract and the rostral spinocerebellar tract. Afferent fibers from C2 to T5 travel up the dorsal funiculus in the fasciculus cuneatus to synapse on neurons in the **accessory (or lateral) cuneate nucleus** (Fig. 7–1) in the lower medulla. This nucleus is the upper-extremity counterpart of the nucleus dorsalis and gives rise to the ipsilateral **cuneocer-**

ebellar tract (dorsal arcuate fibers). This pathway mediates information chiefly from muscle spindles, cutaneous touch receptors, and joint receptors.

The **rostral spinocerebellar tract** is the upper-limb equivalent of the ventral spinocerebellar tract. It originates in the cervical enlargement from cells of the intermediate zone of the spinal cord gray area (Fig. 7–1). Axons of these cells project to the cerebellum and terminate with fibers of the ventral spinocerebellar tract. This pathway mediates information chiefly from Golgi tendon organs and from pressure and pain receptors.

The ascending fibers of the dorsal spinocerebellar, cuneocerebellar, and rostral spinocerebellar pathways enter the cerebellum through the inferior cerebellar peduncle, whereas those of the ventral spinocerebellar tract continue through the pons and ascend into the cerebellum through the superior cerebellar peduncle. All four of these tracts terminate primarily in the midline (vermis and intermediate zone) portions of the cerebellum ipsilateral to the cells of origin of the tracts. These tracts project especially heavily to the anterior lobe but also to the caudal part of the posterior lobe and are concerned with processes that govern standing and walking.

Pathways to the Cerebral Cortex

The **spinal lemniscal system** carries to the cerebral cortex proprioceptive information from receptors for position sense, kinesthesia, and tactile discrimination. Two other pathways mediate tactile sensation. The **spinothalamic tract** of the anterolateral system subserves light touch sensation in addition to pain and temperature. This pathway is described in Chapter 6. In addition, the **lateral cervical system** (spinocervicothalamic pathway) mediates tactile, vibratory, and proprioceptive sensation.

Spinal Lemniscal System

Afferent fibers from muscle spindles, Golgi tendon organs, and mechanoreceptors in joints and skin provide inputs to the spinal lemniscal system. These inputs contribute to conscious position and movement sense. Other fibers in this system convey information about touch, pressure, and flutter-vibration. Many of these fibers are dorsal root afferents that ascend in the posterior funiculi without synapsing in the spinal cord and end in relay nuclei in the lower part of the medulla (Fig. 7–2). Other fibers in this system are axons of dorsal horn cells that receive synapses from mechanoreceptor afferents. (These cells are not shown in Fig. 7–2.)

The posterior funiculus consists of two large bundles of fibers called **fasciculi.** Fibers from the leg ascend adjacent to the dorsal median septum and form the **fasciculus gracilis.** Fibers from the arm ascend lateral to the leg fibers and constitute the **fasciculus cuneatus.** Fibers from the foot enter this system in the lower segments of the spinal cord, followed in ascending order by those from the leg, thigh, trunk, hand, arm, and neck. Thus, the fibers of the posterior funiculus maintain a somatotopic (or ''body map'') organization in relation to one another. The fasciculus gracilis and the fasciculus cuneatus ascend to the lower medulla, where they end in the **nucleus gracilis** and **nucleus cuneatus,** respectively. Clinicians often refer to these tracts as the dorsal column pathways and to the nuclei as the dorsal column nuclei. Additional fibers of the spinal lemniscal system travel within the dorsal part of the lateral funiculus and accompany the lateral cervical system (Fig. 7–3). Thus the term **dorsolateral pathway** can be used for the entire lemniscal pathway in the spinal cord.

The cells of the dorsal column nuclei give rise to the **internal arcuate fibers** (see Fig. 10–8), which promptly cross to the opposite side of the medulla in the **decussation of the medial lemniscus.** They then ascend as the **medial lemniscus** to the thalamus and terminate in the **ventral posterolateral nucleus** (VPL). These fibers maintain a somatotopic organization in both the medial lemniscus and the VPL. In the medulla, medial lemniscus fibers from the nucleus gracilis, conveying information from the leg, lie ventral to fibers from the nucleus cuneatus. In the pons and midbrain, these gracile fibers are lateral to the cuneate fibers. In contrast to the anterolateral system discussed in Chapter 6, few, if any, of the fibers in this system synapse in the reticular formation.

Thalamocortical fibers from the VPL continue to the postcentral gyrus of the parietal lobe. The band of cerebral cortex that receives these terminals is the **primary somatosensory cortex** (Fig. 7–2), where topographic representation of the body areas is similar to that of the motor strip that lies parallel to it on the opposite side of the

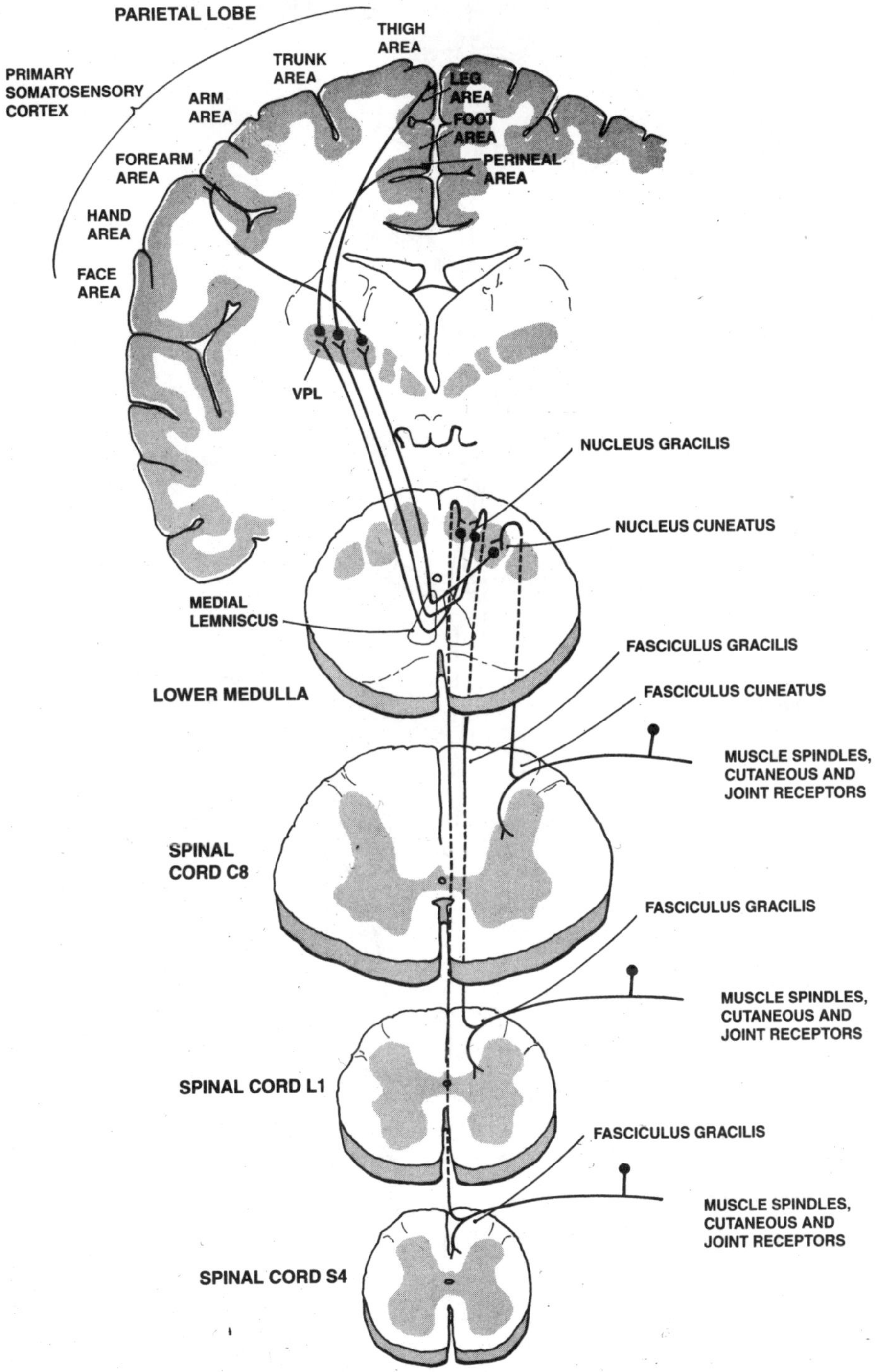

■ **FIGURE 7–2.** The fasciculus gracilis and the fasciculus cuneatus of the spinal lemniscal system mediate proprioception, flutter-vibration, and tactile discrimination. VPL = ventral posterolateral nucleus of the thalamus.

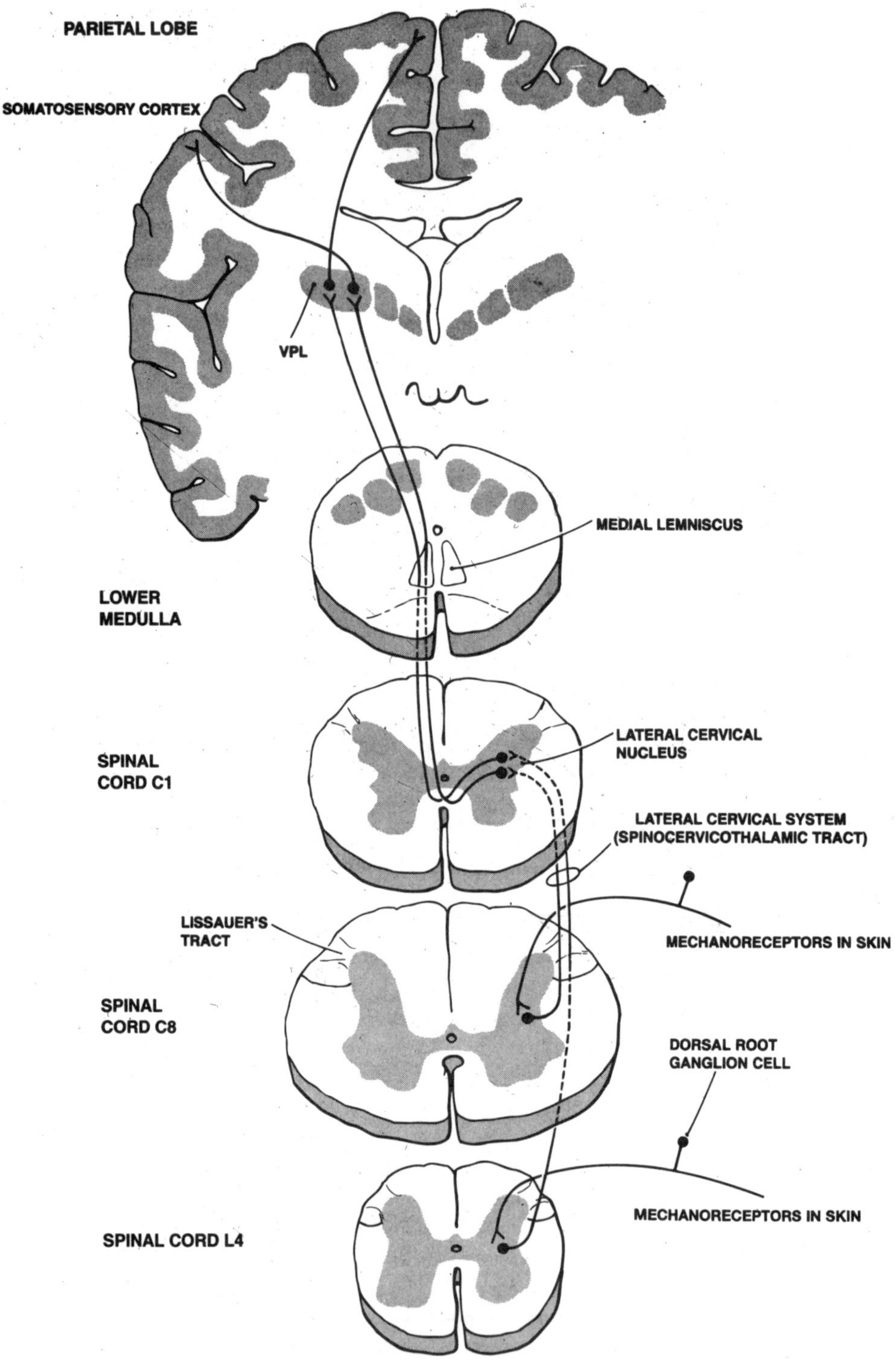

■ **FIGURE 7–3.** The lateral cervical system (spinocervicothalamic tract) mediates touch sensation. VPL = ventral posterolateral nucleus of the thalamus.

central sulcus. The primary somatosensory area includes Brodmann's areas 3, 1, and 2 (see Figs. 20–1 and 20–2).

The spinal lemniscal system mediates the sense of limb position and movement, including the sense of steady joint angles, the sense of motion produced by active muscular contraction (kinesthesis) or passive movement, the sense of tension exerted by contracting muscles, and the sense of effort. The conscious recognition of body and limb posture requires cortical participation. In addition, the lemniscal pathway provides important information about the place, intensity, and temporal and spatial patterns of neural activity evoked by mechanical stimulation of skin, particularly moving stimuli on the skin. Thus, this pathway to the cerebral cortex is necessary for discriminative tactile sensation. It also appears to be important in recognition of flutter-vibration.

Lateral Cervical System

Almost all neurons of the lateral cervical system respond to light mechanical stimulation of the skin on the ipsilateral side of the body, but a few are activated by noxious stimuli. Peripheral nerve fibers entering this system make synaptic connections in the dorsal horn, primarily in lamina IV, throughout the length of the spinal cord. Heavily myelinated axons from the second-order neurons arise in this lamina and ascend ipsilaterally in the most dorsal corner of the lateral funiculus to terminate in the **lateral cervical nucleus.** This nucleus is located just lateral to the dorsal horn of the first four cervical segments (Fig. 7–3). Projections from this nucleus cross the spinal cord in the ventral white commissure to join the contralateral medial lemniscus and proceed with it to terminate in the thalamus. Projections from the thalamus reach the somatic sensory areas of the cerebral cortex. The fibers of the entire lateral cervical system conduct very rapidly.

Physiologic Aspects of Tactile Discrimination

In the various relay nuclei of the pathways mediating tactile discrimination, each neuron receives synaptic input from many afferent fibers, and each afferent fiber ends on many relay cells. Thus, the relay cells receive sensory information that undergoes both **convergence** and **divergence.** In addition, afferent fibers reaching relay nuclei activate not only relay cells but also excitatory and inhibitory interneurons. Consequently, the sensory pathways both transmit information and modulate and transform the information as it moves along to higher levels of the nervous system.

In the somatic sensory system, synaptic inhibition occurs not in the peripheral receptor, but in the first synaptic site in the dorsal horn or dorsal column nuclei and in subsequent synaptic sites along the pathway. Two types of inhibitory processes have been described: (1) **local feedback inhibition** and (2) **distal feedback inhibition.** Local feedback inhibition (also called **lateral inhibition**) involves the inhibition of dorsal horn and dorsal column relay cells that surround the relay cells activated by incoming sensory volleys. This inhibition is mediated by collaterals of the activated cells synapsing on inhibitory interneurons in the relay nucleus. Distal feedback inhibition consists of the inhibition of presynaptic activity **(presynaptic inhibition)** in the terminals of dorsal root ganglion cells in dorsal horn and dorsal column nuclei. This inhibition comes from the axons of neurons in the motor and somatosensory areas of the cerebral cortex and in the brain stem. Local feedback inhibition limits the extent of excitation among adjacent neurons and thereby functionally decreases the divergence of excitation and sharpens the localization of signals. Distal feedback inhibition allows higher levels of the nervous system to regulate the information that moves upward.

Neurons in each of the nuclei along the lemniscal pathway, including the dorsal column nuclei, the VPL, and the somatosensory area of the cerebral cortex, have specific **receptive fields.** The receptive field of each neuron is the area on the body surface that, when stimulated, either excites or inhibits that neuron. The size of the receptive fields of individual neurons varies considerably. The tips of the fingers, the lips, and the tongue are the regions of the body that are most sensitive to touch because they contain the highest density of sensory nerve endings per unit area. This increased density of afferent fibers serving a given region transmits information to larger numbers of relay cells with smaller receptive fields than the parts of the system serving less sensitive areas of the body, such as the arm and back. The more sensitive regions therefore also have the largest areas of representation in the postcentral gyrus.

Stimulation of skin within the receptive field of a neuron usually excites the neuron, and stimulation of skin surrounding the excitatory area usually inhibits the neuron. This process is termed **inhibitory surround.** The result of this arrangement is maximal firing of a neuron in response to a stimulus limited to the area of its receptive field. If the stimulus impinges equally on the receptive field and the inhibitory surround, the neuron will show little or no response; however, neurons with receptive fields at the edges of this larger stimulus become activated. This and other inhibitory processes in sensory systems enhance information about contrasts at the edges of stimulated areas.

The somatosensory cortex consists of narrow vertical **cortical columns** of neurons extending from the pial surface to the white matter. The neurons within each column are interconnected, and each of these neurons responds to the same type of sensory stimulus. Thus, some columns are activated by afferents from the thalamus conveying touch, some by joint position, and some by movement of hair on the skin. Neurons within each column also have receptive fields in the same location on the body. Moreover, there are specific cutaneous, direction-sensitive (for spatial discrimination), and displacement frequency–sensitive (for temporal discrimination) neurons in the somatosensory cortex. These cortical neuronal response properties reflect the integration of multiple inputs from other levels of sensory processing. (See also Chapter 20.)

Effect of Spinal Cord Lesions on Touch Sensation

Simple touch is the least likely of all types of skin sensibility to be impaired by spinal cord lesions, because both major ascending pathways mediate this sensation. Thus, a lesion of the dorsal columns usually abolishes ipsilateral tactile discrimination of the direction of movement of a cutaneous stimulus, but recognition of light touch decreases only slightly or not at all, because the spinothalamic tract also transmits light touch sense. Conversely, after transection of the spinothalamic tract, pain perception is lost on the opposite side of the body, but light touch generally persists because the dorsolateral pathways can also mediate this function (Fig. 7–4).

Complete loss of **proprioceptive sensation** from a spinal lesion requires bilateral interruption of the dorsolateral pathway (both dorsal columns and the lateral cervical system in the dorsal part of the lateral columns). Lesions in this location cause deficits in position sense, vibration sense, and tactile discrimination. The symptoms occur prominently on the same side of the body after unilateral injury of a dorsolateral pathway (Fig. 7–4). Symptoms of varying degrees also result from lesions of the gracile and cuneate nuclei, the medial lemniscus, the thalamus, and the postcentral gyrus. Lesions of the lemniscal pathway leave preserved the sensations of simple touch, pain, and temperature. Interruption of the dorsal columns without injury to the lateral columns results in loss of tactile discrimination of the direction of a moving stimulus on the skin, but appreciation of touch and joint position sense remains intact.

Clinical signs of injury to the lemniscal (dorsolateral) pathways, which are frequently tested in a neurologic examination, include the following:

1. Inability to recognize limb position. In the absence of vision, the patient cannot determine whether a joint has been flexed or extended. The patient also cannot detect the direction of joint or limb displacement during a movement.
2. Astereognosis. The patient loses or shows impairment of the ability to recognize common objects, such as keys, coins, blocks, and marbles, by touching and handling them with the eyes closed.
3. Loss of two-point discrimination. Normally, two light-touch stimuli applied simultaneously to the skin a few millimeters apart can be distinguished from a single stimulus. This ability is greatly decreased. The two points of a compass with blunt tips are usually used for testing.
4. Loss of vibratory sense. The normal person perceives as mild tingling the sensation evoked by application of a vibrating tuning fork to a bony prominence. When this sensory ability is lost, the patient cannot differentiate a vibrating fork from a silent one.
5. A positive Romberg sign. In this test, the patient stands with the feet placed closely together, and the examining physician notes the amount of body sway with the patient's eyes open. The physician then compares the amount of sway when the patient's eyes are closed. An abnormal accentuation of sway or an actual loss of balance with the patient's eyes closed is a positive result. Visual sense is able to compensate in part for a deficiency in conscious recognition of muscle and joint position; therefore, patients with dorsolat-

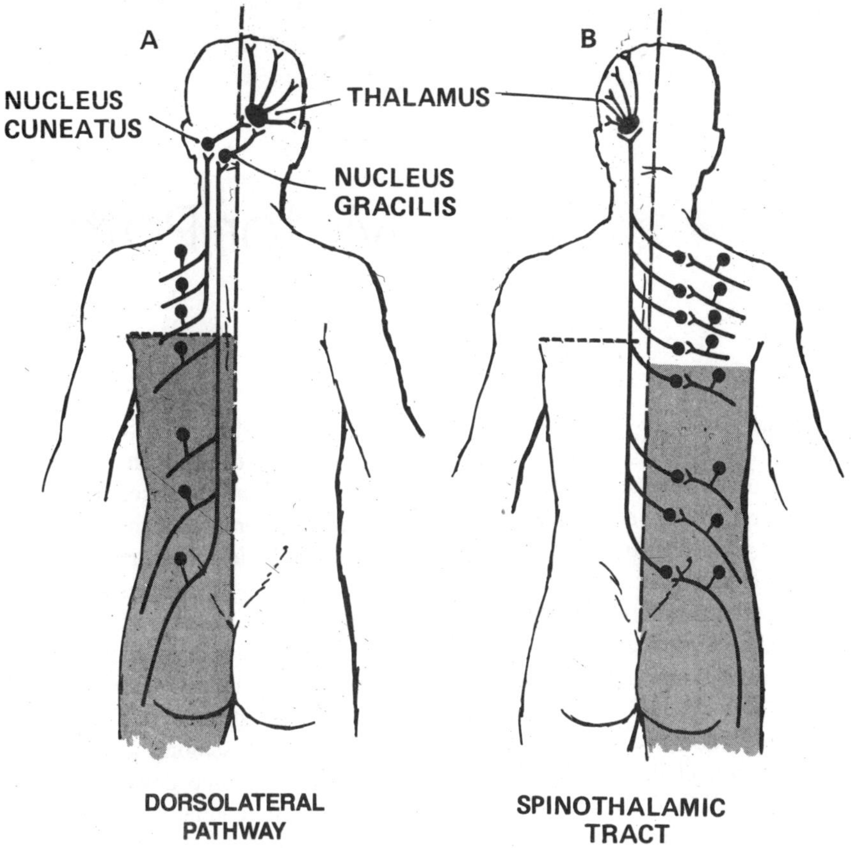

■ **FIGURE 7–4.** The effects of a single lesion on the left side of the spinal cord. The *dashed line* indicates the segmental level of the lesion. **(A)** and **(B)** The effects of this single lesion on the dorsolateral pathway and the spinothalamic tract, respectively. **(A)** The proprioceptive disturbance affects the ipsilateral side of the body because the ascending fibers cross above the level of the lesion, in the medulla, where fibers from the nucleus cuneatus and nucleus gracilis form the medial lemniscus. **(B)** The loss of pain and temperature sensation affects the contralateral side of the body one or two segments below the level of the lesion. This is because fibers entering the spinothalamic tract ascend one or two segments as they cross to the opposite side of the spinal cord.

eral pathway lesions may be able to maintain their balance if they are allowed to keep their eyes open, but they lose their balance when they close their eyes.

Case Follow-up

The patient described at the beginning of this chapter has Friedreich's ataxia, a recessively inherited neurologic disorder resulting from a mutation affecting the triplet repeat GAA on chromosome 9. The disorder leads to progressive degeneration of the dorsal root ganglia with secondary degeneration of the dorsal and ventral spinocerebellar tracts that accounts for the progressive disorder of coordination and ambulation with frequent falls. There is secondary degeneration also in the spinal lemniscal system, the spinothalamic tract, and the lateral cervical system, causing marked impairment of sensation, particularly position sense and vibration sense, which further impair ambulation. The corticospinal pathway also degenerates progressively, with consequent limb weakness. (The corticospinal pathway is discussed in Chapter 8.) The absent deep tendon reflexes result from the loss of afferent fibers originating in muscle spindle receptors. There is no treatment available that will alter the course of this disorder, but research into the fundamental basis of the disease is progressing rapidly.

8

Motor Pathways

Case Study

A 55-year-old woman develops sudden weakness of her left arm and leg, and over the next 30 minutes these limbs become even weaker. When she looks at herself in a mirror, she finds that the lower left half of her face appears to sag, and with vocalization, there is less movement on the lower left than on the lower right side of her face. The woman has hypertension (high blood pressure), diabetes mellitus, and hypercholesterolemia (elevated serum lipids). When she is seen in an emergency room 1 hour later, she has almost complete paralysis of the lower part of the left side of her face and left arm and leg, with an approximately equal degree of weakness in the face, arm, and leg.

What has happened to this woman? Where is the lesion that is responsible for her symptoms? Is treatment available?

Motor Areas of the Cerebral Cortex

Primary Motor Cortex

Based on differences in cytoarchitecture in the cerebral cortex, Brodmann designated 52 anatomic areas. The **primary motor area, Brodmann's area 4,** lies in the precentral gyrus and paracentral lobule of the frontal lobe. It extends from the lateral fissure upward to the dorsal border of the hemisphere and a short distance beyond on the medial surface of the frontal lobe in the rostral aspect of the paracentral lobule (see Figs. 1–2, 1–3, 20–1, and 20–2). The left motor strip controls the right side of the body, and the right strip controls the left side. Neurons in the lowest lateral part of this strip influence the larynx and tongue, followed in upward sequence by neurons affecting the face, thumb, hand, forearm, upper arm, thorax, abdomen, thigh, leg, foot, and perineal muscles. The neurons controlling leg, foot, and perineal muscles are in the paracentral lobule. In humans, areas for the hand, tongue, and larynx are disproportionately large and conform to the development of elaborate motor control of these muscle groups. A functional map of the motor cortex resembles a distorted image of the body turned upside down and reversed left for right. This functional map is termed a **homunculus** (see Fig. 20–7).

Motor Association Areas of the Cortex

Immediately rostral to the primary motor area lies the **premotor cortex,** which is in **Brodmann's area 6** on the lateral surface of the hemispheres (see Fig. 20–1). The premotor area contains a homunculus similar to the one in area 4. The most medial aspect of area 6 can be observed on a midsagittal section of the brain just rostral to the paracentral lobule (see Fig. 20–2). This part of area 6 is the **supplementary motor area,** which also contains a functional map of body movements.

Additional regions of cerebral cortex that can influence movement include Brodmann's areas 3, 1, and 2 on the **postcentral gyrus** and the **secondary motor area,** located where the precentral and postcentral gyri are continuous at the base of the central sulcus. This last area overlaps the **secondary somatosensory cortex.** Brodmann's area 8 in the middle frontal gyrus also influences motor control. This region, termed the **frontal eye fields,** contains neurons that specifically influence eye movements.

Integration of the Motor Cortices and Lower Motor Sites in Directing Movement

Movements result from the actions of neuronal networks at many different levels of the nervous system. The brain stem and spinal cord contain pattern generators for complex movements such as locomotion and other rhythmic activities. The descending pathways of the nervous system have the important task of interacting with and controlling lower-level neuronal patterns of discharge in a hierarchical manner. At the level of the cerebral cortex, individual neurons can control the contractions of individual muscles and can determine the force of these contractions. Nevertheless, **populations** of motor cortical neurons act together to specify the **direction** of movements and the **force** of movements. These functions pertain not only to neurons in the primary motor cortex but also to those in the premotor, supplementary, and postcentral regions. The premotor and supplementary motor areas are important in planning movements. The supplementary motor area appears to have a special role in integrating movements performed simultaneously on both sides of the body.

Descending Fibers from the Cerebral Cortex and Brain Stem Influence Motor Activity

Lower Motoneurons Innervate Muscles

Skeletal muscle activity results from the net influence of higher nervous system structures on motoneurons of the spinal cord and cranial nerve nuclei. Collectively, these spinal cord and brain stem neurons provide the final direct link with muscles through neuromuscular junctions (motor end plates). These neurons are termed **lower motoneurons.** Their cell bodies reside within the central nervous system, and their axons make synaptic contact with extrafusal and intrafusal muscle fibers of somatic and branchiomeric origin. **Somatic muscle fibers** derive from the myotomes of true somites in the developing embryo. **Branchiomeric muscles** develop from the branchial arches of the embryo. The branchiomeres are not true somites, but the muscles that develop from them, like somatic muscles, are striated and are under voluntary control. They include the muscles of mastication and facial expression, as well as the muscles of the pharynx and larynx.

Upper Motoneurons Regulate Activity in Lower Motoneurons

Many descending motor pathways regulate lower motoneuron activity. The cerebral cortex, cerebellum, and basal ganglia control these descending pathways either directly or indirectly. In the strictest sense, the neurons in all such pathways should be termed **upper motoneurons.** Upper motoneurons synapse directly, or through interneurons, on alpha, beta, and gamma motoneurons in the spinal cord and cranial nerve nuclei. They are contained completely within the central nervous system. Clinicians usually use the term upper motoneuron only when referring to the corticospinal tract or, to a lesser extent, the corticobulbar tract (Fig. 8–1).

Corticospinal Tract

The **corticospinal tract,** also termed the pyramidal tract, controls primarily skilled movements of the distal muscles of the limbs and facilitates the alpha, beta, and gamma motoneurons that innervate distal flexor musculature. Approximately one-third of the axons in the corticospinal tract originate in primary motor cortex (area 4). About 10% of these fibers (or 3% of the corticospinal tract fibers) originate in unusually large pyramidal cells called **Betz cells,** which are located in the fifth layer of areas 4 and 6. Another one-third of the fibers in the corticospinal tract arise in the premotor and supplementary motor regions in area 6, and the remaining one-third of the fibers originate in the parietal lobe, primarily areas 3, 1, and 2 of the postcentral gyrus. Taken together, these areas of cortex that contribute to the corticospinal and corticobulbar pathways are called the **sensorimotor cortex.**

The corticospinal tract passes through the posterior limb of the internal capsule and the middle of the cerebral peduncle, or crus cerebri (Fig. 8–1). It then breaks up into bundles in the basilar portion of the pons and finally collects into a discrete bundle, to form the pyramid of the medulla. This pathway bears the name of **pyramidal tract** because of its passage through the

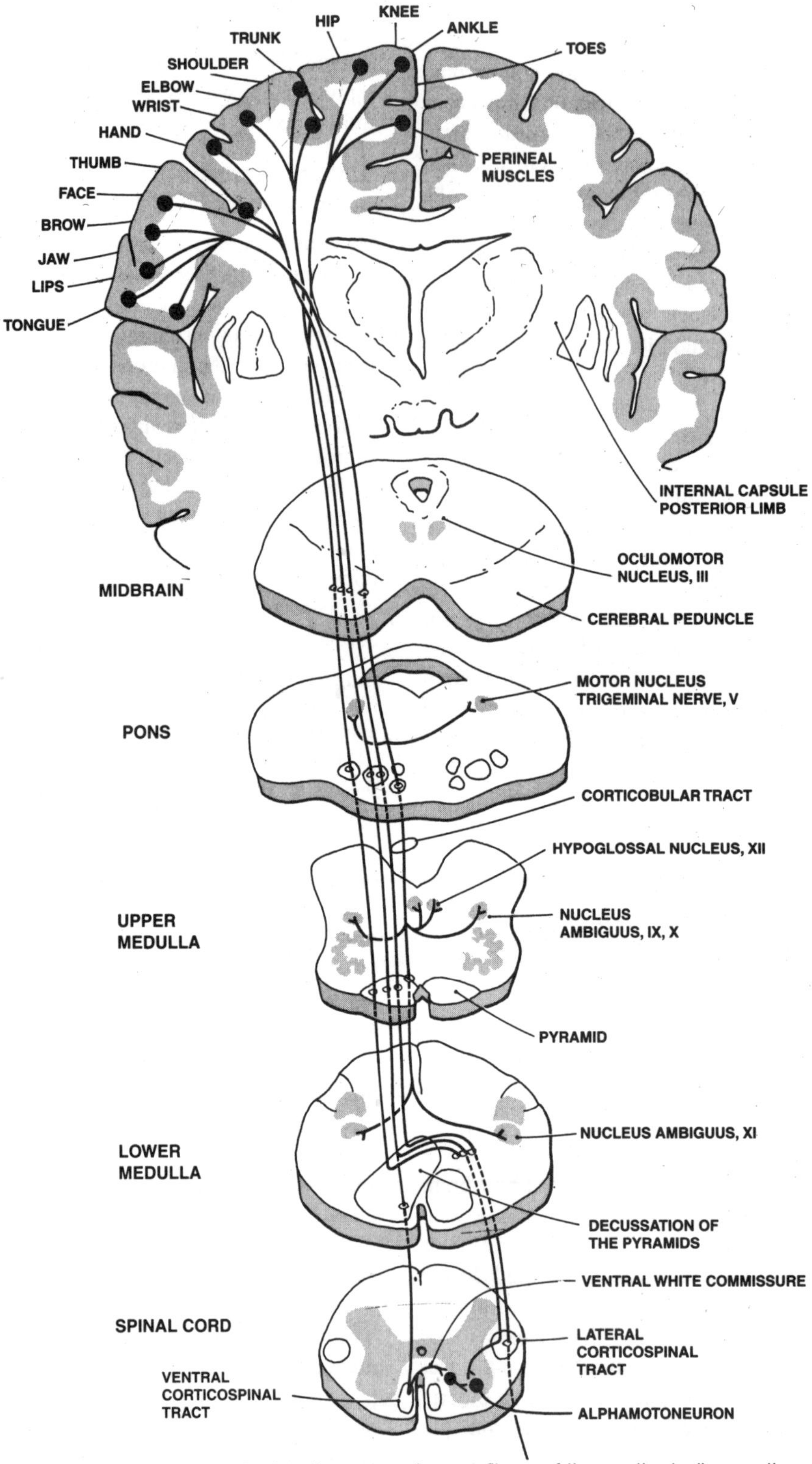

■ **FIGURE 8–1.** The corticospinal pathways and some fibers of the corticobulbar pathways.

medullary pyramid, not because of its origin from pyramidal cells in the cortex. In the lower levels of the medulla, most of the corticospinal tract crosses (decussates) to the opposite side. This region is termed the **level of the motor or pyramidal tract decussation.** Approximately 90% of the fibers cross at this level and descend through the spinal cord as the **lateral corticospinal tract,** which passes to all spinal cord levels in the lateral funiculus and synapses in the lateral aspects of laminae IV through VIII. Many of the cells in laminae VII and VIII are interneurons that synapse on alpha and gamma motoneurons in lamina IX. In primates, a few fibers (perhaps those arising from Betz cells) synapse directly on the alpha, beta, and gamma motoneurons in lamina IX. These motoneurons innervate the muscles in the distal parts of the extremities (i.e., hands and feet).

The 10% of corticospinal fibers that do not decussate in the medulla descend in the anterior funiculus of the cervical and upper thoracic cord levels as the **ventral corticospinal tract.** This tract does not extend below the upper thoracic spinal cord. At their individual levels of termination, however, most fibers in this pathway decussate through the ventral white commissure (Fig. 8–1) before they synapse on interneurons and motoneurons of the contralateral side. The number of fibers in both lateral and ventral corticospinal tracts decreases in successively lower spinal cord segments as more and more fibers reach their terminations.

The corticospinal tract fibers that synapse on interneurons in the base of the dorsal horn (laminae IV, V, and VI) can influence local reflex arcs and cells of origin of ascending sensory pathways. Through this system, the cerebral cortex can control reflex motor output and can also modify sensory input reaching the brain.

The cortical neurons that give rise to the corticospinal tracts use glutamate as a neurotransmitter and excite the neurons on which they synapse. Nevertheless, the corticospinal tract can exert either excitatory or inhibitory effects on motoneurons. **Excitatory effects** result from direct (monosynaptic) connections with motoneurons, and **inhibitory effects** occur through synaptic connections on inhibitory interneurons. Many of the interneurons mediating inhibitory effects use glycine as a neurotransmitter. Activation of the corticospinal tract generally evokes excitatory postsynaptic potentials in motoneurons of flexor muscles and inhibitory postsynaptic potentials in those of extensor muscles.

Corticobulbar Tract

The fibers of the corticobulbar tract arise from neurons in the ventral part of the sensorimotor cortex on the lateral surface of the hemisphere and from Brodmann's area 8. The axons start out in company with the corticospinal tract but take a divergent route at the level of the midbrain. This pathway terminates in the brain stem, where it influences the motor nuclei of cranial nerves III (oculomotor), IV (trochlear), V (trigeminal), VI (abducens), VII (facial), IX (glossopharyngeal), X (vagus), XI (accessory), and XII (hypoglossal). Fibers from cortical area 8 in the middle frontal gyrus, also termed the **frontal eye fields,** influence eye movements indirectly by synapsing on cells in the pontine reticular formation that, in turn, project to the nuclei of cranial nerves III, IV, and VI. (See Chapter 19.) Corticobulbar fibers from the facial region of areas 4 and 6 terminate on interneurons adjacent to the motoneurons that innervate the remaining (nonextraocular) striated musculature, either of somatic or branchiomeric origin. (Some of these connections are shown in Fig. 8–1.) The cranial nerve motor nuclei receive innervation from both cerebral hemispheres, and, in most cases, the muscles they control cannot be contracted voluntarily on one side only. Both the lower facial nucleus, which innervates facial musculature below the eye, and the hypoglossal nucleus receive innervation from the opposite cerebral cortex that is much heavier than the innervation from the ipsilateral cortex. Thus, these muscles can be controlled rather independently on the two sides, and a lesion of one cerebral hemisphere results in weakness primarily on the contralateral (opposite) side.

Like the corticospinal tract, the **corticobulbar tract** contains fibers that terminate on sensory "relay" neurons. In the brain stem, these relay nuclei include the nucleus gracilis and nucleus cuneatus, the sensory trigeminal nuclei, and the nucleus of the solitary tract.

Corticotectal and Tectospinal Tracts

Some authors use the term corticomesencephalic tracts to identify the pathways that arise from cerebral cortical areas in the occipital and inferior parietal lobes and project to the upper parts of the brain stem to influence extraocular muscle activity. In this text, these fibers are termed the **corticotectal tract.** Many of these fibers synapse in the superior colliculus, the interstitial nucleus of Cajal, or the nucleus of Darkschewitsch. These nuclei project to the pontine reticular formation and from there through the **medial longitudinal fasciculus (MLF)** to synapse on the oculomotor, trochlear, and abducens nuclei (see Fig. 19–1).

Corticotectal fibers make connections in the deep layers of the superior colliculus with neurons that give rise to the **tectospinal tract.** Axons of these cells cross the midline in the **dorsal tegmental decussation** (see Fig. 10–13) and descend through the brain stem ventral to the MLF (see Figs. 10–8 through 10–11). In the spinal cord, the tectospinal tract becomes incorporated into the MLF, with which it travels through the ventral funiculus. The tectospinal fibers extend only through the cervical segments of the spinal cord, where they influence neurons innervating muscles of the neck, including the neurons of the spinal accessory nucleus (cranial nerve XI).

The corticotectal-tectospinal projections are concerned with turning movements of the head and eyes, possibly combined with reaching movements of the arm. Corticotectal fibers have a greater influence on reflexive than on voluntary eye movements.

Corticorubral and Rubrospinal Tracts

The corticorubral and rubrospinal tracts represent an indirect route from the cerebral cortex to the spinal cord. Fibers originating from the same cortical areas that give rise to the corticospinal tract also form the **corticorubral tract.** This tract projects to the ipsilateral red nucleus in the tegmentum of the midbrain. Neurons of the red nucleus (in its magnocellular part) give rise to the **rubrospinal tract,** which crosses the midline in the **ventral tegmental decussation** and descends through the lateral tegmentum of the pons, midbrain, and medulla (see Fig. 9–2). In the spinal cord, this crossed pathway lies just anterior to the lateral corticospinal tract in the lateral funiculus. Its fibers synapse at all spinal cord levels in the lateral aspect of laminae V, VI, and VII and thus overlap part of the termination of the corticospinal tract. The rubrospinal tract is functionally similar to the corticospinal tract in that generally it facilitates flexor and inhibits extensor alpha, beta, and gamma motoneurons, particularly those innervating the distal parts of the arms.

Corticoreticular and Reticulospinal Tracts

The reticular formation consists of a matrix of nuclei in the core of the brain stem that receives sensory information from numerous systems and interconnects heavily with the cerebellum and the limbic system. It is described further in Chapter 10. The reticular formation receives a large input from **corticoreticular fibers,** which accompany the corticospinal and corticobulbar fibers. Like the majority of the corticobulbar fibers, the corticoreticular fibers from each hemisphere terminate bilaterally in the brain stem. Unlike the corticospinal and corticobulbar fibers described earlier, the corticoreticular system arises from cells outside, as well as within, the sensorimotor cortex. Important corticoreticular projections originate in medial prefrontal cortex (frontal lobe areas anterior to the sensorimotor cortex) and the limbic lobe, including the amygdala. These cortical areas integrate somatic and visceral components of complex reflex systems such as micturition and genital function. In addition, as part of a much larger network of pathways, the corticoreticular-reticulospinal pathway integrates these reflexes into complex emotional and social behaviors.

Two areas of the reticular formation send major projections into the spinal cord. The pontine reticular formation gives rise to the uncrossed **pontine (medial) reticulospinal tract.** In the medulla and the cervical segments of the spinal cord, this pathway travels within the MLF. In the thoracic spinal cord, where the MLF ends, the medial reticulospinal tract continues through the ventral funiculus to all cord levels. Its fibers synapse in laminae VII and VIII. This pontine tract is mainly excitatory for extensor alpha motoneurons, particularly those innervating the midline musculature of the body and the proximal parts of the extremities (see Fig. 9–2). It also provides an important input to gamma motoneurons. Through these connections the pontine reticulospinal tract influences posture and locomotion.

The medullary reticular formation gives rise to the **medullary (lateral) reticulospinal tract,** which is primarily uncrossed but has a small crossed component. This tract passes to all spinal cord levels in the lateral funiculus immediately anterior to the rubrospinal tract (see Fig. 1–9). It synapses in laminae VII and IX. The tract conveys **autonomic information** from higher levels to the preganglionic sympathetic and parasympathetic neurons to influence respiration, circulation, sweating, shivering, and dilation of the pupils, as well as the function of the sphincteric muscles of the gastrointestinal and urinary tracts in the pelvis. Hypothalamic projections to the spinal cord from the paraventricular and other hypothalamic nuclei also influence these autonomic processes directly, particularly cardiovascular functions.

Raphe-Spinal and Ceruleus-Spinal Projections

The **raphe nuclei** constitute a special subgroup of the larger group of nuclei that make up the reticular formation. Projections from the raphe nuclei are serotonergic (see Fig. 23–4); however, most of the serotonergic neurons also produce other neurotransmitters or neuromodulators. Fibers arising from neurons within the caudal raphe nuclei project to the spinal cord, where they influence transmission of incoming sensory signals and motor responsiveness. These fibers pass down the entire length of the spinal cord near the surface of the lateral funiculus and terminate within laminae I, II, V, and VII. In laminae I and II, fibers from the nucleus raphe magnus exert important influences on the transmission of pain information from peripheral nerves. In the deeper laminae, raphe-spinal projections (from nucleus raphe pallidus and nucleus obscurus) affect both preganglionic autonomic and somatic motoneurons.

The **nucleus locus ceruleus** and nucleus subceruleus give rise to a projection descending into the spinal cord through the ventrolateral funiculus and terminating in laminae I, II, V, VII, IX, and X. This projection is noradrenergic.

Neither the raphe-spinal fibers nor the ceruleus-spinal fibers evoke movement, but depending on the inputs they receive, they can produce either general excitatory or general inhibitory effects that greatly influence motoneuron responsiveness to reflex or corticospinal inputs. Thus, they function as a gain-setting system that determines overall motoneuron responsiveness. In this way, they may be particularly important in modulating the responsiveness of the motor system in different phases of sleep-waking cycles and with changes in emotional state.

Vestibulospinal Tracts

The vestibulospinal tracts are also discussed in Chapter 15. They arise from neurons in the vestibular nuclei of the medulla. Both of these pathways, the **lateral vestibulospinal tract** and the **medial vestibulospinal tract,** pass into the anterior funiculus and synapse on cells in laminae VII and VIII. The lateral vestibulospinal tract extends the entire length of the cord. The medial vestibulospinal tract becomes incorporated into the MLF and ends with the MLF in upper thoracic levels. Stimulation of the lateral vestibulospinal tract evokes **excitatory postsynaptic potentials** in extensor motoneurons innervating the neck, back, forelimb, and hindlimb muscles. These excitatory postsynaptic potentials are monosynaptic for neck motoneurons and some back and leg motoneurons. Stimulation of the lateral vestibulospinal tract also evokes reciprocal inhibition in flexor motoneurons through disynaptic or polysynaptic connections. Stimulation of the medial vestibulospinal tract evokes monosynaptic inhibition and excitation in neck and back motoneurons but does not influence limb motoneurons. The vestibulospinal pathways affect postural adjustments of the body accompanying head movements and the maintenance of postural tone.

Medial Longitudinal Fasciculus

The MLF consists not of a single tract, but of a bundle of several tracts in the midline of the brain stem and the ventral funiculus of the spinal cord. The descending portion of the MLF in the spinal cord contains the **pontine (medial) reticulospinal tract** and the **medial vestibulospinal tract,** which have been discussed. The **interstitiospinal tract,** which arises from the interstitial nucleus of Cajal (an accessory oculomotor nucleus), is also part of the MLF. The interstitiospinal tract supplies only the upper cervical levels, where it synapses in laminae VII and VIII. In the spinal cord (but not in the brain stem), the MLF also contains the **tectospinal tract.** The MLF modulates reflex movements of the head and neck in response to visual and vestibular stimuli.

The ascending MLF in the brain stem also consists of a mixed bundle of fibers of varying origins. It includes fibers interconnecting the vestibular nuclei and the extraocular nuclei (III, IV, and VI). This pathway coordinates eye movements and integrates head movements with eye movements. Damage to this bundle causes internuclear ophthalmoplegia. (See Chapter 13.)

Role of the Lateral, Medial, and Propriospinal Pathways in Spinal Cord Function

Figure 8–2 summarizes the distribution of fibers to the spinal cord that control movement and visceral function. The motor system pathways arising in the cerebral cortex and brain stem that reach the spinal cord appear on the left of this figure. As described previously in this chapter, the **lateral and ventral corticospinal tracts** provide the capacity for control of finely fractionated movements, such as independent movements of the fingers. The remaining pathways descending from the brain that regulate movement can be described as two general projection systems from the brain stem: lateral and ventromedial.

The **lateral brain stem system** consists of fibers arising in the contralateral magnocellular red nucleus that project to the spinal cord through the rubrospinal tract and fibers from the ventrolateral portion of the contralateral pontine and medullary tegmentum that project through the lateral column of the spinal cord. This pathway terminates in the lateral aspect of the dorsal and ventral horns of the spinal cord, including laminae V, VI, VII, and IX. Like the corticospinal tracts, the lateral brain stem system participates in the control of fine manipulative, independent movements of the limbs, particularly of the hands and feet and with discrete motor patterns. This pathway generally facilitates the activity of mo-

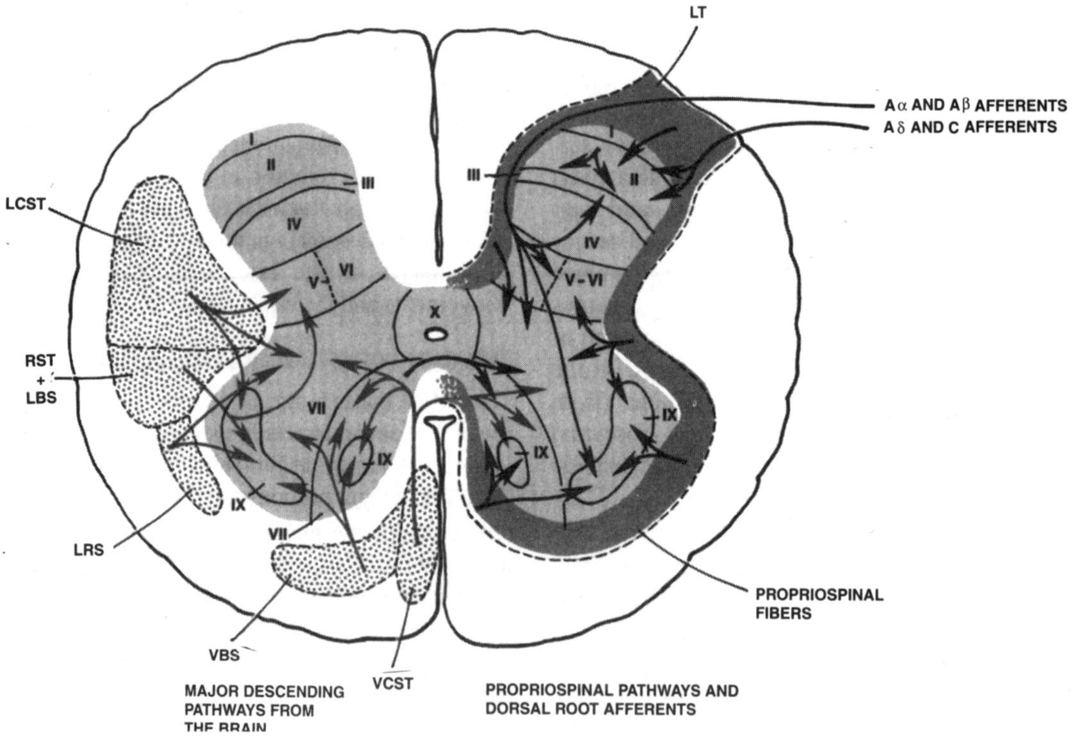

■ **FIGURE 8–2.** Afferents to Laminae I–X of the spinal cord gray matter. (*Left*) Major descending pathways from the brain. LBS = lateral brain stem system (from the pontine tegmentum); LCST = lateral corticospinal tract; LRS = lateral reticulospinal tract; RST = rubrospinal tract; VBS = ventromedial brain stem system (interstitiospinal, tectospinal, medial reticulospinal, and vestibulospinal tracts); VCST = ventral corticospinal tract. (*Right*) Propriospinal fibers surrounding the gray matter, including the posterolateral fasciculus, or Lissauer's tract (LT). Dorsal root afferents: large-diameter (Aα and Aβ) afferents; small-diameter (Aδ and C) afferents.

toneurons projecting to flexor muscles and inhibits the activity of motoneurons projecting to extensors.

The **ventromedial brain stem system** consists of fibers arising in the following: the interstitial nucleus of Cajal (interstitiospinal); the superior colliculus (tectospinal); the mesencephalic, pontine, and medullary reticular formation (including the pontine or medial reticulospinal system); and the vestibular nuclei (lateral vestibulospinal tracts). The ventromedial brain stem system fibers terminate in the ventral and medial aspects of the anterior horn of the spinal cord, including laminae VII, VIII, and IX, which contain motoneurons innervating the axial and girdle musculature. The ventromedial pathways participate in maintenance of the erect posture, integrated movements of the body and limbs, and progression movements of the limbs. These pathways generally facilitate the activity of motoneurons projecting to extensor muscles and inhibit the activity of motoneurons projecting to flexors. The final descending system illustrated on the left side of Figure 8–2 is the **lateral (medullary) reticulospinal system,** which participates in the regulation of autonomic motoneurons in the intermediolateral cell column of lamina VII.

In addition to the major descending pathways from supraspinal levels, **propriospinal pathways** play an essential role in spinal cord function (Fig. 8–2, right). These intersegmental projections arise from both dorsal and ventral horn neurons. Their axons travel in the white matter immediately surrounding the gray matter and link both nearby and distant segments of the spinal cord to integrate local reflexes into coordinated body movements and visceral function. Axonal projections of neurons in the substantia gelatinosa (lamina II) and in lamina VIII do not travel within the propriospinal white matter, but rather, they stay within the gray matter of their respective laminae.

Case Follow-up

The woman described at the beginning of this chapter has an approximately equal degree of weakness in the left lower face, left arm, and left leg. The most likely location of the lesion responsible for these findings is in the right internal capsule. This is because corticobulbar and corticospinal fibers innervating the contralateral face, arm, and leg are close together in this location. These fibers are also close together in the upper brain stem, but the patient has no clinical signs suggesting brain stem disease. The lesion is less likely to be in the cerebral cortex, because the representation of the face, arm, and leg are distributed over a very large region. Clinical evaluation led to the diagnosis of ischemic infarction (stroke) because of cerebrovascular disease resulting from diabetes mellitus and hypertension. A magnetic resonance imaging study verified the localization and diagnosis. Because the woman was seen within 3 hours of the onset of her stroke, she was treated with tissue plasminogen activator in an attempt to dissolve the clot in blood vessels perfusing the internal capsule. The attempt was successful, and the patient's strength gradually improved over the next several hours. She was prescribed medications to maintain better control of her hypertension and to lower her serum cholesterol, and she was instructed to control her diabetes more carefully. She has had no further difficulties since then.

9

Lesions of the Peripheral Nerves, Spinal Nerve Roots, and Spinal Cord

Case Study

A gunman shoots a 25-year-old policeman in the abdomen during an armed robbery. The policeman is quickly transported to hospital, where he is awake and alert. Physical examination reveals moderate blood loss from the wound but a stable blood pressure and pulse. Neurologic examination reveals marked weakness of the right leg with decreased deep tendon reflexes in the leg and no response to plantar stimulation of the right foot. He has loss of position sense and vibration sense in the entire right leg and loss of pain and temperature sensation in the left leg and left lower abdomen. An x-ray of the abdomen reveals that the bullet has lodged in his lower thoracic spine. He is taken to surgery, where the abdominal wound is explored and the bleeding is stopped. No major organ injury has been sustained, and no attempt is made to remove the bullet. Over the next several months, the patient recovers most of his strength in the right leg, but it is stiff when he moves. Examination 6 months postoperatively reveals increased deep tendon reflexes in the right leg, a right extensor plantar response, diminished position sense and vibration sense in the right leg, and diminished pinprick sensation in the left leg and lower abdomen.

What structures in this man's spinal cord have been damaged to cause the neurologic abnormalities observed on examination? What can be done to assist him in rehabilitation?

Degeneration and Regeneration of Nerve Cells and Fibers after Injury

Transection or permanent destruction of an axon leads to complete degeneration of the part that has been separated from the nerve cell body, including loss of the myelin sheath. This process is called **wallerian degeneration.** Degenerated fibers can be studied histologically by obtaining a series of microscopic sections, staining them appropriately, and reconstructing the course of the fibers.

In addition to causing permanent destruction of the disconnected portion, severing an axon harms the nerve cell body itself. For several weeks after the injury, the Nissl bodies (chromophilic substance) in the cell undergo **chromatolysis,** a process in which the ribosomes (RNA) lose their staining characteristics and seem to dissolve in the surrounding cytoplasm. Some of the affected cells disintegrate, but others recover with restoration of Nissl substance. Those cells that recover participate in the process of regeneration.

In the peripheral nervous system, completely severed nerves have some capacity to repair themselves. Schwann (neurolemma) cells, which previously formed the myelin of the central end of the nerve stump, proliferate and attempt to bridge the gap with the distal end of the nerve. The axis cylinders in the central end of the cut nerve divide longitudinally and soon begin to sprout from the end of the nerve. Many sprouting axons go astray in random directions, but some of them cross the gap and enter neurolemmal tubes leading to the peripheral endings. They grow at a rate of 1 to 2 mm per day. Chance apparently determines whether a regenerating motor fiber enters a neurolemmal tube leading to a motor or to a sensory terminal. If suitably matched, connections can be reestablished and function can be restored. Considerable recovery can occur with partial injury to peripheral nerves, provided the neurolemmal tubes remain intact.

In the central nervous system, completely severed nerve fibers do not regenerate effectively. Nevertheless, some partial injuries can prevent conduction of nerve impulses without causing irreversible fiber degeneration. The pressure of brain or spinal cord tumors, herniated intervertebral discs, blood clots, or swelling and edema after trauma may cause partial interruption of function and may produce symptoms that can be alleviated by treatment. The prospect of recovery depends on the severity and duration of the pressure.

Clinical Consequences of Peripheral Nerve Lesions

Injury of an individual peripheral nerve (Fig. 9–1, lesion 1) leads to paralysis of muscles and loss of sensation distal to the lesion involving only muscles and skin areas supplied by the injured nerve. The paralyzed muscles are flaccid (i.e., severely hypotonic) and gradually undergo severe atrophy. All forms of sensation, including proprioception, are lost. The diagnosis of specific peripheral nerve lesions requires knowledge of the sensory and motor innervation patterns for individual nerves (see Figs. 6–1 and 6–2, right sides, for sensory innervation).

The term **polyneuropathy** describes the clinical syndrome resulting from widespread peripheral nerve disease. The lesions commonly occur bilaterally, affecting the distal parts of the extremities much more than the proximal. Muscular weakness and atrophy accompanied by sensory loss in the distal portions of the extremities (often in a ''glove-and-stocking'' distribution) are characteristic of this disorder. The muscle stretch reflexes usually are diminished or absent in the affected portions of the limbs. Frequent causes of polyneuropathy include diabetes mellitus, nutritional deficiencies (often associated with alcoholism or vitamin B_{12} deficiency), paraneoplastic effects of remote malignant disease, and the Guillain-Barré syndrome.

Lower Motoneuron Lesions: Hypotonic Paralysis of Muscles

The term **lower motoneuron** refers to the anterior horn cells of the spinal cord, which innervate the skeletal muscles of the body, and the motor nerve cells of the brain stem, which innervate muscles supplied by the cranial nerves. Destruction of these neurons (Fig. 9–1, lesion 4), their axons in ventral roots (Fig. 9–1, lesion 3), or motor fibers of peripheral nerves (Fig. 9–1, lesion 1) abolishes both the voluntary and reflex responses of muscles. In addition to **paralysis,** the affected muscles show **hypotonia** (i.e., diminished resistance to passive manipulation of the limbs) and absence of the deep tendon reflexes.

Within a few weeks after injury of motoneurons, ventral roots, or peripheral nerves, the fibers of the affected muscles begin to **atrophy.** More profound atrophy occurs in muscle fibers deprived of their motoneurons than in muscles rendered inactive. This is because the anterior horn cells exert a trophic influence on muscle fibers that is essential for maintaining their normal state. Muscles undergoing early stages of atrophy display **fibrillation** potentials. These result from fine twitchings of single muscle fibers that generally cannot be seen on clinical examination but can be detected on electromyographic examination. These differ from **fasciculation** potentials, which result from brief contractions of **motor units** that can be seen in skeletal muscle through the intact skin. Fasciculations can occur in neurologically normal persons and do not necessarily indicate motoneuron disease.

Lesions of Dorsal Roots

Local tumors, infections, or injuries can damage the dorsal (posterior) roots (Fig. 9–1, lesion 2). Herniation of the nucleus pulposus (''slipped disc'') frequently injures dorsal roots by protruding laterally between adjacent vertebral bodies and compressing one or more dorsal roots. The results are **pain and paresthesias** (sensations of

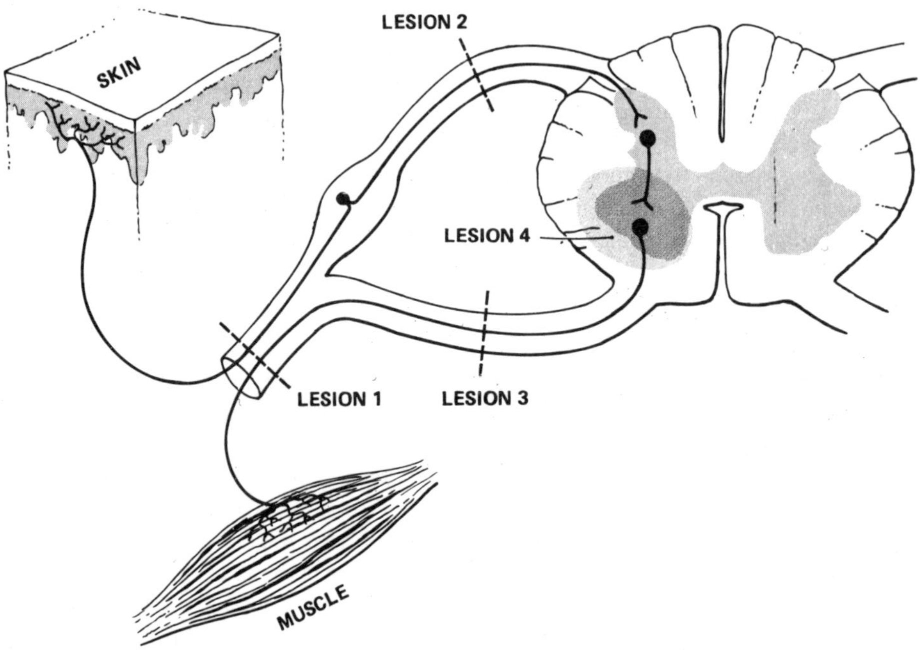

■ **FIGURE 9–1.** A cross section of the spinal cord, dorsal and ventral roots, and peripheral nerve. Lesion 1 affects the peripheral nerve; lesion 2, the dorsal root; lesion 3, the ventral root; and lesion 4, the anterior horn cells.

numbness and tingling) that characteristically occur in the distribution of the affected roots. Examination usually reveals decrease or loss of sensation in a dermatomal distribution (see Figs. 6–1 and 6–2, left sides).

Lesions that damage sensory fibers in the dorsal roots or their cell bodies in spinal ganglia also disrupt the stretch reflex pathway (see Fig. 4–1) and cause **hypotonia and loss of the deep tendon reflexes of the affected segment.** In this instance, the lower motoneurons remain intact, and voluntary muscle strength remains preserved. The trophic influence of anterior horn cells persists, and neither muscle atrophy (except that of disuse if pain interferes with muscle functioning) nor fibrillation potentials appear. Coordination may deteriorate because of the loss of sensory feedback to the nervous system.

Upper Motoneuron Lesions: Spastic Paralysis of Muscles

The term **upper motoneuron** refers to nerve cell bodies that originate in high levels of the central nervous system and send their axons into the brain stem or spinal cord. There the axons synapse, directly or indirectly, on motor nuclei of the cranial nerves and anterior horn cells in the spinal cord. Examples of upper motoneuron pathways include the corticospinal, corticobulbar, reticulospinal, vestibulospinal, and rubrospinal tracts.

A lesion in the **posterior limb of the internal capsule** (Fig. 9–2, lesion 1) disrupts the influence of the cerebral cortex on lower motoneurons on the contralateral side of the body. In addition to the corticospinal and corticobulbar tracts, the lesion also interrupts connections between the cerebral cortex and the origin of the rubrospinal and reticulospinal pathways. Immediately after such a lesion, paralysis affects the face, arm, and leg (hemiplegia) of the opposite side of the body, with hypotonia and decreased deep tendon reflexes. After an interval varying from a few days to a few weeks, muscle strength begins to improve, the deep tendon reflexes recover on the affected side and then progress to become more active than normal, and **hypertonia of the spastic type** develops. The deep tendon reflexes may become so hyperactive that they show **clonus** (i.e., a sustained series of rhythmic jerks). In addition to spastic weakness with hyperreflexia, internal capsule lesions result in the appearance of the **Babinski sign.** This sign, also known as an extensor plantar reflex, is an abnormal response to

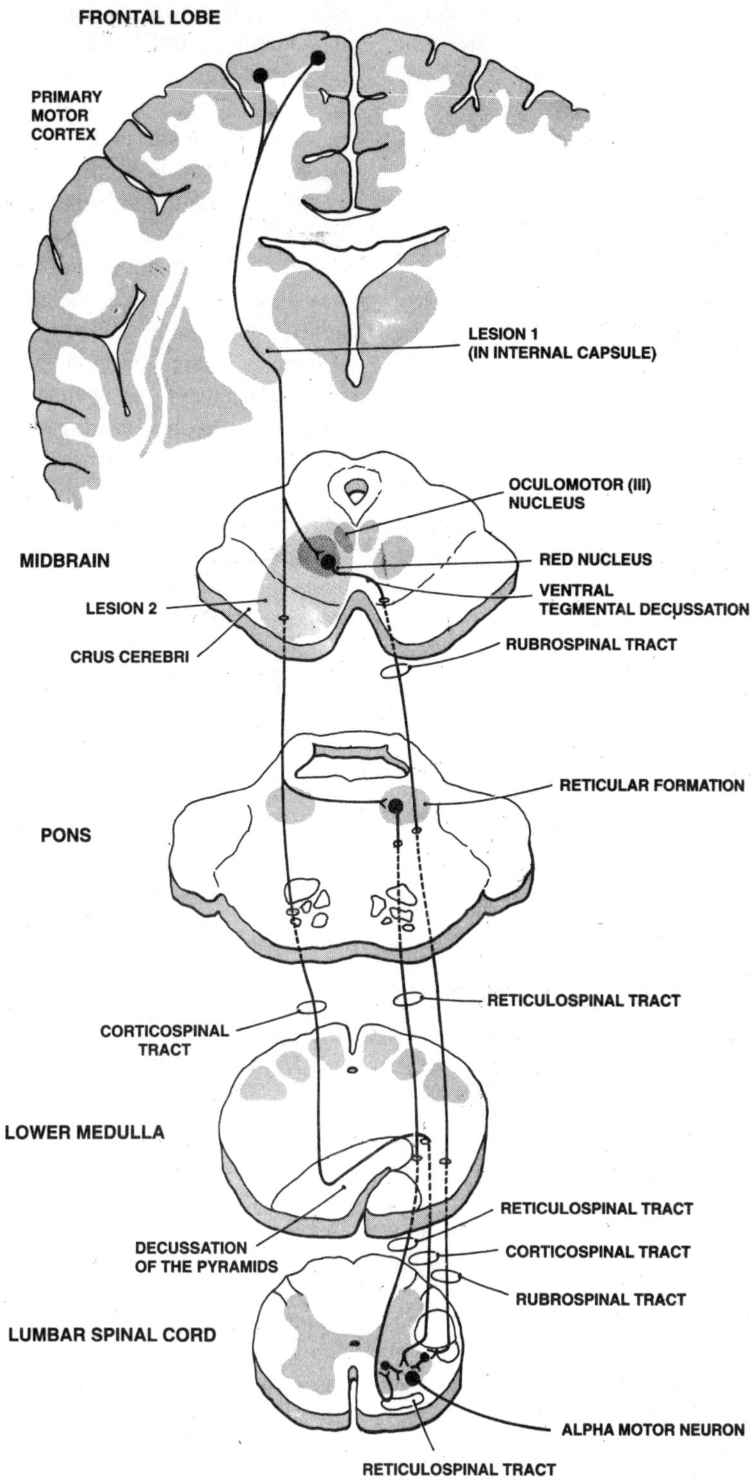

■ **FIGURE 9–2.** Several of the major motor pathways of the central nervous system. Lesion 1 affects the internal capsule and causes a contralateral hemiplegia affecting the lower muscles of the face and the arm and leg; the pathways to the facial nucleus and cervical cord are not shown. Lesion 2 causes an ipsilateral cranial nerve disorder (loss of function of the third cranial nerve) and a contralateral hemiplegia affecting the lower portion of the face and the arm and leg (see Fig. 13–4).

stroking the plantar surface of the outer border of the foot with a blunt object such as a key. The normal response is plantar flexion of the great toe. The Babinski sign consists of dorsiflexion of the great toe, at times accompanied by fanning of the other toes.

As indicated in the previous chapter, the **corticospinal (pyramidal) tract** consists of upper motoneurons in the cerebral cortex with axons coursing through the pyramidal tract in the medulla and terminating on anterior horn cells or interneurons in the spinal cord. In humans, chronic corticospinal tract lesions result in signs of upper motoneuron disease (e.g., paresis or paralysis, spasticity with a characteristic clasp-knife response to passive movements of the limbs, increased deep tendon reflexes, clonus, the Babinski sign, hypertonus, and lack of muscle atrophy except for disuse atrophy). These findings have been verified in a small number of patients whose brains, when examined after death, showed lesions restricted to the pyramidal tract in the medulla. Experimentally placed pyramidal tract lesions in the monkey, however, do not cause spasticity; these lesions result in limb hypotonia. In most humans with spasticity, multiple upper motoneuron projections are affected in addition to the corticospinal tract.

There has been considerable debate about the lower motoneurons that mediate spasticity, with some evidence implicating the gamma (or beta and gamma) motoneurons and other evidence implicating the alpha motoneurons. Hypersensitive gamma and beta fibers can stimulate muscle spindles to a higher rate of discharge, and this results in enhanced responses to muscle stretch. Hypersensitive alpha motoneurons can react excessively to normal levels of proprioceptive input from muscle stretch receptors. Currently, the bulk of evidence suggests that hyperactive alpha motoneurons account for the abnormalities.

The **Babinski sign** is an important finding on neurologic examination, because it indicates a lesion of the corticospinal tract. A lesion of this tract rostral to the pyramidal decussation in the lower medulla causes **contralateral** spasticity, muscle weakness, hyperreflexia, and a Babinski sign. A lesion of this tract caudal to the pyramidal decussation (i.e., in the spinal cord) causes these signs on the **ipsilateral** side of the body.

Lower motoneuron lesions affect only the muscles they innervate, but a small lesion that interrupts the corticospinal tract removes voluntary motor control from the whole sector of the body that lies downstream from the level of the injury. Thus, a lesion of the posterior limb of the internal capsule (Fig. 9–2, lesion 1) paralyzes the contralateral face, arm, and leg. Involvement of the face is limited to the lower facial musculature. (See Chapter 12 for the explanation.) A lesion on one side of the brain stem usually involves at least one of the cranial nerves on the side of the lesion (e.g., the third nerve in the instance of lesion 2 in Figure 9–2). Consequently, the lesion causes loss of function of one or more cranial nerves **ipsilateral** to the lesion, with hemiplegia on the **contralateral** side.

As described earlier, paralysis affecting the arm and leg of one side of the body is termed **hemiplegia. Paraplegia** refers to paralysis of both legs, as, for example, after a transverse lesion of the spinal cord that injures the upper motoneurons of both sides of the cord. **Monoplegia** refers to paralysis of a single extremity, and **quadriplegia** refers to paralysis that includes all four extremities. Weakness without total paralysis is called **paresis.**

Abnormal Reflexes Associated with Lesions of the Motor Pathway

Certain reflexes that cannot be elicited in neurologically normal persons may be found after injuries of the corticospinal tract. The **Babinski sign** is an important example of an abnormal reflex. As mentioned earlier, when found, the Babinski sign strongly indicates a disorder of the corticospinal tract. Many similar pathologic reflexes have been described. The **Hoffmann sign** can be elicited by flicking the nail of the patient's middle finger. Prompt reflexive adduction of the thumb and flexion of the index finger constitutes a positive sign. The Hoffmann sign is commonly associated with injury of the corticospinal tract, but it can be found in neurologically normal persons.

Superficial reflexes, which normally can be evoked by stroking certain areas of the skin, may be absent after injury of the corticospinal tract. Gentle scratching of the skin of the abdominal wall evokes local contraction of the abdominal musculature and causes the umbilicus to deviate momentarily in the direction of the stimulus. In male patients, stroking the upper inner aspect of the thigh normally induces reflex contraction of the cremaster muscle, with elevation of the testicle on the stimulated side. Loss of the **abdominal** or **cremasteric** reflexes confirms the presence of a corticospinal tract lesion, but absence of these reflexes bilaterally in an otherwise normal individual may have no significance.

Transection of the Spinal Cord

Complete transection of the spinal cord causes immediate loss of all sensation and all voluntary movement below the level of the lesion. The finding of a level on the trunk with loss of sensation and motor function below and preserved function above the level provides strong clinical evidence of a spinal cord disorder. Control of the bladder and bowel is also lost. If the spinal cord lesion occurs between cervical levels C1 and C3, respirations stop. After acute spinal transection, **spinal shock** appears; that is, the paralysis is flaccid, the deep tendon reflexes are absent, and plantar stimulation gives no response. Signs of an upper motoneuron lesion appear only after several weeks. Eventually, extensor plantar responses (the Babinski sign) can be detected, followed by the gradual appearance of hyperactive deep tendon reflexes, clonus, and spasticity of the affected limbs. Flexor spasms of the legs may appear intermittently, often triggered by local cutaneous stimulation. Bladder and bowel function usually becomes automatic, with these structures emptying as a reflex response to filling.

Partial injury to the spinal cord results in damage to some ascending and descending pathways and sparing of others. The symptoms and signs of partial spinal injury vary, depending on the location of the injury.

Hemisection of the Spinal Cord (Brown-Séquard Syndrome)

Lateral hemisection of the spinal cord (e.g., from a bullet or knife wound) causes the **Brown-Séquard syndrome** (Fig. 9–3B). The specific effects in a patient with a chronic lesion can be understood by considering the fiber tracts and roots affected by the lesion.

1. Lateral column damage results in paralysis of muscles on the same side of the body below the injury, with spasticity, hyperactive reflexes, clonus, loss of superficial reflexes, and a Babinski sign.
2. Dorsal column damage, along with the lateral column injury, causes loss of position sense, vibration sense, and tactile discrimination on the same side of the body below the level of the injury. Because of the paralysis, sensory ataxia, which may otherwise occur, cannot be demonstrated readily.
3. Damage to the anterolateral system results in loss of the sensations of pain and temperature on the side opposite the lesion beginning one or two dermatomes below the level of the injury (see Fig. 7–4).

Simple touch sensation may be unimpaired. This is because the dorsal columns and anterolateral system remain intact on the side contralateral to the lesion. The dorsal columns carry touch sensation from the ipsilateral side of the body, and the anterolateral system carries touch sensation from the contralateral side of the body below the level of the lesion.

Spinal cord lesions cause symptoms both by interrupting the long ascending and descending tracts of the spinal cord and by injuring dorsal and ventral nerve roots at the level of the injury. The symptoms of root injury occur on the side of the lesion, and when present, give valuable localizing information.

1. Irritation of fibers in the dorsal root zone leads to paresthesias or radicular pain in a band over the affected dermatomes.
2. Destruction of dorsal roots results in a band of anesthesia over the dermatomes supplied by the involved roots.
3. Destruction of ventral roots evokes a flaccid paralysis affecting only the muscles innervated by fibers that have been destroyed.

Few lesions are precisely localized to one lateral half of the spinal cord. More often, spinal lesions involve one sector of the cord and cause a partial, or incomplete, Brown-Séquard syndrome.

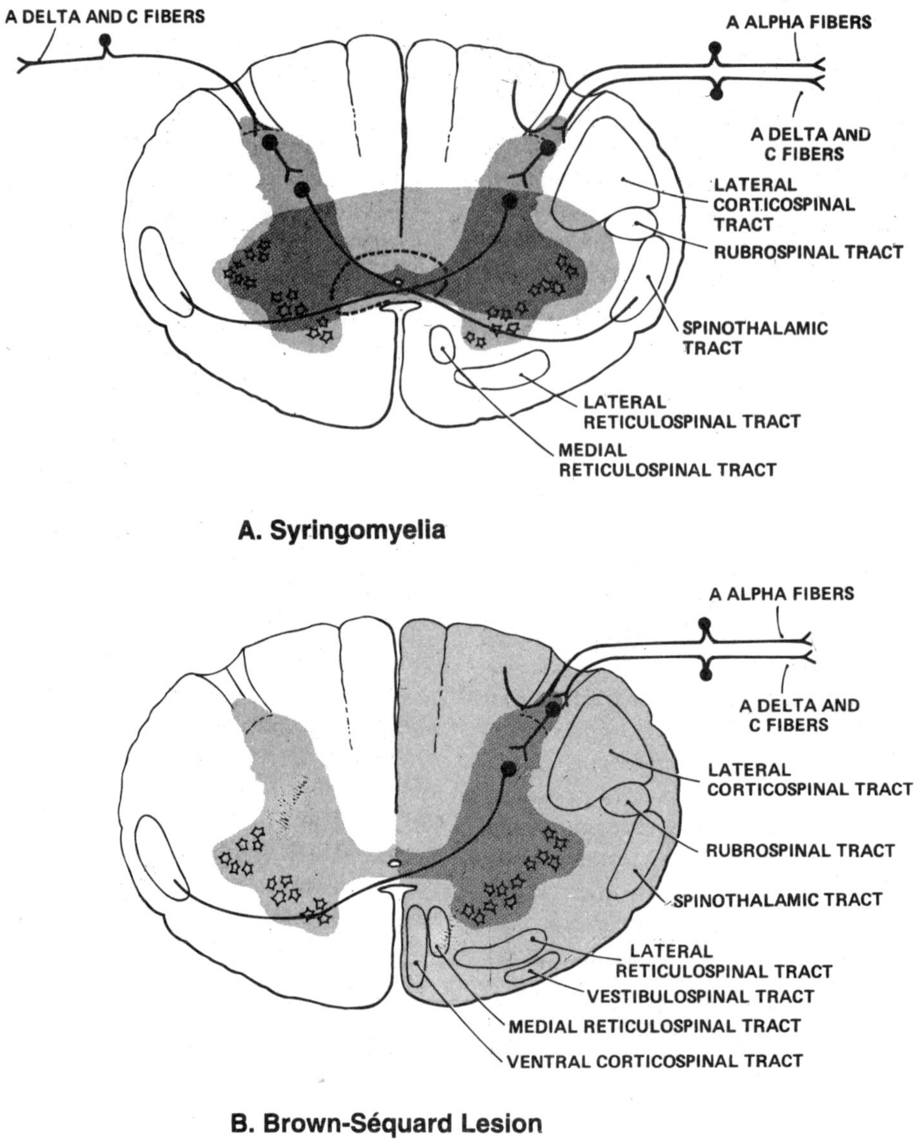

■ **FIGURE 9–3.** **(A)** A cross section of the spinal cord showing the pathways interrupted by a cavitating lesion of a small syringomyelia (*dotted line*) and a larger syringomyelia (*shaded area*). **(B)** A cross section of the spinal cord showing the pathways interrupted by hemisection of the cord (Brown-Séquard lesion).

The position and extent of the lesion determine the particular symptoms and signs in each case. The Brown-Séquard syndrome results more often from lesions compressing the spinal cord from the outside than from lesions within it.

The sensory pathways of the spinal cord show a characteristic layering, with the sacral segments represented in the outer layers and progressively higher segments represented in sequential order from outer layers to inner. Consequently, lesions affecting the central part of the spinal cord, such as tumors or traumatic injury, can result in **sacral sparing.** With sacral sparing, sensation below the level of the lesion is lost, except in the sacral dermatomes, where it is preserved.

Current evidence indicates that patients with traumatic injury to the spinal cord regain function more effectively if they are treated soon after the injury with corticosteroids. Therefore, the rapid diagnosis of a spinal cord disorder is critical after traumatic injury.

Lesions of the Central Gray Matter of the Spinal Cord

Syringomyelia is a progressive disorder of uncertain origin that produces tissue destruction with cavitation around the central canal of the spinal cord, most commonly in the cervical enlargement. A small lesion in this position interrupts the lateral spinothalamic fibers that pass through the ventral white commissure as they cross from one side to the other (Fig. 9–3A, lesion enclosed by dotted line). Because these fibers mediate pain and temperature sensation from dermatomes on both sides of the body, the results are loss of pain and temperature sensibility in a segmental distribution affecting the upper extremities on both sides. The spinothalamic tracts from the lumbosacral segments remain intact; hence sensation in the lower extremities remains preserved. Position sense, vibration sense, and simple touch sensation are spared in the affected dermatomes. This condition, loss of some sensory modalities with preservation of others, is termed **sensory dissociation.** In later stages of the disease, as the lesion enlarges, degeneration often extends to the anterior gray horns (Fig. 9–3A, entire shaded area) and causes paralysis with atrophy of muscles innervated by the segments involved. Signs of upper motoneuron disease may affect the lower extremities from compression of the lateral corticospinal tracts by the cystic cavity.

Lesions Involving the Ventral Horns and the Corticospinal Tracts

Amyotrophic lateral sclerosis (ALS) is a progressive, fatal disease of unknown cause characterized by neuronal degeneration in the motor nuclei of the cranial nerves and in the anterior gray horns of the spinal cord, with degeneration of the corticospinal and corticobulbar tracts bilaterally. Sensation remains preserved in this disorder. Weakness and atrophy affect some muscles, and spasticity and hyperreflexia affect others. The disease commonly presents with limb weakness and atrophy in an asymmetrical distribution. The classic form of this disease begins with weakness, atrophy, and fasciculations of hand and arm muscles, followed later by spastic paralysis of the limbs. Difficulty in speaking and swallowing results from involvement of corticobulbar tracts or nuclei of the lower cranial nerves or both.

Lesions Involving Dorsal and Lateral Funiculi

Subacute degeneration of the spinal cord (combined systems disease) occurs most often in **pernicious anemia,** but it can accompany other types of anemia or nutritional disturbances. The dorsal and lateral columns of the spinal cord degenerate, but the gray matter ordinarily remains preserved. Degeneration of the dorsal and lateral columns results in difficulty in walking, with tingling sensations in the feet. Examination reveals loss of position sense and vibration sense in the legs and a positive Romberg sign. Degeneration of upper motoneuron projections in the lateral columns leads to weakness in the legs, with spasticity, hyperactive muscle stretch reflexes, and bilateral Babinski signs. Later in the course of the disease, the muscle stretch reflexes may disappear because of the development of peripheral neuropathy.

Thrombosis of the Anterior Spinal Artery

The anterior spinal artery courses along the anterior median sulcus and sends terminal branches to the ventral and lateral funiculi and most of the gray matter of the spinal cord. The artery supplies the anterior horns, lateral spinothalamic tracts, and corticospinal tracts. A pair of posterior spinal arteries supplies the dorsal funiculi and posterior part of the dorsal horns (Fig. 9–4). Thrombosis of the anterior spinal artery in the cervical spinal cord produces bilateral atrophy, fasciculations, and flaccid paralysis at the level of the lesion because of destruction of anterior horn cells. An accompanying spastic paraplegia results from bilateral corticospinal tract involvement, and usually loss of pain and temperature sense occurs below the lesion because of bilateral spinotha-

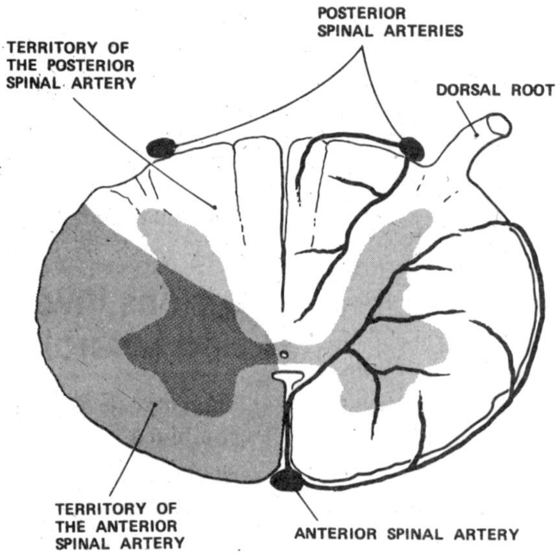

■ **FIGURE 9-4.** A cross section of the spinal cord showing the locations of the anterior and posterior spinal arteries and their branches *(right)* and the territories supplied by these arteries *(left)*.

lamic tract damage. Symptoms begin abruptly, often accompanied by severe pain.

Tumors of the Spinal Cord

Tumors that arise within the vertebral canal but outside the spinal cord (extramedullary tumors) gradually impinge on the cord as they enlarge. Compression of nerve roots often occurs first and accounts for pain distributed over the dermatomes supplied by these roots. This is followed by gradual involvement of the tracts within the spinal cord until a Brown-Séquard syndrome, or some modification of the syndrome, occurs. The order in which symptoms appear may furnish a clue to the site of the tumor. For example, losses of pain and temperature sense involving all segments below a certain level on the left side followed by spastic paralysis on the right suggest that the tumor has arisen from the ventrolateral region of the spinal cord on the right side. Loss of proprioception on the right side followed by extension of the proprioceptive deficit to the left side and the development of spastic paralysis on the right indicate that the tumor is compressing the spinal cord from the dorsomedial region on the right side.

Case Follow-up

The policeman described at the beginning of this chapter received an injury to the right lateral part of the lower thoracic spinal cord that partially interrupted the right lateral column and right dorsal column. The lateral column lesion involved the right lateral corticospinal tract and caused the initial **right leg** weakness with decreased deep tendon reflexes and the later partial recovery of strength along with spasticity and hyperreflexia. Injury of the right lateral column also interfered with the lateral spinothalamic tract and accounted for the initial loss and later decrease of pain and temperature sensation in the **left leg and left lower abdomen.** The injury also interfered with the continuity of the right dorsal column, which resulted in the initial loss and later decrease of the sensations of position and vibration in the **right leg.** Hence the policeman had a Brown-Séquard lesion affecting the right side of his lower thoracic spinal cord. Intensive rehabilitation along with medication to reduce the spasticity greatly improved his neurologic status, and he was able to return to work approximately 1 year after the injury, although he needed to be reassigned to a physically less demanding position.

SECTION 4

Brain Stem and Cerebellum

10

Organization of the Brain Stem and Cranial Nerves

Case Study

While seated at breakfast, a 62-year-old woman suddenly develops a feeling of light-headedness, followed within about 1 minute by severe vertigo, with the perception that the visual environment is in constant motion to the left. She becomes intensely nauseated, and then she vomits. Attempting to walk, she staggers and almost falls to the left. She has a past history of poorly controlled hypertension (high blood pressure) and takes medication for this. She is taken to hospital, where a general physical examination reveals high blood pressure (170/110 mm Hg) and a rapid resting pulse rate (100 per minute). The remainder of the physical examination is normal. Neurologic examination reveals nystagmus (regularly beating movements of the eyes) at rest and with gaze to the right or left and markedly decreased sensation to pinprick and temperature testing on the left side of the face. She has poorly coordinated (ataxic) movements of the left arm and leg and walks with her legsspread apart, tending to stagger to the left.

What part of the nervous system is affected? What kind of pathologic process is responsible? Is treatment available?

Surface Anatomy of the Brain Stem

Medulla

The **medulla (medulla oblongata or bulb)** constitutes the most caudal part of the brain stem. Continuous with the spinal cord at the foramen magnum, it extends rostrally for 2.5 cm to the caudal border of the pons. The central canal of the spinal cord continues through the caudal half of the medulla and then, at a point called the **obex,** flares open into the wide cavity of the fourth ventricle. The rostral part of the medulla thus occupies the floor of the fourth ventricle. The roof of the ventricle consists of the **tela choroidea** (a thin sheet of apposed ependyma and pia mater), the **choroid plexus** (tela choroidea with blood vessels between the ependyma and pia), and the cerebellum. Figures 10–1, 10–2, and 10–3 represent specimens of the brain from which the cerebral cortex, cerebellum, and tela choroidea of the fourth ventricle have been removed.

Anterior (Ventral) Aspect

The **pyramids,** formed by the **pyramidal (corticospinal and corticobulbar) tracts,** form two longitudinal ridges on either side of the ventral median fissure (Fig. 10–1). The decussation of the pyramids can be seen as bundles of fibers crossing and obliterating the fissure at the extreme caudal end of the medulla.

Lateral Aspect

Two longitudinal grooves run along the lateral aspect: the ventrolateral sulcus and the dorsolateral sulcus (Fig. 10–2). The ventrolateral sulcus extends along the lateral border of the pyramid, and the rootlets of the **hypoglossal nerve (XII)** exit from this groove. Radicles of the **cranial portion of the accessory nerve (XI), vagus nerve (X),** and **glossopharyngeal nerve (IX)** emerge in line along the dorsolateral sulcus. The **spinal portion of the accessory nerve (XI)** originates in the gray matter of spinal cord segments C2 to C5. Its rootlets exit through the lateral funiculus of the cord, join, and then ascend along the lateral surface of the medulla. The prominent oval swelling of the lateral area of the medulla between the ventrolateral and dorsolateral sulci, the **olive** (Figs. 10–1 and 10–2), marks the site of the inferior olivary nuclear complex inside the medulla (Fig. 10–9).

Posterior (Dorsal) Aspect

In Figure 10–3, low ridges in the spinal cord indicate the locations of the fasciculus gracilis and fasciculus cuneatus. The fasciculus gracilis forms the ridge between the dorsal median and dorsal intermediate sulci. The fasciculus cuneatus lies between the dorsal intermediate and dorsolateral sulci. Two small eminences, the **clava** and

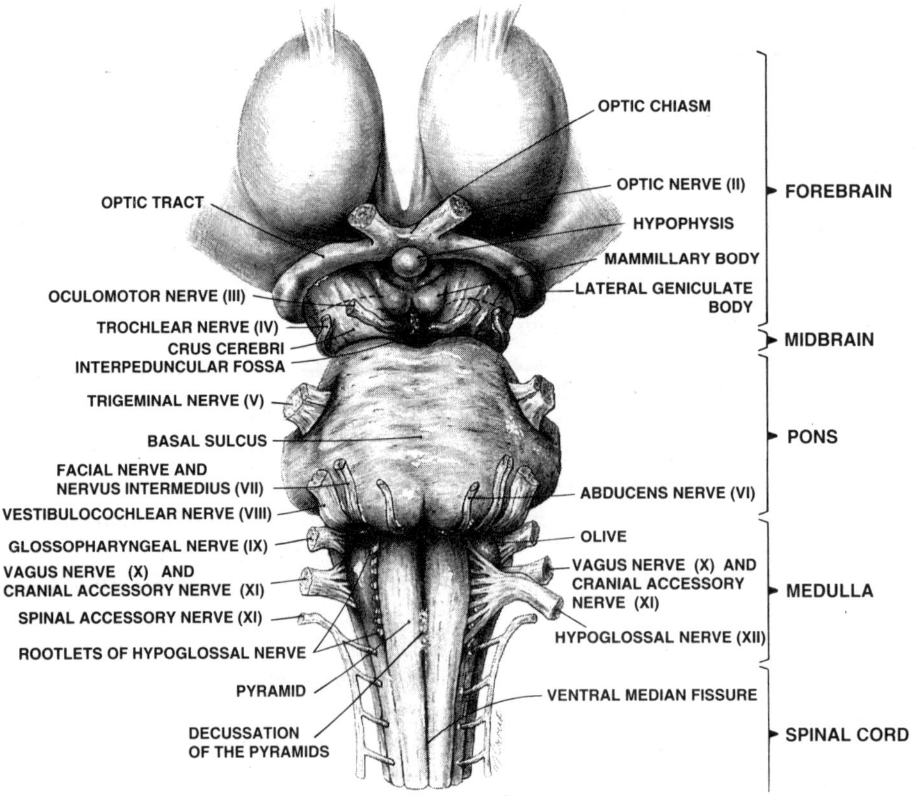

■ **FIGURE 10–1.** The ventral surface of the human brain stem and upper cervical spinal cord.

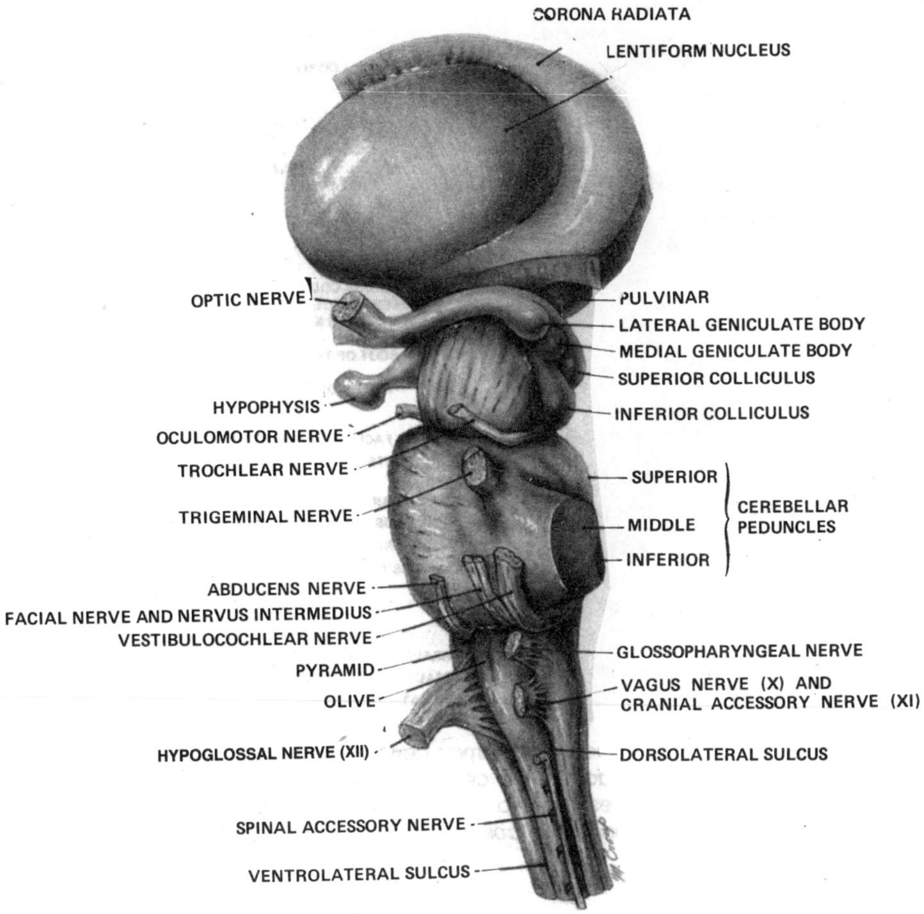

■ **FIGURE 10–2.** The lateral surface of the upper cervical spinal cord, brain stem, lentiform nucleus, and corona radiata.

the **cuneate tubercle,** mark the site of termination of these two tracts in the nucleus gracilis and nucleus cuneatus, respectively. The axons of neurons in the nucleus gracilis and nucleus cuneatus extend ventrally into the tegmentum (floor) of the medulla. Thus, at the rostral end of these nuclei, the dorsal area "opens up," exposing the floor of the fourth ventricle rostral to the **obex** (Fig. 10–4).

Two pairs of small swellings can be seen in the floor of the ventricle. The lateral ridges constitute the **vagal trigone;** the medial ridges constitute the **hypoglossal trigone.** These trigones consist of bulges that indicate the locations of underlying nuclei, the **dorsal motor nucleus of the vagus** and the **hypoglossal nucleus,** respectively. Ridges formed by fibers passing toward the cerebellum demarcate the **striae medullares of the fourth ventricle.** Laterally, these fibers mark the location of the **lateral recesses,** where openings in the fourth ventricle (the **foramina of Luschka**) allow cerebrospinal fluid to flow from the fourth ventricle into the subarachnoid space. Cerebrospinal fluid also leaves this ventricle through a single, midline opening at the obex, the **foramen of Magendie** (see Fig. 25–1).

Pons

The pons consists of a large tissue mass rostral to the medulla. On the ventral surface of the brain stem, the cerebral peduncles pass into the pons from above, and the pyramids emerge from its caudal margin.

Anterior (Ventral) Aspect

A band of thick transverse fibers, which constitutes the pons (or "bridge") proper, occupies the entire anterior aspect (Fig. 10–1). A shallow

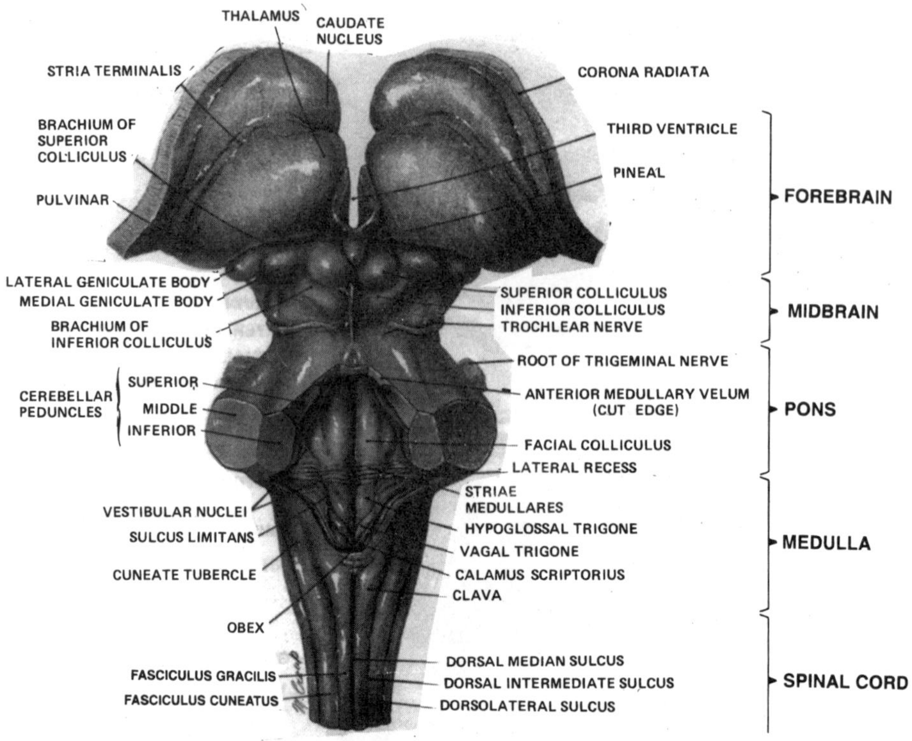

■ **FIGURE 10–3.** The dorsal surface of the human cervical spinal cord, brain stem, thalamus, caudate nucleus, and corona radiata. The cerebellum has been removed by cutting through the cerebellar peduncles. The tela choroidea also has been removed; its line of attachment to the medulla is indicated in *color.*

furrow (the **basal sulcus**) extends along the midline and coincides with the course of the basilar artery. The **abducens nerves (VI)** exit from the inferior pontine sulcus at the caudal border of the pons close to the pyramids.

Lateral Aspect

The transverse fibers of the pons converge to form compact lateral bundles—the **middle cerebellar peduncles (brachia pontis)**—that attach the pons to the overlying cerebellum (Figs. 10–2 and 10–3). The **cerebellopontine angle** consists of the triangular space formed between the caudal border of the middle cerebellar peduncle, the adjoining part of the cerebellum, and the upper part of the medulla. The **facial nerve (VII)** and the **vestibulocochlear nerve (VIII)** emerge from the brain stem in this niche (Fig. 10–2). The **trigeminal nerve (V),** one of the largest of the cranial nerves, penetrates the brachium pontis near the middle of the lateral surface of the pons.

Posterior (Dorsal) Aspect

The posterior surface of the pons forms the rostral part of the floor of the fourth ventricle (Fig. 10–3). At its widest point, this triangular area contains the pontomedullary junction and the lateral recesses of the ventricle. The **facial colliculus** lies rostral to the lateral recess in the floor of the ventricle. The abducens nucleus (VI) and the fibers of the facial nerve (VII) that cross over the nucleus of VI form this colliculus (i.e., "little hill") (Fig. 10–10). Two fiber bands, the **superior cerebellar peduncles (brachia conjunctiva),** form the walls of the fourth ventricle at this level. The cerebellar vermis in the caudal pons (Fig. 10–10) and the **anterior medullary velum** rostrally join these peduncles in the midline and complete the roof of the ventricle (Figs. 10–3 and 10–11).

Midbrain

The **midbrain** consists of a short segment of brain stem between the pons and the diencepha-

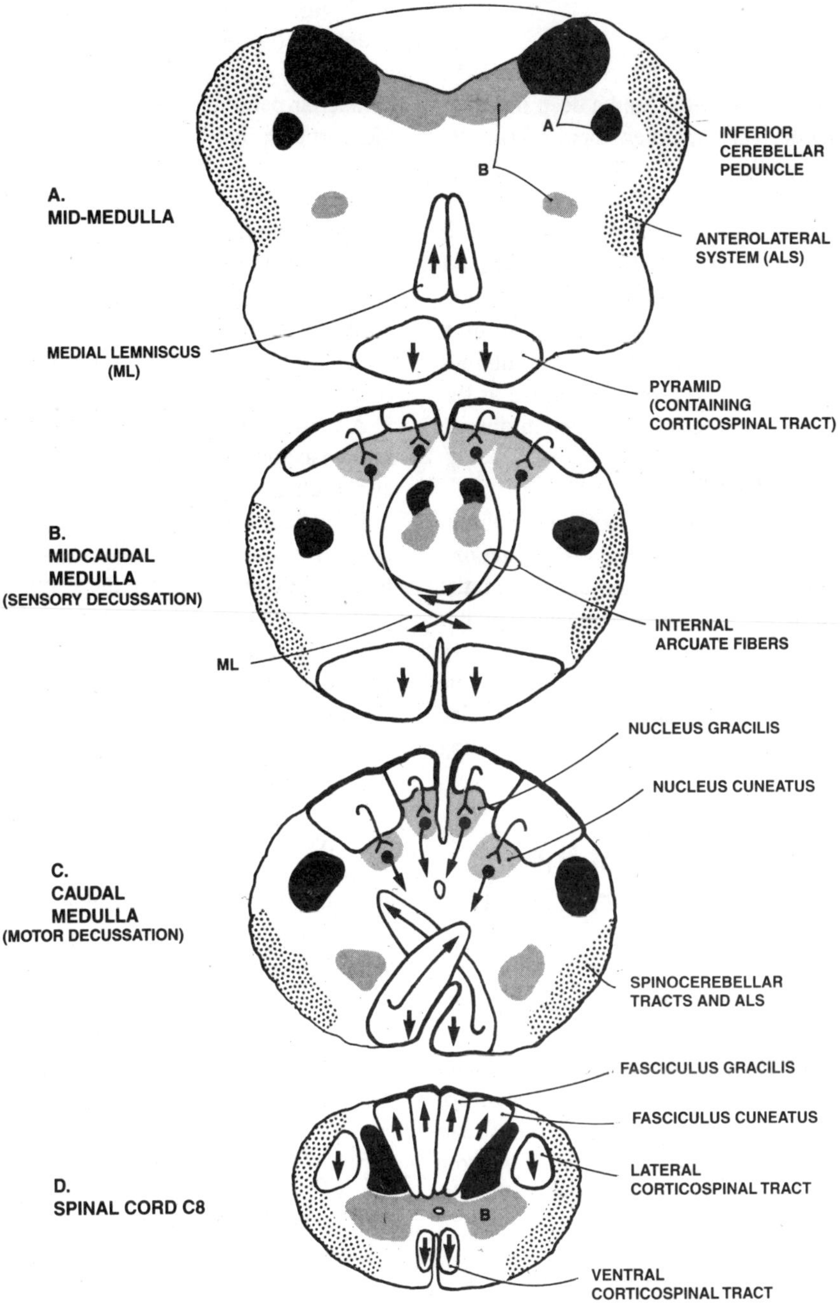

■ **FIGURE 10–4.** Schematic representation of transverse sections through the cervical spinal cord and medulla to highlight anatomic differences between these areas that result from the decussations of the corticospinal tracts and the spinal lemniscal system. The spinocerebellar and spinothalamic tracts lie on the lateral surface in both spinal cord and medulla.

lon. The **cerebral aqueduct,** a markedly narrow tubular passage connecting the third ventricle with the fourth, traverses it longitudinally.

Anterior (Ventral) Aspect

Two ropelike bundles of fibers, the **cerebral peduncles** or **crura cerebri,** and a deep **interpeduncular fossa** that separates them, form the inferior surface (Fig. 10–1). The optic tract, a continuation of fibers in the optic nerves (II), skirts around each cerebral peduncle just before it disappears into the cerebral hemisphere above. At its caudal end, the peduncle passes directly into the basilar portion of the pons. The **oculomotor nerves (III)** exit from the sides of the interpeduncular fossa and emerge on the surface at the transverse groove between the pons and midbrain.

Posterior (Dorsal) Aspect

The posterior surface (**tectum**) of the midbrain contains four rounded elevations—the **corpora quadrigemina.** The rostral pair are called the **superior colliculi,** and the somewhat smaller caudal pair are the **inferior colliculi** (Fig. 10–3). The **trochlear nerves (IV),** the smallest of the cranial nerves, emerge from the posterior surface just behind the inferior colliculi after decussating in the anterior medullary velum.

Internal Structures at the Transition from Spinal Cord to Brain Stem

The internal anatomy of the brain stem appears more complex than the simple arrangement of internal gray matter surrounded by white matter in the spinal cord. Examining the brain stem for both continuities and changes in position of fiber tracts and cell columns across the transition from spinal cord to medulla assists in understanding the internal structure of the brain stem.

Corticospinal and Spinal Lemniscal Systems Cross the Midline; Anterolateral and Spinocerebellar Systems Continue up the Same Side

Two of the major fiber systems of the spinal cord, the **corticospinal tract** and the **spinal lemniscal system** (dorsal columns), undergo shifts that radically change the arrangement of gray and white matter in the medulla as compared with the spinal cord. The corticospinal tracts descend through the ventral part of the brain stem. In the midbrain, they lie on the surface in the cerebral peduncles (crura cerebri), but in the pons, they are covered by the pontine fibers that form the middle cerebellar peduncles on the sides of the pons. As the corticospinal fibers emerge from the caudal part of the pons, they form the pyramids on the ventral surface of the medulla. Just before entering the spinal cord, most of these fibers turn dorsally and cross to the opposite side to take up a lateral position in the white matter of the spinal cord (the lateral corticospinal tract). This crossing is called the **motor, or pyramidal, decussation** (Fig. 10–4C).

A major bundle of fibers from the spinal cord, known as the **dorsal columns** (fasciculus gracilis and fasciculus cuneatus), terminates in the medulla, where the fibers synapse in the gracile and cuneate nuclei (Fig. 10–4B and C). Axons from neurons in these nuclei then migrate ventrally around the central gray matter of the medulla, cross the midline, collect together to form the medial lemniscus, and begin their ascent to the thalamus. In their course around the central gray matter, these fibers are called **the internal arcuate fibers** (Fig. 10–4B). This constitutes the sensory decussation of the medulla.

In contrast to the shift in position of the corticospinal tract and spinal lemniscal system, the spinothalamic tracts of the anterolateral system remain near the lateral surface of the brain stem as they ascend toward the thalamus. Situated dorsal to the anterolateral system, the spinocerebellar fibers ascend through the medulla (Fig. 10–4C) to enter the inferior cerebellar peduncle (Fig. 10–4A).

Sensory and Motor Cell Columns of the Spinal Cord Continue into Medulla

The sensory and motor cell columns of the spinal cord, which receive sensory inputs and give rise to motor axons of peripheral nerves, continue into the medulla and maintain their positions relative to one another (Fig. 10–4). With the disappearance of the dorsal column fibers and nuclei in the caudal medulla, and the opening of the central canal of the spinal cord into the fourth ventricle, the gray matter of the dorsal and ventral horns becomes exposed on the floor of the ventricle. Despite the new location, the relationship of the major sensory and motor cell columns with each other does not change. The sensory cell columns, derived from the embryonic alar plate, remain dorsolateral to the motoneuron cell groups, which develop from the basal plate. (See Chapter 1.) These cell columns, located near the ventricle, become the sensory and motor cell groups of the cranial nerve nuclei. During brain stem development, however, some cell groups migrate away from the ventricle and become "displaced" cranial nerve nuclei (Fig. 10–4A). In addition, some alar plate cell groups migrate to form integrative nuclei (e.g., dorsal column nuclei).

Throughout the brain stem, as in the spinal cord, neurons in the sensory columns receive sensory nerve fiber synapses, and the motor column neurons give rise to the motor fibers of the cranial nerves. Ten of the 12 pairs of cranial nerves in the human nervous system (III through XII) serve as components of the brain stem. This includes the cranial (or bulbar) part of cranial nerve XI. (A separate part of cranial nerve XI, the spinal accessory nerve, arises from cells in the upper cervical segments of the spinal cord.)

Classification of Cranial Nerve Nuclei and Fibers according to Their Functions

The adjective **general** pertains to cells and fibers of cranial nerves with functions similar to those of the spinal nerves. This includes sensory fibers from the body wall and viscera and motor innervation to the viscera and to skeletal muscles of somitic myotome origin. The classification **special** applies to cranial nerves that have specialized functions or target tissues, including those from the retina and inner ear, those conveying olfactory and gustatory impulses, and those innervating striated muscle derived from the embryonic branchial (pharyngeal) arches. With one exception, both general and special categories include sensory neurons and motoneurons. The exception is that there are no special somatic motoneurons; the innervation to the branchiomeric muscles is classified as special visceral motor.

Afferent Fibers of Cranial Nerves

General afferent fibers have their cells of origin in cranial sensory ganglia.

- **General somatic afferent (GSA)** fibers carry exteroceptive (i.e., pain, temperature, and touch) and proprioceptive information from sensory receptors in skin, muscle, tendons, and joints.
- **General visceral afferent (GVA)** fibers transmit impulses from visceral structures (i.e., hollow organs and glands) within the head and neck and in the thoracic and abdominal cavities.

Special afferent fibers arise from neurons found only in the ganglia of certain cranial nerves.

- **Special somatic afferent (SSA)** fibers convey sensory information from special sense organs in the eye and ear (i.e., vision, hearing, and equilibrium).
- **Special visceral afferent (SVA)** fibers carry impulses from olfactory and gustatory receptors.

Efferent Fibers of Cranial Nerves

General efferent fibers arise from motoneurons in the brain stem and autonomic ganglia. Collectively, general efferent fibers innervate all musculature of the body, except the branchiomeric muscles that develop in the pharyngeal arches of the embryo.

- **General somatic efferent (GSE)** fibers convey motor impulses to somatic skeletal muscles (myotomic origin). In the head, the somatic musculature consists exclusively of tongue muscles and extraocular muscles.
- **General visceral efferent (GVE)** fibers control smooth muscle and cardiac muscle and regulate glandular secretion. Parasympathetic preganglionic and postganglionic cells and fibers are components of four cranial nerves.

Special efferent fibers innervate the musculature of branchiomeric origin. They arise from selected cranial nerve nuclei in the brain stem.

- **Special visceral efferent (SVE)** fibers consist of nerve components that innervate striated muscles derived from the branchial (pharyngeal) arches. These include muscles of the jaw, of facial expression, and of the pharynx and larynx. SVE fibers are not part of the autonomic nervous system.

Functionally Distinct Cranial Nerve Cell Columns

Functionally Distinct Cell Columns Are Organized Mediolaterally in the Brain Stem

Each of the seven functional groups of fibers in the cranial nerves connects to a corresponding cell column within the brain stem tegmentum, and the individual cell columns are discontinuous. The nuclear cell groups that make up the individual cell columns have discrete names. As described earlier, the sensory cell columns lie lateral to the motoneuron cell groups throughout the brain stem.

For example, the midbrain, pons, and medulla contain the GSE column. Located consistently close to the midline and directly beneath the ventricle, the cells of this column consist of motoneurons innervating muscles derived from myotomes. Rather than forming a continuous column of cells, these neurons are distributed in four discrete nuclei. Three of these nuclei innervate muscles of the orbit. These include the oculomotor nucleus through cranial nerve III and the trochlear nucleus through IV, which arise in the midbrain, and the abducens nucleus through cranial nerve VI, which originates in the pons. The fourth GSE cell group is a large nucleus in the medulla that innervates the tongue muscles through cranial nerve XII (Fig. 10–5).

In order from medial to lateral, the cell columns consist of the GSE, GVE, SVE, GVA, SVA, GSA, and SSA. Figure 10–5 shows the locations of the motor and sensory cranial nerve cell columns in the brain stem and the individual

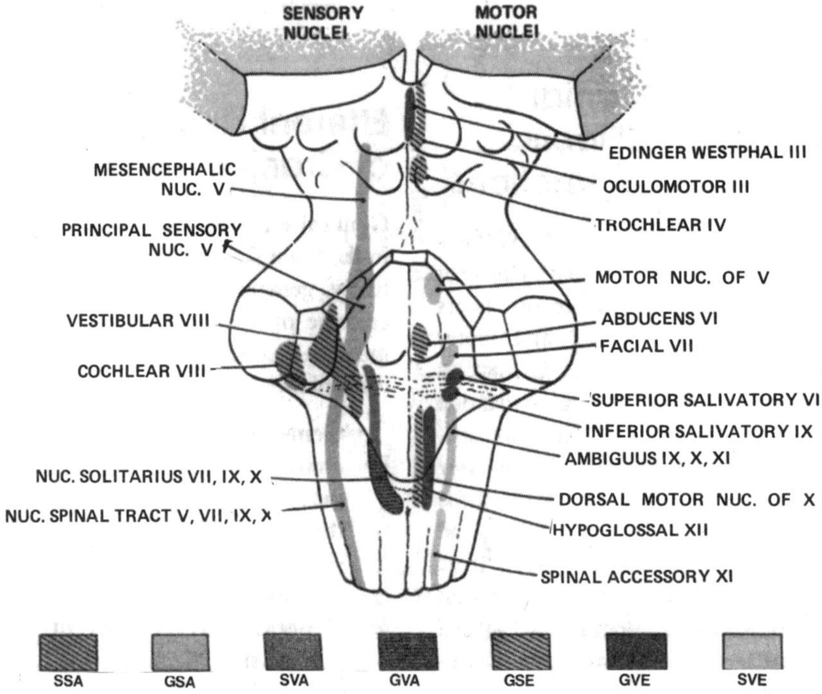

■ **FIGURE 10–5.** Dorsal surface of the brain stem that shows the relative mediolateral positions of the nuclear columns (functional cell columns) associated with cranial nerves III to XII. For clarity, motor nuclei are shown on the *right* and sensory nuclei on the *left*. Compare this illustration with Figure 10–6.

nuclei that belong to each column. Figure 10–6 provides a cross section at the level of the rostral medulla that shows the internal positions of the individual cranial nerve nuclei of the medulla and the functional columns to which they belong.

Motor Nuclei Give Rise to Efferent Fibers

As noted earlier, the **GSE** fibers of cranial nerves III, IV, VI, and XII arise from nuclei arranged as a discontinuous column of cells adjacent to the midline (Fig. 10–5). Situated in line with the anterior horn cells of the spinal cord and homologous to the anterior horn cells, these nuclei innervate musculature derived from myotomes.

The **GVE** nuclei include the superior and inferior salivatory nuclei with fibers entering nerves VII and IX, respectively, and the dorsal motor nucleus of X. These three nuclei form a column lateral to the somatic efferent column. The GVE nucleus of III, the Edinger-Westphal nucleus, lies "misplaced" medially. These four nuclei comprise the parasympathetic cranial nerve nuclei.

The most lateral motor cell column consists of the **SVE** nuclei of cranial nerves V (motor nucleus of V), VII (facial nucleus), IX, X, and XI (the nucleus ambiguus). These three nuclei innervate the branchiomeric musculature, with the exception of a specific subnucleus of the nucleus ambiguus, which provides preganglionic parasympathetic innervation to the heart.

Sensory Nuclei Receive Input from Afferent Fibers Originating in the Sensory Ganglia

The sensory fibers of cranial nerves V, VII, VIII, IX, and X arise from cell bodies in their respective cranial nerve sensory ganglia. Like the central processes of cells in the dorsal root spinal ganglia, they enter the central nervous system and terminate in sensory nuclei. All **visceral afferent**

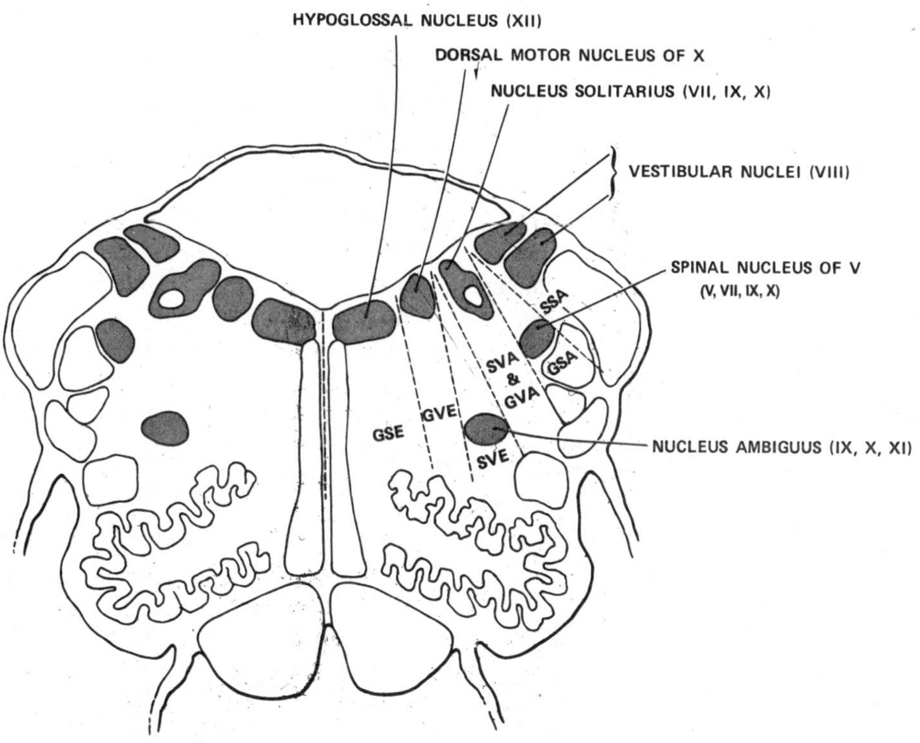

■ **FIGURE 10–6.** Schematic cross section of the upper medulla showing the anatomic organization of the functional cell columns *(in color)* that contribute motoneurons to, and receive sensory input from, the cranial nerves. GSA = general somatic afferent; GSE = general somatic efferent; GVA = general visceral afferent; GVE = general visceral efferent; SSA = special somatic afferent; SVA = special visceral afferent; SVE = special visceral efferent. Refer to Figure 10–9 for identification of unlabeled structures.

fibers in the cranial nerves terminate in the **nucleus of the tractus solitarius,** a nuclear area adjacent to the visceral efferent column. The nucleus of the tractus solitarius receives **GVA fibers** in its caudal part and gustatory **SVA fibers** in its cephalic or rostral portion.

The **GSA** column of nuclei receives somatosensory fibers primarily from cranial nerve V. This column extends from the midbrain through the caudal extent of the medulla and into the cervical spinal cord. It consists of the **mesencephalic nucleus,** the **principal sensory nucleus,** and the **nucleus of the spinal tract of V.** The nucleus of the spinal tract receives most of its input from the face over nerve V and a few fibers from the skin of the ear that travel over cranial nerves VII, IX, and X. This nucleus is continuous with the substantia gelatinosa in the spinal cord and, like the substantia gelatinosa, processes primarily pain and temperature sensations. Figure 10–6 indicates that the **SSA fibers** of nerve VIII from the ear terminate in the most dorsolateral portion of the brain stem.

Cranial Nerves Containing More than One Functional Component Are Connected to More than One Cell Column

Some cranial nerves contain fibers of more than one functional type; thus, these cranial nerves originate in more than one functional cell column in the brain stem. For example, the vagus nerve contains fibers that arise from, or terminate in, five of the seven functional cell columns. It includes motor fibers that originate within a GVE nucleus, the dorsal motor nucleus of X, and an SVE nucleus, the nucleus ambiguus. It also has groups of both GVA and SVA fibers that synapse on separate cell groups in the nucleus solitarius, as well as GSA fibers that end in the spinal nucleus of V (Fig. 10–6).

As an overall principle of the organization of cranial nerve fibers, each functional group of sensory nerve fibers (GVA, SVA, GSA, or SSA), regardless of the nerves over which the fibers travel, converges onto the corresponding cell column, which consists of one to several nuclei. In a corollary manner, motoneurons from individual motor cell columns (GSE, GVE, or SVE) diverge into multiple cranial nerves to distribute to their targets.

Reticular Formation

The reticular formation consists of a collection of nuclei that forms the central core of gray matter throughout the brain stem. Although as many as 20 nuclei can be differentiated by their cytoarchitecture, connections, and functions, they belong to two fundamentally different longitudinal zones, medial and lateral.

The Lateral Zone of the Reticular Formation Is Receptive and Integrative

The lateral zone of the reticular formation contains many interneurons with short axons. These interneurons integrate reflex connections between the sensory and motor cranial nerve nuclei and receive inputs from long tracts from the spinal cord and the forebrain. In this capacity, the lateral zone of the reticular formation can be viewed as the rostral extension of the interneuronal pool of the spinal cord.

The Medial Zone of the Reticular Formation Gives Rise to Ascending and Descending Tracts

The medial zone contains many large neurons with extensive axonal projections. Collectively, these cells receive information from the lateral zone interneurons and project to the spinal cord, cerebellum, hypothalamus, and cerebral cortex, especially the limbic lobe cortex. Some very large neurons with bifurcating ascending and descending axons reach both the hypothalamus and the spinal cord. Other neurons with only ascending or descending axonal projections nonetheless interconnect with each other within the reticular formation, so they also contribute to the distribution of its influence along the entire neuraxis.

Nuclei of the reticular formation function prominently in the processing of pain (see Chapter 6), visceral function (see Chapters 5 and 21), posture and muscle tone (see Chapter 8), and eye movements (see Chapter 19). Nuclei of the reticular formation also contribute to behavioral arousal and participate in controlling cycles of sleep and wakefulness.

Ascending Reticular Activating System and Arousal

The reticular formation participates with a larger system, the **ascending reticular activating sys-**

tem, in processes required for alertness or **arousal.** Specific nuclei of the anatomically defined reticular formation, most of which use acetylcholine as a neurotransmitter, belong to the ascending reticular activating system. Through their projections to the glutamatergic thalamocortical neurons in the **intralaminar nuclei of the thalamus,** these reticular formation nuclei activate the cerebral cortex and initiate or increase arousal.

The cholinergic neurons of the reticular formation also project to other cholinergic nuclei in the forebrain, including the basal nucleus of Meynert, that, in turn, excite the cortex. Finally, monoaminergic neurons of the brain stem contribute to arousal by direct stimulation of the cerebral cortex. These include dopaminergic projections from the ventral tegmental area, noradrenergic projections from the locus ceruleus, and serotonergic fibers from the raphe nuclei. (See the discussion later in this chapter and Figures 23–2, 23–3, and 23–4.) Thus, five different neurotransmitter systems (glutamatergic, cholinergic, dopaminergic, noradrenergic, and serotonergic) contribute to cerebral cortical excitation in behavioral arousal.

Serotonergic and Noradrenergic Cell Groups

Two neurochemically defined groups of nuclei within the central core of the brain stem function as part of the reticular formation. These include the **serotonergic nuclei,** located along the midline **raphe** of the brain stem, and the **noradrenergic cell groups,** which include the **locus ceruleus** and cell groups in the medial reticular zone of the pons and medulla. These two monoaminergic systems originate in the brain stem and in no other part of the central nervous system.

Similar to other medial reticular formation neurons, both serotonergic and noradrenergic neurons give rise to very long axons. In addition, both these neuronal groups distribute fibers to all parts of the neuraxis, from the caudal spinal cord to the cerebral cortex. Nevertheless, selective projections arise within each group of nuclei. Within the serotonergic nuclei, for example, the most rostral cell groups send axons to the cerebrum, the most caudal send axons to the spinal cord, and the intermediate nuclei influence cranial nerve nuclei and the cerebellum (see Fig. 23–4). In the noradrenergic nuclei, the locus ceruleus sends axons to far rostral and far caudal central nervous system targets as well as the brain stem and cerebellum. The pontine and medullary noradrenergic cells have more limited projections, with notably less influence on the cerebral cortex (see Fig. 23–3).

The monoaminergic projections serve many different functions, which are as diverse as modulating sensory transmission, states of alertness, and mood. In all their target tissues, the monoamines play a modulatory role, by enhancing or decreasing the responsiveness of the neuron pools they innervate. More information about these cell systems can be found in Chapter 8 (Raphe-spinal and ceruleus-spinal projections) and in Chapter 23.

Sleep and Waking

Sleep consists not simply of the absence of arousal. It is an actively induced behavioral state essential for life. In addition, sleep occurs in cycles that have different phases, each of which includes a particular pattern of physiologic states. In humans, two general phases of sleep, **slow-wave sleep** and **rapid-eye-movement (or REM) sleep,** differ dramatically in their characteristic levels of electroencephalographic activity, skeletal muscle tone, parasympathetic tone, and ease of reversibility (ease with which the individual can be awakened). Further, both these phases of sleep differ from the physiologic pattern of waking state functions.

Numerous neuroanatomic sites regulate specific aspects of sleep and waking. These sites are located primarily in the hypothalamus, the midbrain and pontine reticular formation, and the aminergic cell groups of the brain stem.

The activity of cholinergic and associated noncholinergic neurons in the midbrain reticular formation maintains the **waking state.** These neurons project to the thalamus, where they interfere with a slow-wave-sleep bursting pattern of firing in the thalamus and cortex. The slow-wave-sleep bursting pattern blocks the transmission of sensory information to the cortex. A group of histaminergic neurons in the posterior hypothalamus also becomes active during wakefulness.

The nucleus reticularis pontis oralis, which extends from the pons into the caudal midbrain, assumes particular importance in both **waking**

and REM sleep states. Several functional groups of neurons within this nucleus interact with nearby histamine neurons in the posterior hypothalamus, serotonergic raphe neurons, and noradrenergic cells of the locus ceruleus. The interactions of these cell groups influence waking and also control the visual system spiking activity, rapid eye movements, and loss of skeletal muscle tone that characterize REM sleep. Gamma-aminobutyric acidergic neurons in the region of the anterior hypothalamus induce **slow-wave sleep** by inhibiting histaminergic neurons of the posterior hypothalamus and cell groups in the nucleus reticularis pontis oralis that sustain wakefulness.

Atlas of the Brain Stem: Transverse Sections

Figures 10–7 through 10–13 present drawings of histologic sections of the human brain stem. These thin slices of tissue were cut perpendicular to the long axis of the brain stem and were stained with the Weigert method, in which chemicals in the stain bind to components of myelin. Thus, the dark areas on the left side of each of these cross sections represent myelinated fibers, and the light areas represent areas free of such fibers. The light areas are filled with neuronal cell bodies forming the various nuclei of the brain stem.

Internal Structures of the Medulla

Caudal Half of the Medulla

A **central gray area** surrounds the **central canal** and merges at its perimeter with a zone containing a network of fibers and cells known as the **reticular formation.** The corticospinal tracts descend through the most anterior part of the medulla in the pyramids. At the caudal end of the medulla, most of these fibers cross in the prominent **motor (or pyramidal) decussation** (Fig. 10–7) that brings them to the lateral position that they maintain in the spinal cord.

On the posterior side at this level, the fasciculus gracilis and fasciculus cuneatus remain present, but the nuclei in which their fibers terminate appear. Axons of the cells in these nuclei take an anterior, arched course, to form the **internal arcuate fibers** that cross the midline as the **decussation of the medial lemniscus** (Fig. 10–8).

The **accessory cuneate nucleus** appears lateral to the rostral part of the cuneate nucleus (Fig.

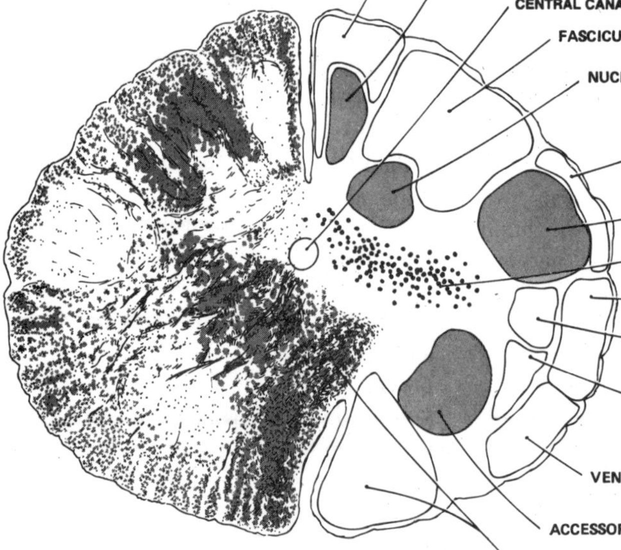

■ **FIGURE 10–7.** Cross section of the lowest level of the medulla, through the decussation of the pyramids. The *left* side represents the general appearance of this level in a myelin-stained histologic preparation. On the *right,* the major nuclei *(color)* and tracts *(white)* are outlined and labeled.

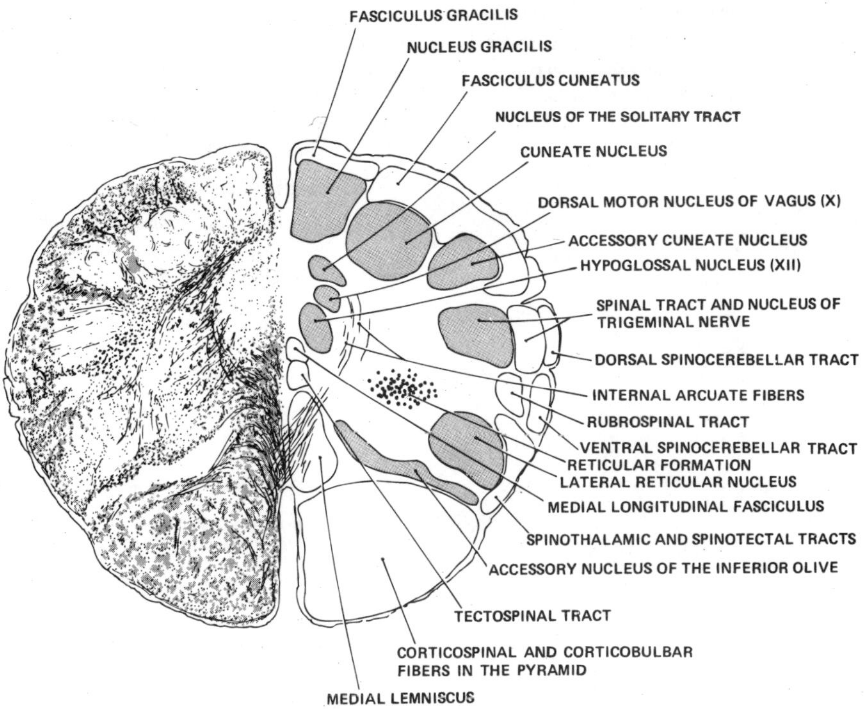

■ **FIGURE 10–8.** Cross section of the lower medulla at the level of the decussation of the internal arcuate fibers forming the medial lemniscus.

10–8). Cells in this nucleus do not contribute axons to the medial lemniscus. Their axons ascend laterally into the inferior cerebellar peduncle as the cuneocerebellar tract (see Fig. 7–1).

In the posterolateral region, a clear nuclear area capped by a peripheral zone of fine fibers represents the **spinal nucleus and spinal tract of the trigeminal nerve.** These two structures extend from the pontine region through the medulla to the second segment of the cervical spinal cord. The spinal tract contains fibers of the trigeminal ganglion cells that transmit pain, temperature, and simple touch information to the adjacent spinal nucleus neurons.

Rostral Half of the Medulla

The principal nucleus of the **inferior olivary nuclear complex,** a prominent structure in the anterolateral region, resembles a crinkled sac with an opening (hilum) directed toward the midline (see Fig. 10–9). Many efferent fibers of the complex cross the midline and stream toward the posterolateral corner of the medulla to join dorsal spinocerebellar and cuneocerebellar fibers in the thick **inferior cerebellar peduncle (restiform body).**

Several distinct, symmetrically paired cellular areas occupy the posterior part of the medulla close to the floor of the ventricle. These nuclear columns extend longitudinally through the upper medulla (Fig. 10–5). The **nucleus of the hypoglossal nerve (XII)** is nearest the midline. Fibers from this nucleus pass anteriorly and emerge between the pyramid and the olive (Fig. 10–9) as the rootlets of the hypoglossal nerve, which innervates the striated muscles of the tongue. The **dorsal motor nucleus of the vagus nerve (X)** lies at the side of the hypoglossal nucleus and contains neurons that form an important part of the parasympathetic division of the autonomic nervous system. The most lateral nuclear column, separated from the motor nuclei by the sulcus limitans, contains the **vestibular nuclei** (medial and inferior at this level of the medulla), which receive afferent fibers from the vestibular division of the vestibulocochlear nerve (VIII). This nerve brings information to the brain concerning position and movement of the head in space, as well as auditory information.

The **nucleus ambiguus,** seen indistinctly in Weigert-stained preparations, is located in the anterolateral part of the reticular formation. Its fibers course posteromedially at first, but they arch back and leave the medulla anterior to the

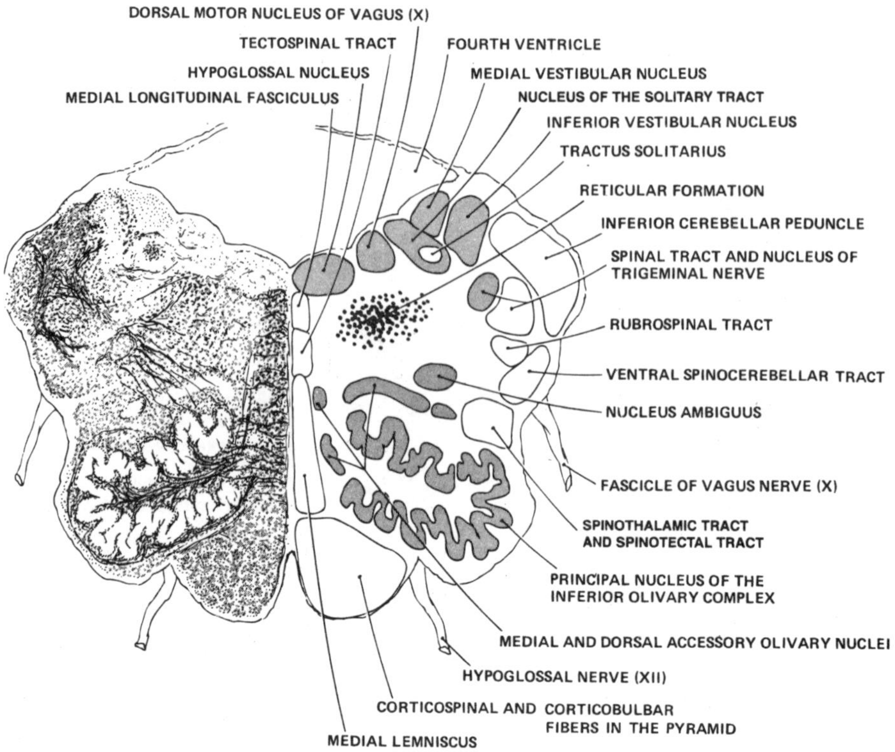

■ **FIGURE 10–9.** Cross section of the upper medulla.

inferior cerebellar peduncle as fibers of the glossopharyngeal (IX), vagus (X), and cranial portion of the accessory (XI) nerves (see Figs. 10–9 and 11–1). These nerve fibers control the branchiomeric muscles of the pharynx and larynx and thus control swallowing and vocalization. An isolated bundle of longitudinal fibers accompanied by a small nucleus appears in the posterior part of the reticular formation. This bundle is known as the **solitary tract** and is composed of afferent root fibers from the facial, glossopharyngeal, and vagus nerves. The cells of the **nucleus of the solitary tract** surround the tract and receive fibers from it that carry information about taste and visceral sensations. The spinal tract and nucleus of cranial nerve V continue rostrally in a lateral position, somewhat ventral to the other nuclei surrounding the ventricle.

The anterolateral fiber system from the spinal cord (including the spinothalamic tract) appears adjacent to the nucleus ambiguus on its anterolateral side. Two large bands of fibers lie vertically at either side of the midline. The extreme posterior portion of each band contains the **medial longitudinal fasciculus (MLF),** a structure that extends from the upper thoracic spinal cord to the midbrain. At this level in the medulla, the MLF contains several descending pathways, including the **medial vestibulospinal, interstitiospinal,** and some of the **pontine reticulospinal tracts.** The **tectospinal pathway,** which descends through the brain stem anterior to the MLF, joins the fibers of this fasciculus in the caudal medulla and extends into the spinal cord as part of this tract. The **medial lemniscus** comprises the most ventral and largest portion of this vertically situated band of fibers.

Internal Structures of the Pons

Examination of histologic sections of the pons reveals two evident subdivisions: a posterior portion, known as the **tegmentum,** and an anterior part, called the **basilar portion.** In this region of the brain stem, the roof portion (tectum), overlying the cavity of the ventricle, becomes expanded and specialized to form the cerebellum.

Caudal Portion of the Pons

The corticospinal tracts appear in a central location in the basilar portion. The gray matter that surrounds them contains cells of the **pontine**

nuclei. Transverse pontine fibers (i.e., the pontocerebellar tract) crossing from one side to the other, posterior and anterior to the corticospinal tracts, consist of axons from cell bodies in the pontine nuclei (Fig. 10–10). The fibers from the pontine nuclei of one side form the contralateral **middle cerebellar peduncle** and terminate in the cerebellar cortex. The pontine nuclei receive input from the ipsilateral cerebrum, and their projections to the cerebellum constitute a major route by which the cerebral cortex communicates with the cerebellar cortex.

The **medial lemniscus** appears as an ellipsoid bundle of fibers. In the medulla, the long axis of this ellipse becomes oriented in the anterior-posterior axis. In the tegmentum of the pons, these fibers shift, and the long axis of the ellipse extends transversely along the boundary with the basilar portion of the pons.

The **MLF** retains its position near midline in the floor of the fourth ventricle. At this level of the pons, the MLF consists primarily of ascending fibers. These fibers arise in the vestibular nuclei and project to the nuclei supplying the extraocular muscles. The descending **interstitiospinal and pontine reticulospinal tracts** become partially intermingled with the MLF at this level.

The **trapezoid body,** an auditory relay structure, appears as a prominent band of decussating fibers in the anterior part of the tegmentum. Its fibers interlace at right angles with the rostrocaudally oriented fibers of the medial lemniscus (Fig. 10–10). The **superior olive** consists of a small nucleus that lies lateral and slightly posterior to the trapezoid body. It also belongs to the auditory system.

The **central tegmental tract** consists of an isolated bundle in the anterior part of the reticular formation that contains descending pathways (mainly **rubro-olivary tracts**) and part of the important **ascending reticular formation projections** to the thalamus and hypothalamus. At this level, the central tegmental tract also carries **ascending taste fibers** from the solitary nucleus to the ventral posteromedial nucleus of the thalamus. The spinal nucleus and tract of the trigeminal nerve have not changed their position, but fibers of the middle cerebellar peduncle cover the lateral side.

The **motor nucleus of the facial nerve (VII)** lies immediately posterior to the superior olive and medial to the nucleus of the spinal tract of the trigeminal nerve (V). Before leaving the brain stem, the fibers of the facial nerve form an internal loop **(internal genu of the facial nerve).** The first segment of this loop courses posterome-

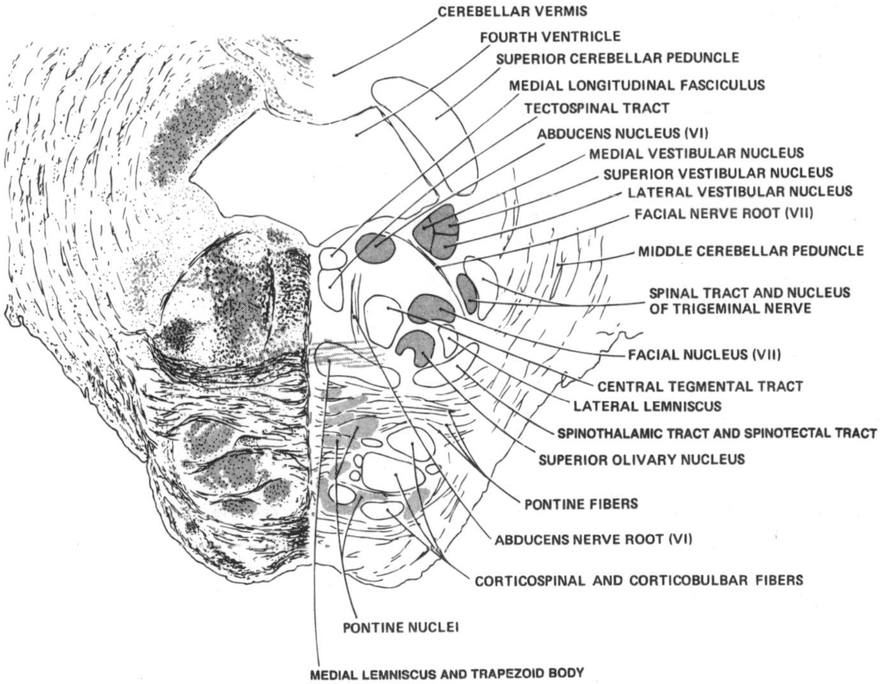

■ **FIGURE 10–10.** Cross section of the pons at the level of the nuclei of cranial nerves VI and VII.

dially toward the floor of the fourth ventricle and passes close and just caudal and medial to the **nucleus of the abducens nerve.** The facial nerve then courses rostrally and laterally around the abducens nucleus. After completing this "hairpin" bend, the nerve takes a direct course anterolaterally and slightly caudally (facial nerve root in Fig. 10–10) to its exit at the pontomedullary junction. Peripherally, its fibers innervate a thin sheet of branchiomeric muscles underneath the skin of the face. These muscles control facial expression.

Fibers of the **abducens nerve** take a straight course through the tegmentum of the pons (Fig. 10–10) and exit close to the lateral border of the pyramidal tract on the anterior aspect of the brain stem (Fig. 10–1). These fibers innervate the lateral rectus muscle in the orbit.

The **vestibular nuclei** continue to occupy a lateral area in the floor of the fourth ventricle. The individual subnuclei at this level include the lateral, superior, and medial subnuclei (Fig. 10–10). The spinal (inferior) nucleus remains confined to the medulla.

Sections through the cerebellum at the lower level of the pons generally show the paired, deep cerebellar nuclei. These nuclei do not appear in Figure 10–10, but they can be seen in Figures 16–3 and 16–4. Most of the neuronal outflow from the cerebellar cortex comes from the deep cerebellar nuclei. They include the following structures:

1. Fastigial nucleus: located in the midline of the roof of the fourth ventricle near the vermis.
2. Globose nucleus: a small group of cells located just lateral to the fastigial nucleus.
3. Emboliform nucleus: a slightly elongated cellular mass located between the globose and dentate nuclei.
4. Dentate nucleus: the largest and most laterally placed of the cerebellar nuclei; it resembles the inferior olivary nuclear complex and is purselike in shape, with an anteromedial hilum.

Middle Portion of the Pons

The basilar portion of the pons appears widened and thickened at the level of the middle pons. Dispersed in separate fascicles, the corticospinal tracts mingle with numerous other scattered longitudinal fibers. These are the **corticopontine fibers** descending from the ipsilateral frontal, temporal, parietal, and occipital lobes to synapse with cells of the pontine nuclei (Fig. 10–11).

Two oval-shaped nuclei lie side by side in the posterolateral part of the tegmentum, the **main**

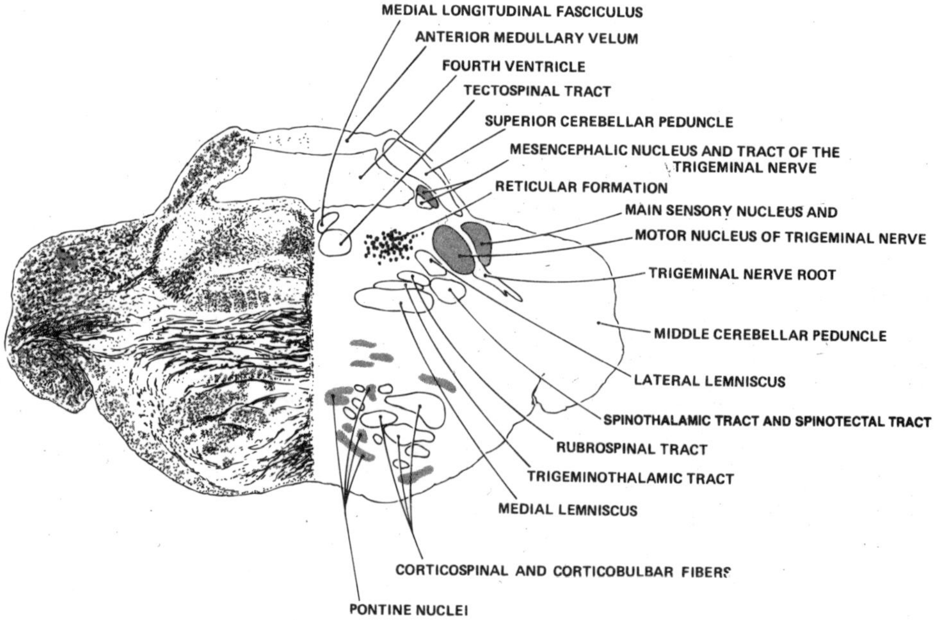

■ **FIGURE 10–11.** Cross section of the pons at the level of the main (principal) sensory and motor nuclei of V.

(principal) sensory nucleus of the trigeminal nerve laterally and the **motor nucleus of the trigeminal nerve** medially. Small filaments of the nerve pass posteriorly and rostrally as the **mesencephalic tract** of the trigeminal nerve. These fibers consist of processes of primary sensory cells ("misplaced" ganglion cells) in the adjacent mesencephalic nucleus. These cells carry signals from stretch receptors in the muscles of mastication. Most make monosynaptic connections with the motor nucleus of cranial nerve V and contribute the afferent signals for the jaw reflex. The main sensory nucleus receives fibers of the trigeminal nerve conveying information from mechanoreceptors that are necessary for tactile discrimination. The motor component of the trigeminal nerve (V) arises from neurons in the motor nucleus and innervates the muscles of mastication. Trigeminal nerve fibers emerging from the surface of the pons pass directly through the middle cerebellar peduncle (Figs. 10–1 and 10–2).

The **superior cerebellar peduncles (brachia conjunctiva)** appear in the walls of the fourth ventricle as large, compact bands (see Figs. 10–10 and 10–11). The anterior medullary velum forms the roof of the ventricle.

Internal Structures of the Midbrain

In cross sections, the midbrain contains three zones: (1) a basal portion, the cerebral peduncle or crus cerebri; (2) the tegmentum, similar to the pontine **tegmentum;** and (3) the tectum, or roof portion, lying above the aqueduct and forming the quadrigeminal plate.

Caudal Half of the Midbrain (Level of the Inferior Colliculus)

Each cerebral peduncle appears in cross section as a prominent, crescent-shaped mass of fibers within which the corticospinal and corticobulbar tracts occupy a central position, flanked at either side by corticopontine fibers (Fig. 10–12). The **substantia nigra** lies between the cerebral peduncle and the tegmentum. In the freshly sectioned brain and in some histologic preparations, the neurons of this area appear brown because of the melanin pigment contained in some of their cell bodies.

The central part of the tegmentum contains a massive interlacement of fibers—the **decussation of the superior cerebellar peduncle.** The **medial lemniscus** has been displaced laterally and ro-

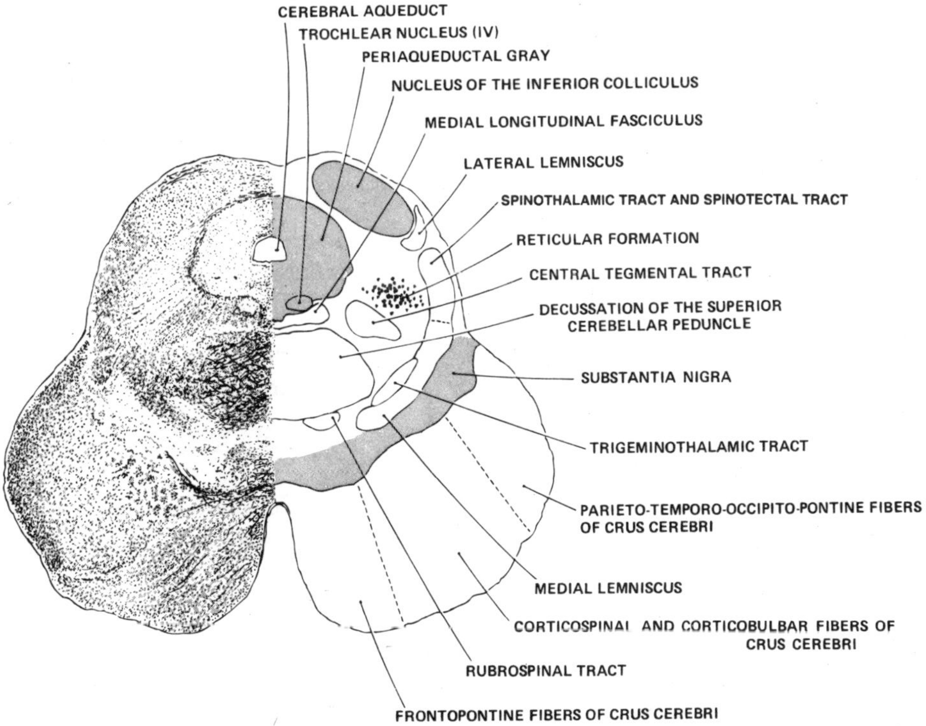

■ **FIGURE 10–12.** Cross section of the lower midbrain at the level of the inferior colliculus and decussation of the superior cerebellar peduncles.

tated slightly. Its outer border lies in close relation to adjacent fibers of the anterolateral system (spinothalamic tracts). The **lateral lemniscus,** containing the ascending auditory fibers, appears well defined in the lateral part of the tegmentum posterior to the anterolateral system. Many of the fibers in the lateral lemniscus terminate dorsally in the **nucleus of the inferior colliculus.** The small, globular **nucleus of the trochlear nerve** lies near the **MLF** in the anterior part of the central gray substance **(periaqueductal gray matter).**

Rostral Half of the Midbrain (Level of the Superior Colliculus)

The cerebral peduncle and the substantia nigra continue to occupy the basal portion of the midbrain. The **red nuclei** appear as conspicuous globular masses in the anterior portion of the tegmentum (Fig. 10–13). The crossed fibers of the superior cerebellar peduncle pass into the red nucleus and around its edges. Many of these fibers terminate in the red nucleus; others pass forward to the thalamus. Together, these structures comprise an important part of the outflow from the cerebellum. The tectospinal and rubrospinal tracts arise from this part of the midbrain. Both tracts cross near their origin: the tectospinal in the **dorsal tegmental decussation** and the rubrospinal in the **ventral tegmental decussation.**

The nuclear complex of the oculomotor nerve lies in the anterior part of the central gray matter, with the **MLF** beside it. The root fibers of the oculomotor nerve stream ventrally through and around the red nucleus before converging at their exit in the interpeduncular fossa (see Fig. 13–4). From there, the root fibers travel to the orbit, where they innervate four of the six muscles that control eye movements and one muscle that elevates the eyelid. This nerve also contains preganglionic parasympathetic fibers, which constrict the pupil and change the shape of the lens within the eye.

In transverse sections through the rostral midbrain, where the midbrain joins the diencephalon, the **medial geniculate nuclei (or bodies)** appear to be protrusions on the lateral surfaces of the midbrain. They are not brain stem structures, but the most ventral, caudal nuclei of the thalamus, where fibers of the brachium of the inferior colliculus synapse on auditory thalamocortical neurons.

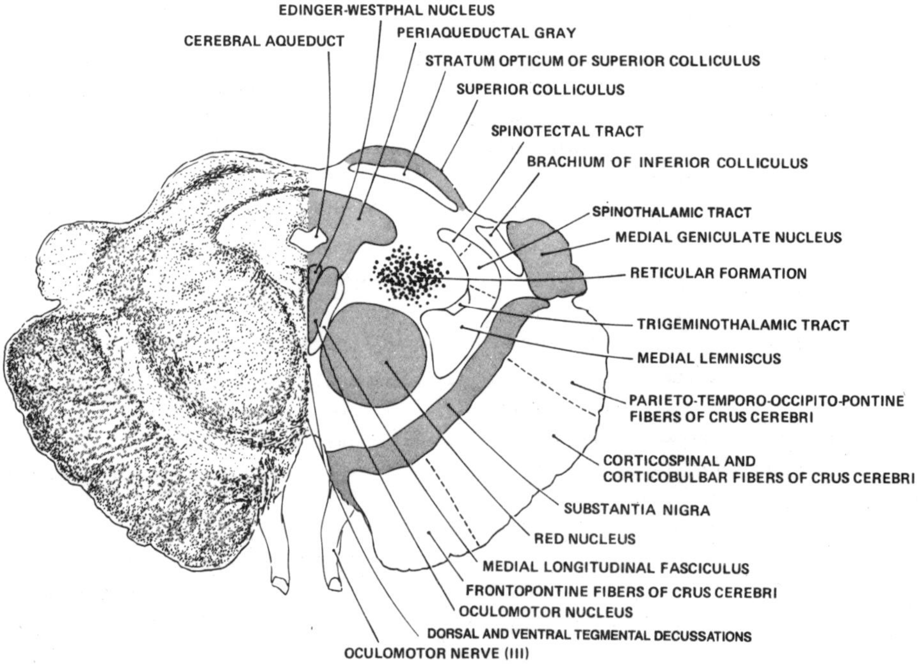

■ **FIGURE 10-13.** Cross section of the upper midbrain at the level of the superior colliculus and red nucleus.

Blood Supply to the Brain Stem and Cerebellum

The **vertebral arteries** provide the primary source of blood to the brain stem. Direct branches of the left and right vertebral arteries supply the anterolateral parts of the medulla. The anteromedial medulla receives blood from the **anterior spinal artery.** At the pontomedullary junction, the two vertebral arteries join to form the **basilar artery,** which supplies branches to the pons and the midbrain (Fig. 10–14). Branches of both the vertebral and basilar arteries wrap dorsally around the brain stem to supply the dorsal aspect of the brain stem and the entire cerebellum. These arteries include the following: the **posterior inferior cerebellar arteries,** which supply the medulla as well as the cerebellum; the **anterior inferior cerebellar arteries,** which provide blood for the pons and the cerebellum; and the **superior cerebellar arteries,** which distribute to both the midbrain and the cerebellum (Fig. 10–14). At the rostral end of the midbrain, the basilar artery terminates by dividing into the right and left **posterior cerebral arteries,** which pass superior to the tentorium cerebelli to supply the posterior and ventral surfaces of the cerebral hemispheres.

Case Follow-up

The woman described at the beginning of this chapter has neurologic abnormalities that point to a disorder in the upper medulla that affects structures in the dorsolateral sector (Fig. 10–14). The structures affected include the left medial and inferior vestibular nuclei, the left spinal tract and nucleus of the trigeminal nerve, and the left inferior cerebellar peduncle. Involvement of the vestibular nuclei causes her nystagmus and probably accounts for the vertigo, nausea, and vomiting. Injury to the spinal tract and nucleus of the trigeminal nerve results in the decrease of pinprick and cold sensation on the left side

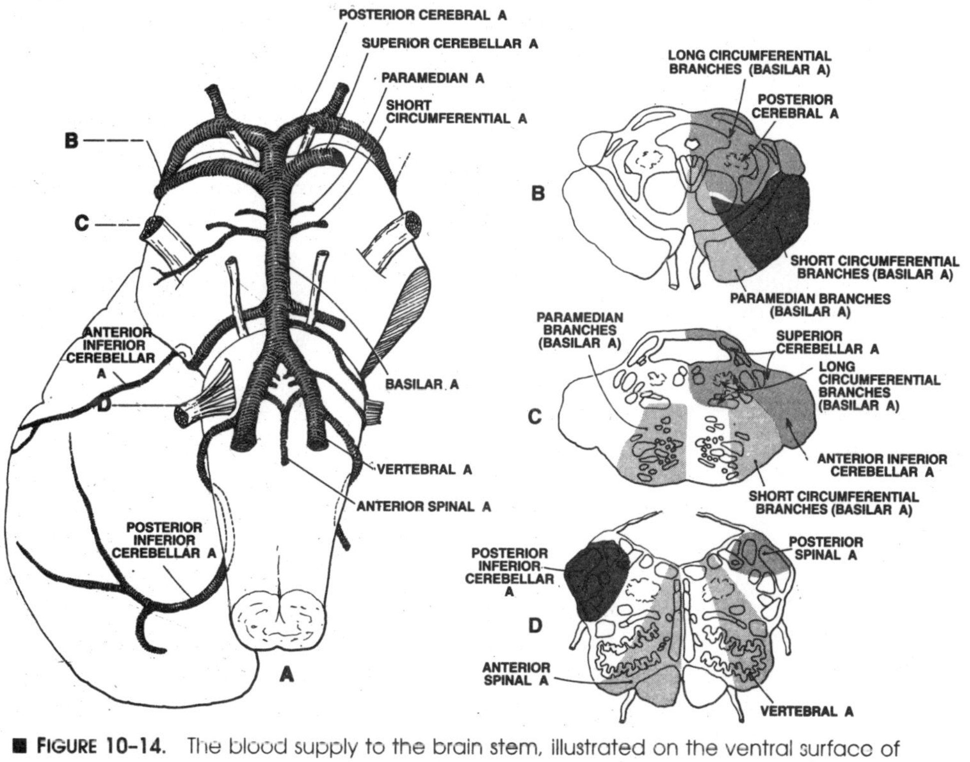

■ **FIGURE 10–14.** The blood supply to the brain stem, illustrated on the ventral surface of the brain stem **(A)** and on the cross sections at three levels through the brain stem **(B, C,** and **D).** In **B, C,** and **D,** the territories of individual arteries, or arterial branches, are *shaded* and labeled. In some cases, these territories overlap. Cross sections in **B, C,** and **D** correspond to Figures 10–13, 10–11, and 10–9, respectively.

of her face. Injury to the left inferior cerebellar peduncle is responsible for the ataxia affecting the left arm and leg as well as the gait abnormality. The patient's history of hypertension suggests the possibility of ischemic vascular disease. A magnetic resonance imaging study is compatible with this diagnosis. Because the patient is evaluated within 3 hours of the onset of her symptoms, she receives tissue plasminogen activator in an attempt to dissolve the clot in blood vessels perfusing the brain stem. She is admitted to hospital, and, over the next 24 hours, she experiences a complete reversal of all her symptoms by the time of discharge from hospital. She receives a new medication to improve the control of her high blood pressure and instructions to take one tablet of 81 mg of aspirin daily as a preventive measure for additional ischemic cerebrovascular events.

11

Cranial Nerves of the Medulla

Case Study

A 50-year-old man sees his dentist for routine care, and on examination the dentist finds that the right side of the patient's tongue is much smaller than the left. The dentist refers him to a neurologist, who finds marked atrophy of the right side of the patient's tongue, and on protrusion, the tongue deviates strongly to the right. The man's speech is unaffected.

What could account for the atrophy of one side of the tongue? Why does the tongue protrude to the right? How can this problem be investigated?

Hypoglossal Nerve (XII)

The **hypoglossal nerve** provides the motor innervation to the tongue. Its general somatic efferent fibers arise from lower motoneuron cell bodies in the **hypoglossal nucleus.** This nucleus consists of a column of cells that extends nearly the entire length of the medulla in a position just under the fourth ventricle close to the midline. Axons of these cells pass between the pyramid and the olive to exit as rootlets of the hypoglossal nerve. They innervate the intrinsic musculature of the tongue as well as muscles at its base. These include the genioglossi, which together draw the root of the tongue forward and cause the tip of the tongue to protrude. The genioglossus muscle of each side causes the tongue, on protrusion, to deviate to the opposite side. Injury to the hypoglossal nucleus or nerve on one side causes a lower motoneuron lesion, with paralysis and atrophy of the muscles on the side of the lesion. On voluntary protrusion, the tongue deviates to the paralyzed side.

Accessory Nerve (XI)

The **accessory nerve** consists of two distinct parts. The **spinal portion** arises from a dorsal group of anterior horn cells **(spinal accessory nucleus)** in cervical cord segments C2 through C5. The nerve exits the spinal cord through the lateral funiculus as a series of rootlets, ascends through the foramen magnum, and courses along the side of the medulla (see Figs. 10–1 and 10–2). Here it joins the **cranial portion** of the same nerve from the medulla. These cranial root fibers consist of visceral efferents that arise from neurons in the **nucleus ambiguus.** After traveling together for a short distance, the two roots again separate. The cranial fibers turn away to join the vagus nerve and, along with the terminal branches of the vagus, innervate the branchiomeric muscles of the larynx and the heart (Fig. 11–1).

The spinal portion of nerve XI passes through the jugular foramen and descends in the neck to end in the sternomastoid and trapezius muscles. Injury to the spinal accessory nerve results in paralysis of the sternomastoid muscle, which causes weakness in rotating the head to the opposite side. Paralysis of the upper part of the trapezius muscle causes downward and outward rotation of the upper part of the scapula, sagging of the shoulder, and weakness in attempts to shrug the shoulder.

Vagal System: Nervus Intermedius (VII), Glossopharyngeal (IX), Vagus (X), and Cranial Accessory (XI) Nerves

Closely related in function, four nerves of the medulla and pons articulate with a common group of cell columns. These are as follows: (1) the **nervus intermedius,** which contains the sensory and parasympathetic fibers of the facial nerve (VII); (2) the **glossopharyngeal nerve** (IX); (3) the **vagus nerve** (X); and (4) the **cranial portion of the accessory nerve** (XI). These nerves are considered collectively as the vagal system.

The vagal system contains special visceral motor, preganglionic parasympathetic, and sensory fibers, but the fiber bundles do not separate into dorsal and ventral nerve roots as in the spinal nerves. All fibers enter and leave the medulla in a series of rootlets arranged in a longitudinal row posterior to the olive (Fig. 11–1).

Four nuclear columns contribute fibers to, or receive fibers from, the four nerves of the vagal system, as follows:

1. The **special visceral motor column** of the medulla, the nucleus ambiguus, innervates the branchial musculature.
2. The **general visceral motor column,** or preganglionic parasympathetic column, consists of the superior and inferior salivatory nuclei, the dorsal motor nucleus of X, and the external subnucleus of the nucleus ambiguus.
3. The **visceral sensory column** consists of the nucleus of the tractus solitarius (solitary

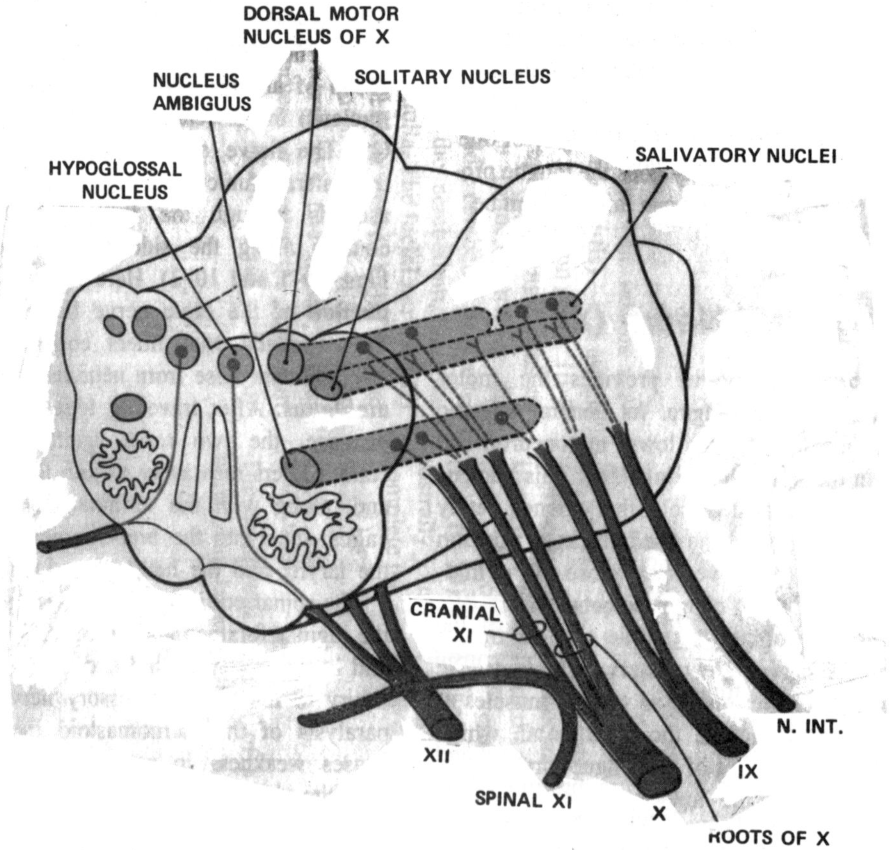

■ **FIGURE 11-1.** The three nuclear cell columns of the vagal system and their connections with the four nerves of that system. The hypoglossal nucleus and nerve root are also shown. N. INT. = nervus intermedius.

nucleus), a sensory cell column that processes both general visceral sensations (from the viscera of the head, neck, thorax, and abdomen) and the special visceral sense of taste.

4. The **general somatic afferent column,** a portion of the spinal nucleus of V, receives pain and touch information from a small area of skin of the auricle.

Innervation of the Branchial Musculature

The cells of the **nucleus ambiguus** consist of special visceral efferent lower motoneurons. Their axons enter the glossopharyngeal and vagus nerves and the cranial root of the accessory nerve to furnish motor innervation to the striated branchiomeric musculature of the soft palate, pharynx, and larynx. All these fibers, except the glossopharyngeal branch to the stylopharyngeus, follow the peripheral branches of the vagus.

A unilateral lesion of the vagus nerve leads to difficulty in coughing, clearing the throat, and swallowing. Frothy mucus collects in the pharynx and overflows into the larynx. The palatal arch droops on the side of the lesion. During phonation, the soft palate rises only on the normal side, and the uvula deviates to the normal side. Bilateral lesions of the vagus nerves result in difficulty in swallowing (dysphagia), with regurgitation of food into the nose on swallowing. Certain vocal sounds become difficult to produce (dysphonia), and the voice develops a nasal quality. A tendency toward mouth breathing occurs, along with snoring at night and difficulty in draining mucus from the nasal passages into the pharynx. One of the recurrent laryngeal nerves, carrying innervation to the larynx, may be injured inadvertently during operations on the thyroid gland, with resulting transient or permanent hoarseness. Paralysis of both recurrent nerves causes stridor and dyspnea, which may necessitate tracheotomy.

Parasympathetic Innervation of the Viscera

The **dorsal motor nucleus of the vagus nerve** consists of preganglionic parasympathetic nerve cell bodies, whose axons leave the medulla and project general visceral efferent fibers to parasympathetic **terminal ganglia** located in the head, neck, thorax, and abdomen. Located near or within the viscera that they innervate, the ganglia send short postganglionic fibers directly to the smooth muscle, cardiac muscle, and gland cells of the organs. Stimulation of vagal parasympathetic fibers slows the heart rate, constricts the smooth muscle of the bronchial tree, stimulates the glands of the bronchial mucosa, promotes peristalsis in the gastrointestinal tract, relaxes the pyloric and ileocolic sphincters, and stimulates the secretion of gastric and pancreatic juices. A separate group of neurons, in the **external subnucleus of the nucleus ambiguus,** contains preganglionic parasympathetic neurons that also innervate the heart. Preganglionic fibers from these neurons leave the medulla in the cranial accessory nerve (XI) and join the branches of the vagus nerve to reach the heart, where they contribute to cardiac slowing associated with the carotid sinus reflex (described later).

The **salivatory nuclei** lie at the rostral end of the general visceral efferent nuclear column. Neuronal activity in these nuclei stimulates secretion by the salivary glands. The cells in the superior salivatory nucleus send preganglionic fibers to the nervus intermedius, and those in the inferior nucleus send preganglionic fibers to the glossopharyngeal nerve (Fig. 11–1). The **nervus intermedius,** a rootlet of the facial nerve (VII), contains the preganglionic parasympathetic and sensory fibers that belong to this cranial nerve, whereas the larger motor root of nerve VII contains only branchiomotor fibers to the muscles of facial expression. Some of the preganglionic fibers entering the nervus intermedius terminate in the **pterygopalatine ganglion,** which sends postganglionic fibers to the lacrimal gland and to the mucosal glands of the palate, pharynx, and posterior nasal chambers. Other preganglionic fibers of the nervus intermedius end in the **submandibular ganglion,** which innervates the submandibular and sublingual salivary glands. Preganglionic fibers of the glossopharyngeal nerve end in the **otic ganglion,** the parasympathetic ganglion that innervates the parotid gland.

Sensory Functions of the Vagal System

Taste System

The visceral sensory fibers of the vagus and glossopharyngeal nerves have cell bodies in the inferior sensory ganglia of nerves IX and X. These ganglia reside near the base of the skull. The geniculate ganglion, located at the external genu of the facial nerve, contains the cell bodies of sensory fibers in the nervus intermedius. After entering the medulla in the dorsolateral sulcus, the sensory fibers of the vagal system pass directly into the **solitary tract.** From this tract, they distribute branches to the adjacent **solitary nucleus.**

Chemical stimulation of receptor cells in taste buds of the tongue initiates impulses mediating the sense of **taste.** Special visceral afferent fibers of the nervus intermedius and the glossopharyngeal nerves conduct this information to the rostral (gustatory) portion of the solitary nucleus. Ganglion cells subserving taste in the **geniculate ganglion** of the facial nerve have peripheral processes in the chorda tympani nerve and central processes in the nervus intermedius. The peripheral processes of these cells receive input from taste buds on the anterior two-thirds of the tongue. The taste buds on the caudal one-third of the tongue receive innervation from peripheral processes of cells in the **inferior ganglion (petrosal) of the glossopharyngeal nerve.** A few taste buds on the epiglottis receive innervation from neurons in the **inferior ganglion (nodose) of the vagus.** This small vagal component of the taste system is not shown entering the gustatory portion of nucleus solitarius in Figure 11–1.

Secondary fibers (the ascending gustatory tract) from cells of the rostral portion of the **solitary nucleus** (sometimes called the gustatory nucleus) ascend **ipsilaterally** through the brain stem in the central tegmental tract to the most medial part of the **ventral posteromedial nucleus** (VPMpc) of the thalamus. In most mammals, but not in primates, these ascending solitarius fibers synapse in the parabrachial nucleus (or pontine taste area), which projects to the VPMpc. From the VPMpc, thalamocortical fibers project to the cerebral cortex, Brodmann's area 43, a taste recognition area located in the opercular cortex at the ventral end of the central sulcus, where the precentral and postcentral gyri meet. This area continues into the anterior insula. It lies adjacent to, but separate from, the primary somatosensory cortical area for the tongue (see Fig. 20–1).

General Visceral Sensory Portion of the Vagal System

The glossopharyngeal and vagus nerves supply the **general visceral afferent** fibers for touch and pain sensations to the mucosa lining the posterior part of the soft palate, middle ear cavity, auditory tube, pharynx, larynx, and trachea. These fibers have nerve cell bodies in the inferior ganglia of nerves IX and X. The fibers enter the solitary tract along with the special sensory fibers of taste, but they terminate in the caudal portion of the nucleus of the solitary tract.

The glossopharyngeal and vagus nerves also conduct action potentials mediating general visceral sensory stimuli from the viscera of the neck, thorax, and abdomen. The glossopharyngeal nerve selectively innervates the carotid sinus baroreceptors and the chemoreceptors in the carotid body, whereas the long vagus nerve distributes to receptors in the heart, bronchi, esophagus, stomach, small intestine, and ascending colon that respond to stretch and pressure. (As described in Chapter 6, the anterolateral system of the spinal cord, which receives input from visceral afferents accompanying the sympathetic nerves, transmits the sensation of pain from the viscera.) Vagal stimulation may be responsible for the sensation of nausea, but most afferent impulses from viscera are not recognized consciously when they are conducted by the vagus.

A chief function of the nontaste afferent fibers of the vagal system concerns the operation of visceral reflexes described at the end of the chapter. Interneurons in the reticular formation mediate all these reflexes polysynaptically.

Visceral sensory information from the nucleus solitarius also projects to a network of structures that integrates visceral and somatic motor responses in complex emotional and social behaviors. The ascending pathways from the nucleus solitarius carry discrete types of visceral sensory input to the parabrachial area of the pons and from here to the medial part of the VPM of the thalamus and to the periaqueductal gray area of the midbrain, the hypothalamus, and the amygdala. The thalamocortical projections of this visceral sensory pathway end in the insular cortex. All these structures form a network of interconnected nuclei that includes the reticular formation, the parabrachial nucleus, the periaqueductal gray area, the hypothalamus, the amygdala, and the limbic cortex. This network integrates visceral function into emotional and social behaviors and is discussed further in Chapter 21.

Somatic Sensory Innervation of the Auricle and External Auditory Meatus

Fibers with cell bodies in the **superior ganglion of IX,** the **superior ganglion of X,** and the **geniculate ganglion** of nerve VII transmit to the brain stem the **general somatic sensations** of pain, touch, and temperature from the skin of the posterior part of the auricle and the external auditory meatus. On entering the brain stem, the central processes of these cells enter the spinal tract of nerve V and terminate, along with the other fibers in that tract, on cells in the adjacent nucleus of the spinal tract. This general somatic afferent component of the vagal system is not illustrated in Figure 11–1.

External Course and Distribution of Nerves of the Vagal System

Nervus Intermedius (VII)

The **nervus intermedius,** the smaller of the two divisions of the facial nerve root, exits from the brain stem at the junction of the medulla and pons. It enters the internal acoustic meatus and proceeds laterally in the facial canal toward the medial wall of the middle ear cavity. The sensory ganglion **(geniculate ganglion),** located on the external genu of the facial nerve at the angle of a sharp bend in the facial canal, contains the cell bodies of taste fibers in nervus intermedius. The preganglionic parasympathetic fibers pass through this sensory ganglion en route to synapses in the more peripheral autonomic ganglia. From the external genu, some peripheral fibers continue as the **greater superficial petrosal nerve** to the **pterygopalatine ganglion.** The rest of the taste and parasympathetic fibers pass downward in the facial canal but leave it abruptly and cross the tympanic cavity as the **chorda tympani nerve.** Leaving the middle ear at the medial end of the **petrotympanic fissure,** the chorda tympani descends between the pterygoid muscles to join the lingual branch of the mandibular division of the trigeminal nerve. Some fibers of the chorda tympani project to the submandibular ganglion, and the rest reach taste receptors in the anterior two-thirds of the tongue.

Glossopharyngeal Nerve (IX)

The **glossopharyngeal nerve** leaves the skull through the **jugular foramen,** which contains its two sensory ganglia, superior and inferior. The nerve passes downward and forward to reach the stylopharyngeus muscle and the mucosa of the palatine tonsil, the fauces, and the posterior one-third of the tongue.

The glossopharyngeal nerve has five branches:

1. The **tympanic branch** enters the tympanic plexus, provides sensory innervation to the membranes of the tympanic cavity, proceeds from the plexus as the **lesser superficial petrosal nerve,** and terminates in the otic ganglion.
2. The **carotid branch** descends along the internal carotid artery to the carotid sinus and the carotid body.
3. The **pharyngeal branch** enters the pharyngeal plexus with the vagus nerve and supplies the mucous membrane of the pharynx with sensory branches.
4. The **stylopharyngeal branch** consists of motor fibers to the stylopharyngeus muscle.
5. The **lingual branch** sends taste and general sensory fibers to the posterior one-third of the tongue.

Vagus Nerve (X)

The two **sensory ganglia** of the vagus nerve, the **superior (jugular)** and **inferior (nodose),** are located near the jugular foramen through which the nerve passes. The nerve courses down the neck within the carotid sheath to enter the thorax; it passes anterior to the subclavian artery on the right and anterior to the aortic arch on the left. Both branches pass behind the roots of the lungs. The left nerve continues on the anterior side and the right nerve on the posterior side of the esophagus to reach the gastric plexus. Fibers diverge from this plexus to the duodenum, liver, biliary ducts, spleen, kidneys, and the small and large intestine as far as the splenic flexure.

The vagus nerve has several branches:

1. The **auricular branch** extends to the skin in the external auditory canal and a small sector of the auricle. The nucleus of the spinal tract of nerve V provides the central connections of this branch.

2. The **pharyngeal branch** extends to the pharyngeal plexus, along with the glossopharyngeal nerve. It supplies the major motor innervation of the pharynx and soft palate.
3. The **superior laryngeal internal branch** mediates sensation from the mucosa of the upper part of the larynx and epiglottis. Its external branch innervates the inferior pharyngeal constrictor and cricothyroid muscles.
4. The **recurrent laryngeal branch** on the left side loops around the aortic arch from anterior to posterior. On the right side, it takes a similar course around the subclavian artery. Both nerves ascend in the laryngotracheal grooves and supply motor fibers to the intrinsic muscles of the larynx and sensory fibers to the mucosa below the vocal cords.
5. The **cardiac (superior and inferior cervical cardiac rami and thoracic) branches** enter the cardiac plexus on the wall of the heart with cardiac nerves from the sympathetic trunks. They terminate in the ganglia of the plexus near the sinoatrial and atrioventricular nodes.
6. The **pericardial, bronchial, esophageal, and other branches** divide to enter the pulmonary, celiac, superior mesenteric, and other plexuses to the thoracic and abdominal viscera.

Cranial Accessory Nerve (XI)

The cranial accessory nerve joins the vagus nerve and contributes to the laryngeal branches of that nerve, particularly the recurrent laryngeal. Additional fibers from a separate (external) part of the nucleus ambiguus follow vagal branches to and innervate the heart.

Reflexes of the Vagal System

Salivary-Taste Reflex

The salivary-taste reflex illustrates the secretory function of the vagal system. Placing a gustatory stimulus such as a drop of lemon juice on the tongue causes the salivary glands to increase their output of saliva. Taste fibers in the facial and glossopharyngeal nerves carry the afferent stimulus to the nucleus of the solitary tract. Connecting fibers from this nucleus project through interneurons in the adjacent reticular formation to parasympathetic neurons in the superior and inferior salivatory nuclei. Parasympathetic preganglionic neurons in the superior salivatory nuclei pass through the facial nerve to the submandibular ganglion, where a synapse occurs, and postganglionic fibers connect with the submandibular and sublingual salivary glands. Parasympathetic preganglionic neurons in the inferior salivatory nuclei project through the glossopharyngeal nerve to the otic ganglion, where a synapse occurs, and postganglionic fibers innervate the parotid salivary glands.

Carotid Sinus Reflex

Increased blood pressure stimulates special **baroreceptors** in the wall of the **carotid sinus** and sends impulses over afferent fibers of the glossopharyngeal nerve to the nucleus of the solitary tract. Second-order neurons in this nucleus project through reticular formation interneurons to the dorsal motor nucleus of nerve X and the external subnucleus of the nucleus ambiguus. Parasympathetic fibers from these nuclei project through the vagus nerve to the sinoatrial and atrioventricular nodes, as well as to the atrial muscle itself. Activating this reflex reduces the heart rate. Simultaneously, stimulation of neurons in the rostral ventrolateral medulla activates a pathway that descends to sympathetic neurons of the spinal cord, dilates peripheral blood vessels, and thereby further reduces blood pressure. Some persons with hypersensitive carotid sinus reflexes develop syncope after light external pressure over the carotid sinus.

Carotid Body Reflex

The **carotid body** contains special chemoreceptors that respond to changes in the carbon dioxide and oxygen content of circulating blood. Activation of these chemoreceptors sends impulses through the glossopharyngeal nerve to the nucleus of the solitary tract. Fibers from the solitary nucleus then go to the **respiratory center of the medulla,** where they influence the respiratory rate. The respiratory center consists of diffusely arranged cells of the ventrolateral reticular formation with reticulospinal fibers descending to the lower motoneurons of the phrenic and intercostal nerves.

Propagation of nerve impulses over **reticulospinal fibers** from the respiratory center produces inspiration. As the lungs become inflated, stretch receptors in the walls of bronchioles discharge impulses that ascend to the medulla through the vagus nerve. Connecting neurons reach the respiratory center and, by inhibition, temporarily arrest the inspiratory phase of respiration. The respiratory center depends on impulses descending from the pons for maintenance of the rhythm. The activity of neurons in the respiratory center can be controlled voluntarily for acts such as singing and talking.

Cough Reflex

Coughing usually occurs as a response to irritation of the larynx, trachea, or bronchial tree, but at times it can be produced by stimulation of vagus nerve fibers in other locations, including the external auditory canal or the tympanic membrane. Afferent impulses reach the solitary nucleus and tract by way of the vagus nerve. Projections to the respiratory center bring about forced expiration. At the same time, fibers going to the nucleus ambiguus cause efferent impulses to the muscles of the larynx and pharynx for their participation in coughing.

Gag Reflex

Touching the posterior wall of the pharynx results in contraction of muscles in the soft palate and pharynx. Sensory fibers of the glossopharyngeal nerve provide the afferent arm of this reflex. After entering the solitary tract, these fibers connect through interneurons with the nucleus ambiguus, which sends efferent fibers through the vagus nerve to the striated muscles of the pharynx.

Vomiting Reflex

Forceful emptying of the stomach requires relaxation of the gastroesophageal sphincter and contraction of the muscles of the anterior abdominal wall, which expels the gastric contents. Simultaneous closure of the glottis prevents inspiration. The stimulus, which may arise in any part of the gut innervated by the vagus nerve, evokes impulses sent to the nucleus of the solitary tract by sensory fibers of the vagus nerve. From here, impulses project to the nucleus ambiguus to close the glottis and to neurons of the medullary reticular formation. Impulses in the reticular formation course through the reticulospinal pathways into the spinal cord and activate the appropriate lower motoneurons to induce contraction of diaphragm and abdominal muscles.

A general elevation of intracranial pressure can cause vomiting. This probably results from transmission of the increased pressure onto the floor of the fourth ventricle. Vomiting can also occur with localized pressure on the medulla from a pathologic process such as a local tumor or hemorrhage.

Initiation of vomiting has also been attributed to the **area postrema,** which lies immediately rostral to the obex, on the floor of the fourth ventricle. This area contains a chemoreceptor region with connections to the nucleus solitarius, through which it can elicit vomiting in response to drugs or other emetic agents in the cerebrospinal fluid.

Case Follow-up

The man described at the beginning of this chapter has paralysis of the right nerve XII, which causes atrophy of muscle fibers on the right side of the tongue. When he protrudes the tongue, it deviates to the right because the action of the left genioglossus muscle is unopposed. He was studied with magnetic resonance imaging, which demonstrated a tumor of the clivus (a portion of the skull base) that had trapped the right nerve XII branches. An operation was performed, and much of the tumor, which proved to be a chordoma, was removed. Postoperatively, the man had double vision on gaze to the right (surgically induced injury to the right nerve VI) and diminished sensation on the right side of the face (surgically induced injury to the right nerve V). Radiotherapy was given, and the patient has had no further growth of tumor in a follow-up period of 20 years.

12

Cranial Nerves of the Pons and Midbrain

Case Study

A 30-year-old man awakens one morning with a feeling of stiffness on the right side of his face. When he looks into a mirror, the entire side of his face seems flattened, with the normal folds of skin around the lips, nose, and forehead appearing ''ironed out.'' When he grimaces to look at his front teeth, the lower facial muscles on the left contract strongly, and those on the right hardly contract at all, pulling his lips forcefully to the left. He attempts to eat breakfast, but he finds that liquids drool from his lips on the right, and food collects on the right side of his mouth. He seeks medical care the same morning, and when he is seen by a neurologist several hours later, examination reveals marked weakness of the right facial muscles, including the brow, eye, lips, and chin. His right eye closes only partially, even with forceful attempts. Saliva drools slightly from the right side of his mouth. The right eye appears dry. In response to a light touch of the right cornea with a wisp of cotton, the left eyelid closes promptly, but the right eyelid does not close at all, even though the patient detects the touch. Hearing is intact in the right ear, but the patient notes that sounds seem excessively loud. The patient cannot taste a solution of salt in water on the right side of the tongue, but he can taste it on the left side.

Where is the lesion responsible for this patient's symptoms and findings? What could account for the lesion? Is treatment available for this? What is the prognosis?

In the first part of this chapter, the three cranial nerves that control the extraocular muscles are described together even though they are anatomically separated in the pons and the midbrain. Chapter 19 describes the reflexes and coordinated eye movements controlled by these nerves.

Abducens Nerve (VI)

Course of the Nerve

Arising from its nucleus beneath the fourth ventricle in the pons (Fig. 10–10), the **abducens nerve** supplies general somatic efferent fibers to the **lateral rectus** muscle of the eye. The nerve leaves the brain stem anteriorly at the junction of the medulla and pons and passes along the floor of the posterior fossa of the skull between two layers of dura mater. It then enters the **cavernous sinus,** passes through the sinus, and enters the orbit through the **superior orbital fissure.**

Consequences of Damage to the Nerve

The abducens nerve has the longest intracranial course of the cranial nerves and can be damaged in the brain stem or, more often, in its intracranial course. In addition, prolonged elevation of intracranial pressure from any cause may damage the nerve.

Complete loss of function of the nerve makes it impossible voluntarily to turn the eye outward beyond the midline. In addition, the unopposed pull of the medial rectus muscle causes the eye to turn inward (adduct), thereby producing an

internal strabismus. Strabismus, or **squint,** is an abnormality of eye position and movement in which the axes of the eyes are not parallel. When strabismus occurs from a nerve VI lesion, visual images do not fall on corresponding points of the left and right retinas, and as a result, the images cannot be fused properly. The result is **diplopia (double vision),** which worsens with attempts to gaze to the side of the lesion. The two images appear side by side; therefore; the disorder causes **horizontal diplopia.** Patients usually attempt to minimize the diplopia by rotating the head so the chin turns toward the side of the lesion. With bilateral abducens nerve paralysis, both eyes become turned inward, and neither eye can be moved in a lateral direction past the midposition.

Trochlear Nerve (IV)

Course of the Nerve

The nucleus of the **trochlear nerve** lies anterior to the periaqueductal gray area in the midbrain, in the region of the inferior colliculus (Fig. 10–12). The general somatic efferent fibers of the trochlear nerve travel caudally a short distance, then curve posteriorly around the central gray area. The fibers decussate in the anterior medullary velum and exit from the posterior surface of the tectum caudal to the inferior colliculus. The trochlear nerve is the only cranial nerve with fibers emerging from the posterior aspect of the brain stem. The nerve then passes around the outside of the brain stem to its ventral surface, courses through a sheath in the lateral wall of the cavernous sinus, and enters the orbit through the superior orbital fissure.

Consequences of Damage to the Nerve

The trochlear nerve innervates the superior oblique muscle on the side opposite to its nucleus of origin. The muscle depresses the eye, especially when it is adducted (turned medially). Thus, an isolated lesion of the trochlear nerve results in loss of downward ocular movement when the eye is turned toward the nose. Patients with an isolated trochlear nerve lesion complain of vertical diplopia, tilt the head to align the eyes, and thereby eliminate the diplopia. Lesions limited to the trochlear nerve occur only rarely.

Oculomotor Nerve (III)

Course of the Nerve

The nucleus of the **oculomotor nerve** lies anterior to the periaqueductal gray area in the midbrain, in the region of the superior colliculus (Fig. 10–13). The fibers course ventrally, and some penetrate the medial portions of the red nucleus and the cerebral peduncle. The nerve exits from the brain stem at the interpeduncular fossa, passes along the brain stem, courses through a sheath in the lateral wall of the cavernous sinus, and enters the orbit through the superior orbital fissure. Shortly after its exit from the brain stem, the nerve passes close to the **circle of Willis,** which is an anastomotic group of arteries at the base of the brain. An **aneurysm** (saccular dilatation) in one of the arteries in this region may compress the oculomotor nerve. Tumor or hemorrhage above the tentorium cerebelli may push the inferior margin of the temporal lobe under the edge of the tentorium and may exert pressure on the oculomotor nerve as it crosses the tentorium. Mass lesions in the cavernous sinus or superior orbital fissure may also compress the nerve.

The oculomotor nucleus provides general somatic efferent innervation to the **medial, superior,** and **inferior recti,** the **inferior oblique,** and the **levator palpebrae superioris** muscles. Each of these muscles receives nerve fibers from its own subgroup of neurons in the oculomotor nuclear complex. The medial rectus, inferior rectus, and inferior oblique muscles receive input only from neurons on the ipsilateral side of the brain stem. The superior rectus muscle receives innervation only from neurons on the contralateral side of the brain stem. The levator palpebrae muscles receive input from neurons on both sides of the brain stem. A special subgroup of general visceral efferent cells in this complex, forming the **Edinger-Westphal nucleus,** contributes **preganglionic parasympathetic fibers** to the **ciliary ganglion,** whose postganglionic fibers innervate the **ciliary muscle** for accommodation and the **sphincter muscle of the iris** for constriction of the pupil.

Consequences of Damage to the Nerve

Lesions of the oculomotor nerve cause ipsilateral lower motoneuron paralysis of the muscles supplied by the nerve resulting in several abnormalities.

1. The eye deviates outward (abduction), resulting in an **external strabismus,** because of the unopposed action of the lateral rectus muscle and the inability to turn the eye vertically or inward.
2. **Ptosis** or drooping of the upper eyelid with inability to raise the lid voluntarily appears because of loss of innervation to the striated fibers of the levator palpebrae muscle.
3. The pupil becomes dilated **(mydriasis)** because of the unopposed action of the radial muscle fibers of the iris, which are supplied by the sympathetic system.

The patient with a lesion of the oculomotor nerve complains of a drooping lid and double vision. Incomplete lesions produce partial effects. There may be some weakness of all functions, or one symptom may appear without the others (e.g., dilation of the pupil without paralysis of eye movements). Patients with diabetes mellitus are prone to develop vascular lesions of the oculomotor nerve with loss of all functions, except pupillary responses.

The pathways mediating conjugate ocular movement are described in Chapter 19.

Facial Nerve (VII)

Functional Components

The seventh cranial nerve, the **facial nerve,** consists of motor, sensory, and parasympathetic divisions. The motor division innervates the **muscles of facial expression** (mimetic muscles), platysma, stapedius, stylohyoid, and posterior belly of the digastric, which originate from the second pharyngeal arch. These motor fibers are thus considered special visceral efferent. The sensory and parasympathetic divisions are parts of the **nervus intermedius.** These components of the nerve convey parasympathetic secretory fibers to the salivary and lacrimal glands and to the mucous membranes of the oral and nasal cavities (general visceral efferent). They also convey taste sensation from the anterior two-thirds of the tongue (special visceral afferent) and general somatic sensation from the auricle and external auditory meatus. The course and distribution of the nervus intermedius are described in Chapter 11 as part of the vagal system.

Course and Distribution of the Nerve

The motor division arises from nerve cell bodies in the facial nucleus of the pontine tegmentum. The neuronal cell groups in this nucleus are subdivided according to the particular muscles that they innervate. The fibers emerging from these neurons pass dorsally, encircle the nucleus of the abducens nerve, and emerge at the lateral aspect of the caudal border of the pons in the angle formed by the junction of the cerebellum and the pons (i.e., the **cerebellopontine angle**). The nerve enters the **internal auditory canal** and then the **facial canal,** leaves the skull by way of the **stylomastoid foramen,** and courses through the substance of the parotid gland behind the ramus of the mandible. The fibers then divide into branches that fan out to the face and scalp. The fibers also supply the stapedius, the posterior belly of the digastric, and the stylohyoid muscles. The nervus intermedius courses together with the facial nerve from the brain stem to the internal auditory meatus and then into the facial canal. The fibers of the nervus intermedius leave the facial nerve during its course through the facial canal.

Consequences of Distal Lesions of the Nerve

Loss of function of the facial nerve from a lesion at the stylomastoid foramen causes total paralysis of the muscles of facial expression on that side. The muscles of the affected side of the face sag, and the normal lines around the lips, nose, and forehead appear "ironed out." When the patient attempts to smile, the corner of the mouth on the paralyzed side does not move, and saliva may ooze from between the lips on the paralyzed side. The cheek may puff out during expiration because of buccinator muscle paralysis. Although corneal sensation persists, the corneal reflex fails on the side of the lesion because the motor fibers to the orbicularis oculi do not function. The inability to close the eye on the side of the paralysis leads to irritation of the cornea and a predisposition to infection; thus, protective eyedrops must be used during the day, and a bandage must be worn over the eye. The facial nerve can lose function overnight without any known cause except for marked swelling with compression of the nerve in the distal part of the bony facial canal, a condition termed **Bell's palsy.** Fortunately, most patients with Bell's palsy recover spontaneously in 1 or 2 months.

Consequences of Proximal Lesions of the Nerve

Disorders that affect the facial nerve in the cerebellopontine angle, within the internal auditory canal, or in the proximal parts of the facial canal, may affect the facial nerve fibers to the stapedius muscle and the fibers of the nervus intermedius. Consequently, these disorders may cause three symptoms in addition to paralysis of facial muscles, as follows: (1) **hyperacusis** (increased sensitivity to sounds) results from paralysis of the stapedius muscle; (2) loss of taste sensation on the anterior two-thirds of the tongue ipsilaterally results from injury to the nervus intermedius; and (3) decreased secretion of tears and saliva occurs ipsilaterally because of damage to the nervus intermedius.

Effects of Damage to Corticobulbar Neurons that Control Facial Nerve Function

As described earlier, lower motoneuron or peripheral nerve lesions affecting the facial nerve usually cause paralysis of muscles in both the upper and lower parts of the ipsilateral face. In contrast, upper motoneuron lesions in the primary motor or primary sensory areas of cerebral cortex or in the course of the corticobulbar fibers cause weakness only of the muscles in the lower part of the face on the contralateral side. The muscles of the brow usually are spared. The brow appears unaffected relative to the lower face because the cerebral cortex provides a small but equal amount of direct bilateral input to the lower motoneurons that innervate the forehead muscles. In contrast, the cerebral cortex densely innervates the lower motoneurons projecting to the contralateral lower facial muscles but provides only modest input to these lower motoneurons ipsilaterally.

When paralysis results from injury to upper motoneurons rather than to the facial nerve itself or its nucleus, involuntary contraction of the muscles of facial expression frequently remains preserved. In response to an emotional stimulus, the muscles of the lower face contract symmetrically when the patient smiles or laughs spontaneously in response to something amusing. The reason for this is that the limbic system of the forebrain controls this and other related types of spontaneous, emotional behavior. The limbic system consists of a network of interrelated nuclei that includes areas of the prefrontal cortex, the limbic cortex, and the amygdala, with projections through locomotor nuclei in the brain stem and the periaqueductal gray to the reticular formation.

Trigeminal Nerve (V)

The fifth cranial nerve received the term **trigeminal** (Latin for triplet) **nerve** because it divides into three major peripheral nerves: **ophthalmic, maxillary,** and **mandibular.** A mixed nerve, the trigeminal includes a large motor root supplying the muscles of mastication and an even larger sensory root distributed to the face, mouth, nasal cavity, orbit, anterior half of the scalp, and dura mater. Sensory branches of the ophthalmic nerve innervate the skin of the forehead and nose, the branches of the maxillary nerve innervate the cheeks and upper lip, and the branches of the mandibular nerve innervate the lateral side of the face and lower jaw (see Fig. 6–1).

Motor Division

Innervation of the Muscles of Mastication and Signs of Denervation

Fibers from the **motor nucleus of nerve V** in the lateral tegmentum of the rostral pons (Fig. 10–11) enter the mandibular branch of the fifth nerve and innervate the **muscles of mastication** (i.e., temporalis, masseter, and medial and lateral pterygoid muscles). Fibers from this nucleus also innervate several other smaller muscles (tensor tympani, tensor veli palatini, mylohyoid, and anterior belly of the digastric muscles). These muscles arise embryologically from the first branchial arch; thus, by definition, the motor fibers innervating them are called **special visceral efferent fibers.** Peripheral lesions of this portion of the fifth nerve cause atrophy and weakness, which can be recognized by observing and feeling the size and tautness of the masseter muscles during clenching of the jaw. Fasciculations can be seen in the muscle fibers after denervation. The pterygoid muscles draw the mandible forward and toward the midline; hence, with denervation, the chin deviates in the direction of the paralyzed side when the jaw opens.

The motor nucleus of each side of the brain stem receives input from upper motoneurons originating in both the left and right motor areas of the cerebral cortex, and supranuclear lesions confined to one side have negligible clinical effects. The motor nucleus also receives monosynaptic inputs from the muscle spindle afferents in the muscles of mastication. These afferents arise from the cells of the mesencephalic nucleus of nerve V (Fig. 12–1). These cells form the afferent side of the reflex arc that mediates the jaw jerk. The **jaw jerk** is a stretch reflex obtained by placing the examiner's index finger over the middle of the patient's chin with the patient's

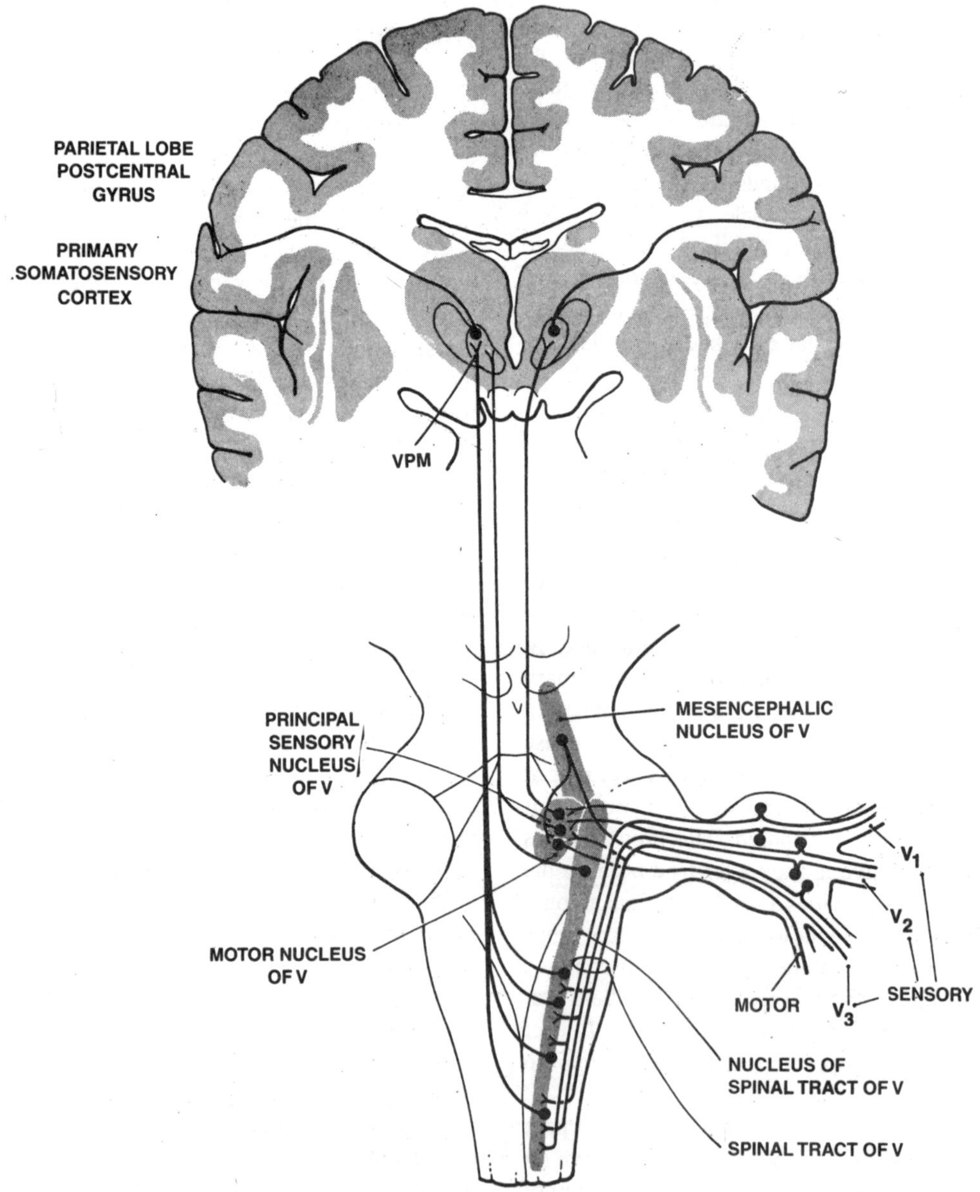

■ **FIGURE 12–1.** Dorsal view of the brain stem showing the connections of the afferent and efferent fibers of the trigeminal nerve. V_1 = ophthalmic nerve; V_2 = maxillary nerve; V_3 = mandibular nerve; VPM = ventral posteromedial nucleus of the thalamus.

mouth slightly open and tapping the finger gently with a reflex hammer. The normal response is a slight contraction of the masseter and temporalis muscles bilaterally, causing the jaw to close slightly. This response can become exaggerated by upper motoneuron lesions rostral to the level of the pons and decreased or absent with lesions that interrupt the reflex arc.

Sensory Division

Primary Sensory Cell Bodies Are in the Trigeminal Ganglion and the Mesencephalic Nucleus

The **trigeminal (semilunar, gasserian) ganglion** contains cell bodies of the afferent fibers of the fifth nerve, with the exception of the proprioceptive fibers from muscle spindles in muscles of the head. These proprioceptive fibers consist of peripheral processes of neuronal cell bodies in the **mesencephalic nucleus,** which is located in the dorsolateral part of the pontine tegmentum and the lateral periaqueductal gray area of the midbrain (see Figs. 10–11 and 12–1). Essentially displaced ganglion cells, the unipolar nerve cell bodies of this nucleus are unique in being located within the central nervous system. The cells of both the trigeminal ganglion and the mesencephalic nucleus of nerve V give rise to the general somatic afferent fibers of the nerve branches.

Trigeminal Nuclei Form the General Somatic Afferent Cell Column of the Brain Stem

The cells of the mesencephalic nucleus form the most rostral part of a general somatic afferent column of cells that stretches caudally to the spinal cord, where it becomes continuous with the substantia gelatinosa (Fig. 12–1). Incoming sensory fibers carrying different somatosensory modalities distribute their terminals to different parts of this cell column.

As described earlier, the most rostral nucleus, the **mesencephalic nucleus,** conveys muscle stretch information to neurons in the motor nucleus of nerve V. Trigeminal afferents from mechanoreceptors for tactile discrimination, joint position sense, and pressure sensation terminate in the **principal, or main, sensory nucleus** of nerve V.

Fibers of trigeminal ganglion cells mediating the sensations of pain, temperature, and light touch turn caudally after entering the pons. They form the **spinal tract of the trigeminal nerve,** which gives off terminal branches to the **nucleus of the spinal tract of nerve V** as it descends through the pons and medulla into the upper cervical segments of the spinal cord.

Trigeminal Pathways to the Cerebral Cortex

Fibers arising from cells of the nucleus of the spinal tract cross to the opposite side of the brain stem, form the **ventral trigeminothalamic tract,** and ascend with the spinothalamic tract through the pons and midbrain to the medial part of the **ventral posteromedial nucleus (VPM)** of the thalamus. In the medulla, the ventral trigeminothalamic tract fibers ascend as they cross; therefore, in the lower medulla, they course near the medial lemniscus, but they gradually shift laterally to join the spinothalamic tract. Thalamocortical fibers project from the VPM to the somatosensory cortex on the postcentral gyrus (see Figs. 12–1 and 6–3).

This system processes inputs from pain, thermal, and touch receptors in the skin throughout the distribution of the trigeminal nerve and from the small area of skin in the auricle innervated by general somatic afferents in cranial nerves VII, IX, and X. (See Chapter 11.) Branches of the fifth cranial nerve mediate pain sensation from the cornea, the mucous membranes of the oral and nasal cavities, the teeth, and the dura in the anterior part of the cranial cavity.

Trigeminal nerve fibers from mechanoreceptors for tactile discrimination project to the **principal sensory nucleus** (see Figs. 12–1 and 10–11) and to the rostral part of the nucleus of the spinal tract. These neurons are functionally similar to those of the gracile and cuneate nuclei, and, like these nuclei, the principal sensory nucleus and the rostral nucleus of the spinal tract send crossed fibers to accompany the contralateral medial lemniscus. These crossed fibers terminate in the VPM, but they project to neurons separate from those receiving projections from the intermediate and caudal parts of the spinal nucleus of nerve V. In addition, the dorsal portion of the principal sensory nucleus gives off a fascicle of uncrossed fibers that ascend to the ipsilateral VPM as part of the central tegmental tract. These fibers have been termed the **dorsal trigeminothalamic tract** (see Fig. 12–1). The term **trigeminal**

lemniscus has been applied to all the trigeminothalamic fibers, although they do not gather into a single distinct bundle.

Corneal Blink Reflex

When a foreign body touches the cornea of one eye, the **corneal blink reflex** evokes prompt closure of both the ipsilateral and the contralateral eyelids. Sensory fibers entering the upper part of the spinal tract of nerve V synapse with cells of the nucleus of the spinal tract, which send axons to the nucleus of the facial nerve. Motor fibers of the facial nerve then activate the orbicularis oculi muscle to close the eye on the side that had been touched. Interneurons in the nucleus of the spinal tract project to the facial nucleus of the opposite side, where they synapse on motoneurons that close the eye on that side as well. The response on the side stimulated is termed the **direct corneal reflex;** the response in the contralateral eye is termed the **consensual corneal reflex.** Interrupting the trigeminal nerve on one side abolishes both the direct response and the consensual response to stimulation of the ipsilateral cornea. With a disorder affecting the facial nerve on one side, however, touching the ipsilateral cornea does not evoke a direct response but does evoke a consensual response. Touching the cornea also activates reflex connections with autonomic neurons in the superior salivatory nucleus to increase lacrimation. These reflex pathways are not illustrated in Figure 12–1.

In clinical examinations, the examiner tests the corneal blink reflex by touching the cornea with a wisp of cotton and observing orbicularis oculi closure. This method assists in evaluating the integrity of both the fifth and the seventh cranial nerves.

Consequences of Damage to the Trigeminal System

Lesions in the lateral part of the medulla or lower pons that damage the spinal tract of nerve V frequently include the spinothalamic tract as well. This damage causes loss of pain and temperature sense on the same side of the face as the lesion and loss of pain and temperature sense on the opposite side of the body beginning at the neck. In the upper pons and midbrain, the fibers mediating pain, temperature, touch, joint position sense, and vibration sense have crossed and ascend in close proximity. Consequently, in these regions, one lesion can cause anesthesia of the entire opposite side of the body, including the face.

Tic douloureux, or **trigeminal neuralgia,** is a disorder characterized by attacks of unbearably severe pain lasting only for seconds over the distribution of one or more branches of the trigeminal nerve. A small **trigger zone** may be present, and its stimulation by light touch, temperature changes, or facial movement may set off a painful paroxysm. The cause of the disorder is unknown, but some investigators attribute it to compression of the trigeminal nerve by a small artery. Separation of the artery from the nerve, which requires a major neurosurgical operation, can relieve the symptoms. Nevertheless, medical therapy relieves the symptoms in most patients.

Case Follow-up

The patient described at the beginning of this chapter developed a peripheral seventh nerve palsy on the right that resulted in severe weakness of the superficial facial muscles on the right. He also had paralysis of the stapedius muscle causing hyperacusis and paresis of the nervus intermedius fibers resulting in loss of taste sensation on the anterior portion of the tongue and decreased secretion of tears on the right. The site affected was in the proximal portion of the facial nerve, as indicated by the involvement of the nerve to the stapedius muscle and the nervus intermedius. Owing to the proximal location of the lesion, he was thoroughly investigated to determine whether he had a tumor, aneurysm, or infection affecting the nerve, but no abnormality was found. The diagnosis was Bell's palsy. He was treated with artificial tears and was provided with a patch over the right eye to protect the cornea. The patient's sense of taste improved about 3 weeks after the onset of this disorder, and the facial weakness resolved completely over the next 4 weeks.

13

Lesions of the Brain Stem

Case Study

A 59-year-old man experiences the sudden onset of light-headedness without vertigo, along with mild weakness of the left arm and leg. He calls 911, and an ambulance arrives within 20 minutes. En route to hospital, his left limbs become completely paralyzed, and he develops double vision. He has hypertension (high blood pressure), type 2 insulin-dependent diabetes mellitus, hypercholesterolemia, and a previous history of myocardial infarction. On examination in the emergency room, his general physical examination reveals a blood pressure of 150/90 mm Hg and a pulse rate of 80 beats per minute. Apart from obesity, the examination is normal. On neurologic examination, he is alert and cooperative. He cannot voluntarily move the left lower face, arm, or leg. His right eyelid is closed, and lifting the eyelid reveals that the right eye deviates outward. He can voluntarily move the right eye fully to the right, but when he attempts to move his eyes to the left, the right eye moves only to the midline. He cannot move the right eye upward or downward. The right pupil is 7 mm in diameter and is poorly reactive to light, and the left pupil is 3 mm in diameter and is briskly reactive to light applied to either the left eye or the right eye. Movements of the left eye are full.

Where is the lesion responsible for these findings? What kind of pathologic process is responsible? Is treatment available?

Principles of Localization

The brain stem contains a compact arrangement of diverse structures; hence even a small single lesion commonly damages several of them simultaneously. Brain stem lesions frequently injure the afferent or efferent components of the cranial nerve nuclei, most of which innervate structures on the ipsilateral side of the body. These lesions also frequently injure the long descending motor and long ascending sensory pathways, both of which innervate structures on the contralateral side of the body. Consequently, a unilateral lesion of the brain stem often causes loss of function of one or more cranial nerves on the ipsilateral side and hemiplegia with hemisensory loss on the contralateral side. Thus, the **lesion is usually on the same side** of the brain stem as the cranial nerve abnormality.

The **rostrocaudal level of the lesion,** whether in the mesencephalon, pons, or medulla, frequently can be determined by the cranial nerve affected. For example, mesencephalic lesions affect cranial nerve III, pontine disorders involve cranial nerve V, and medullary lesions affect cranial nerve XII.

The **mediolateral position of the disease process** within the brain stem can be determined with knowledge of the positions of the long tracts. The corticospinal tract and medial lemniscus remain in relatively consistent positions in the pons and medulla, close to the midline and the base. Thus, unilateral medial lesions of these regions of the brain stem cause contralateral hemiparesis and loss of position and vibratory sensation. In contrast, unilateral lateral lesions spare these structures but affect the spinothalamic tract and cerebellar connections. Thus, lateral lesions cause contralateral loss of pain and temperature sense and ipsilateral limb ataxia without paralysis. The loss of one sensory modality (e.g., pain and temperature with preservation of the others from disease affecting the spinothalamic tract) can occur with discrete medullary or pontine lesions **(dissociated sensory loss).**

In addition to cranial nerves and long pathways, the brain stem contains the **reticular formation,** which includes autonomic components important in controlling respiration, blood pressure, and gastrointestinal functions. The reticular formation also participates in arousal, wakefulness, and sleep. Large brain stem lesions that affect the reticular formation bilaterally can cause coma or even sudden death. Ischemic or hemorrhagic strokes and severe craniocerebral trauma are the leading causes of these extensive brain stem lesions.

Brain stem lesions result from diverse types of pathologic processes, including hemorrhage, vascular occlusion, tumor, and multiple sclerosis. With hemorrhage or vascular occlusion, the territories served by individual branches of the vertebral and basilar arteries may be involved. These territories are illustrated in Figure 10–14. Many of the clinical disorders associated with specific brain stem lesions have been given eponyms, but because there is considerable lack of uniformity in their usage, only the more familiar ones are presented here.

Lesions of the Medulla

Medial Sector

Several of the individual cranial nerves pass close to the pyramidal tract before they emerge from the brain stem. A single lesion that includes the nerve and the tract at this point causes loss of function of the cranial nerve on the side of the lesion and contralateral hemiplegia. For example, a lesion of the right hypoglossal nerve and the right pyramid results in paralysis of the muscles of the right half of the tongue and in left hemiplegia (Fig. 13–1, lesion 1). The paralysis of

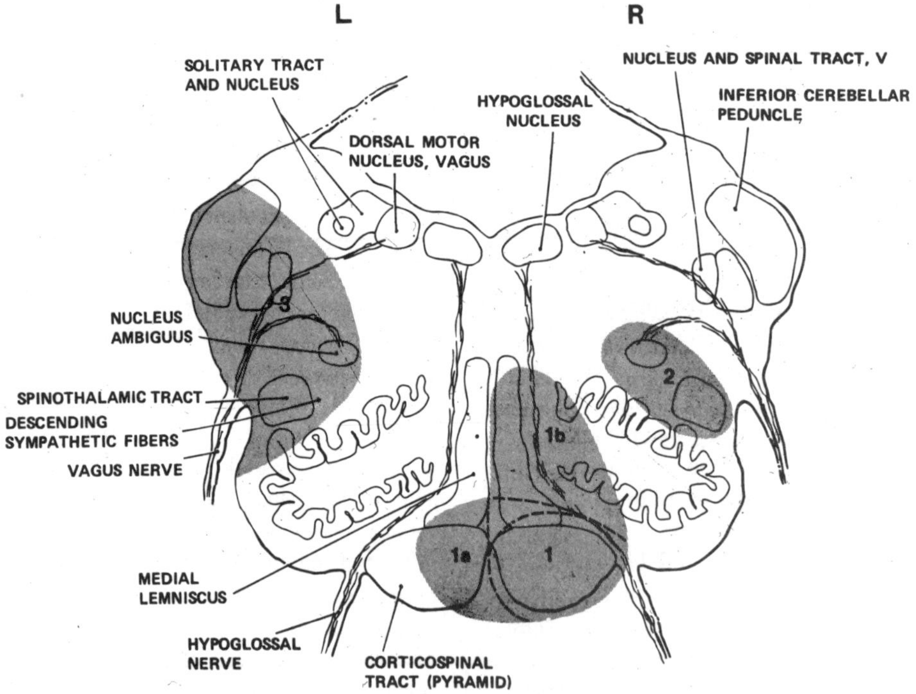

■ **FIGURE 13–1.** A cross section of the medulla. The *shaded areas* indicate the positions of lesions. (Some of the lesions shown in this diagram occur only rarely in actual practice and are presented here for illustrative purposes). **(1)** A lesion affecting the right hypoglossal nerve and right pyramid. **(1a)** An extension of the lesion involving the pyramida tract on the left. **(1b)** An extension of the lesion involving the medial lemniscus on the right. **(2)** A lesion of the nucleus ambiguus and spinothalamic tract. **(3)** A lesion affecting the dorsolateral portion of the medulla and involving the inferior cerebellar peduncle, the spinal tract and nucleus of the trigeminal nerve, the spinothalamic tract, the nucleus ambiguus, the vestibular nuclei (not shown), the descending sympathetic pathways, and the emerging fibers of the vagus nerve. Compare with Figure 10–9.

the arm and leg affects the side opposite the lesion because the pyramidal tract crosses to the left after it has passed caudal to the site of the lesion, at the junction of the medulla and the cervical spinal cord. The muscles of the face are not involved because the lesion affects the brain stem caudal to the connections of the corticobulbar fibers with the facial nerve nucleus. When a lesion occurs acutely, as with vascular occlusion, the arm and leg show hypotonic paresis or paralysis, with weakness, diminished resistance to passive manipulation, decreased deep tendon reflexes, loss of superficial reflexes, and absence of the response to plantar stimulation. Within 4 to 8 weeks after an acute lesion, or with a pre-existing chronic lesion, the arm and leg develop a spastic paralysis, with weakness, "clasp-knife" resistance to passive manipulation, hyperreflexia, loss of superficial reflexes, and an extensor plantar (Babinski) response. The tongue deviates to the right side when protruded, and the right half of the tongue becomes progressively atrophic.

Extension of this lesion across the midline damages the left pyramid and causes right hemiplegia (Fig. 13–1, lesion 1a). In some patients, disease of the anterior spinal artery, which provides the vascular supply to this area of the medulla, results in recurring symptoms with recovery of function between attacks (see Fig. 10–14). If lesions 1 and 1a in Figure 13–1 occur temporarily at different times, the result will be **alternating hemiplegia.** (Alternating hemiplegia also occurs with ischemia of the basal part of the pons.) If the same lesion expands dorsally, it will affect the right medial lemniscus and defects will occur in position sense, vibration sense, and tactile discrimination (Fig. 13–1, lesion 1b). Because the medial lemniscus crosses in the lower part of the medulla caudal to this level, the sensory disorders affect the opposite (left) side of the body.

Lateral Sector

A small lesion in the lateral part of the medullary reticular formation can include the nucleus ambiguus and the lateral spinothalamic tract simultaneously (Fig. 13–1, lesion 2). A lesion on the right side causes loss of pain and temperature sense on the left side of the body, except the face. The sensory loss affects the contralateral side because lateral spinothalamic tract fibers cross the midline near their origin. Destruction of the nucleus ambiguus paralyzes the voluntary muscles in the pharynx and larynx supplied by the right glossopharyngeal, vagus, and cranial accessory nerves. Failure of the right side of the soft palate to contract causes difficulty in swallowing, and, on phonation, the palate and uvula become drawn to the nonparalyzed left side. Loss of function of the right vocal cord results in dysphonia, with hoarseness of the voice.

Dorsolateral Sector of the Upper Medulla (Wallenberg's Syndrome)

The posterior inferior cerebellar artery, a branch of the vertebral artery, supplies the dorsolateral portion of the medulla and the inferior surface of the cerebellar vermis (see Fig. 10–14). Dysfunction in the dorsolateral sector of the upper medulla usually results from occlusion of the vertebral artery leading to thrombosis of small penetrating branches or the **posterior inferior cerebellar artery (Wallenberg's syndrome).** Medullary injury from occlusion of the penetrating branches can occur without cerebellar involvement, or cerebellar injury from occlusion of the posterior inferior cerebellar artery can occur without medullary involvement. Thus, the clinical findings of vertebral artery occlusion vary considerably. **Atherosclerosis** (thickening of the arterial walls with deposits of fatty tissue) or **dissection from injury** (diversion of blood through the inner lining of the artery) of the vertebral artery are the most common causes. The damage in the medulla involves the inferior cerebellar peduncle, spinal tract and nucleus of the trigeminal nerve, spinothalamic tract, nucleus ambiguus, descending sympathetic pathways, and emerging fibers of the vagus nerve (Fig. 13–1, lesion 3). These lesions often affect the vestibular nuclei as well. Loss of function of the spinocerebellar fibers in the inferior cerebellar peduncle results in cerebellar ataxia and hypotonia (i.e., diminished resistance to passive manipulation) of the limbs ipsilateral to the lesion.

Injury to the spinal tract of the trigeminal nerve causes loss of pain and temperature sensation on the face ipsilaterally and loss of the blink reflex after ipsilateral corneal stimulation. In contrast, damage to the lateral spinothalamic tract leads to loss of pain and temperature sensation in the limbs and trunk contralateral to the lesion. Damage to the vestibular nuclei causes nystagmus. Injury to the descending sympathetic pathways produces ipsilateral Horner's syndrome, with pupillary constriction, ptosis (i.e., partial closure of the upper eyelid), enophthalmos, and loss of sweating in the ipsilateral half of the face. Loss of function of the nucleus ambiguus or the peripheral fibers in cranial nerves IX, X, and XI results in ipsilateral paralysis of the soft palate, pharynx, and larynx, with dysphagia (i.e., difficulty swallowing) and dysphonia.

Lesions of the Pons

Medial Sector of the Caudal Part

A lesion that includes the emerging fibers of the right abducens nerve and the right corticospinal tract causes ipsilateral abducens palsy and contralateral hemiplegia (Fig. 13–2, lesion 1). The abducens palsy leads to internal deviation of the right eye from paralysis of the lateral rectus and the unopposed pull of the medial rectus muscle. Immediately after the lesion, the hemiplegic limbs become hypotonic, with diminished resistance to passive manipulation, decreased deep tendon reflexes, and a flexor or equivocal response to plantar stimulation. In the patient with a chronic lesion, the hemiplegic limbs become hypertonic, with spasticity, hyperreflexia, and an extensor plantar response.

Lesions of this part of the brain stem often extend far enough laterally to include fibers of the facial nerve and thereby to produce a peripheral type of facial paralysis. When unilateral loss of function of the abducens and facial nerves ac-

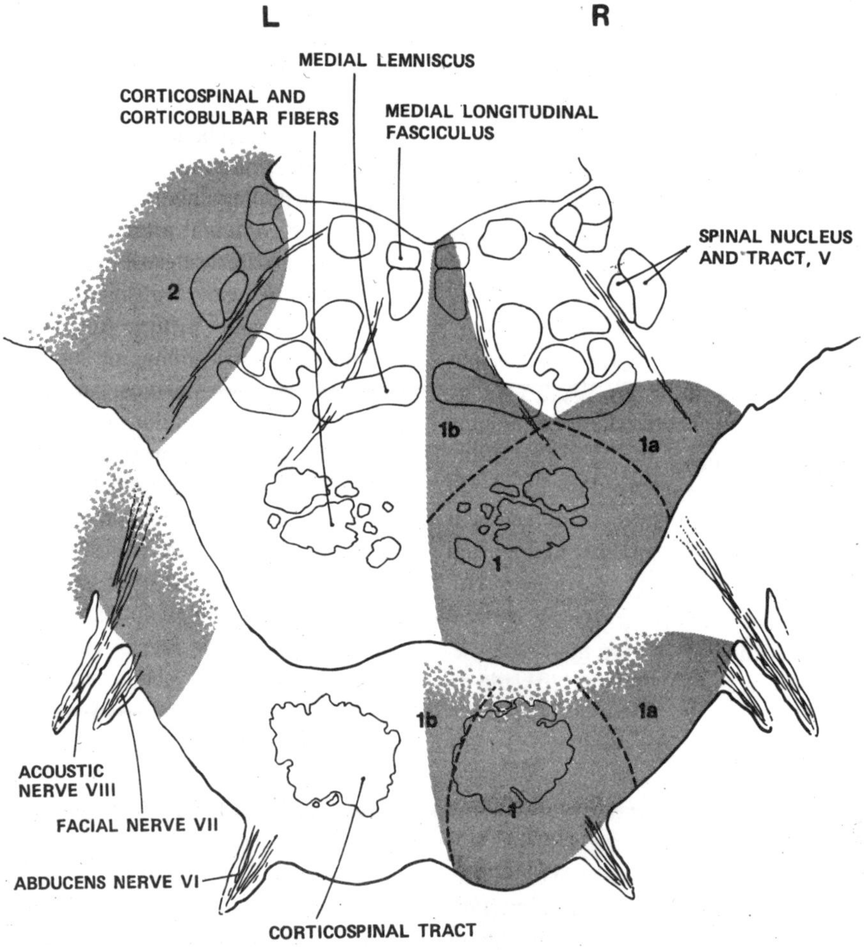

■ **FIGURE 13–2.** A cross section of the caudal portion of the pons. The *shaded areas* indicate the positions of lesions. **(1)** A lesion of the right corticospinal tract and the emerging fibers of the right abducens nerve. **(1a)** An extension of the lesion to include the facial nerve. **(1b)** An extension of this lesion into the pontine tegmentum that involves the right medial lemniscus and the right medial longitudinal fasciculus. **(2)** The region affected by a cerebellopontine angle tumor. For unidentified structures, see Figure 10–10.

companies contralateral hemiplegia, the condition is called the **Millard-Gubler syndrome** (Fig. 13–2, lesion 1a).

A medial pontine lesion with dorsal expansion into the pontine tegmentum involves the right medial lemniscus, the paramedian pontine reticular formation, and the medial longitudinal fasciculus (Fig. 13–2, lesion 1b). Interrupting fibers of the right medial lemniscus causes loss of position sense, vibration sense, and tactile discrimination on the left side of the body. Damage to the neurons responsible for conjugate lateral gaze in the right paramedian pontine reticular formation abolishes the ability to turn the eyes voluntarily to the right and results in paralysis of right lateral gaze. The eyes often become tonically drawn to the left by the predominating influence of the unaffected (left) side of the paramedian pontine reticular formation, but such an effect is temporary. Pathways controlling eye movements are described in Chapter 19. The combination of symptoms produced by this lesion is known as **Foville's syndrome.**

Damage to the medial longitudinal fasciculus bilaterally produces **internuclear ophthalmoplegia,** a disorder commonly found in multiple sclerosis. With attempted gaze to one side, the adducting eye (i.e., the eye moving toward the nose) fails to move beyond the midline, whereas the abducting eye (i.e., the eye moving away from the nose) moves fully outward but develops coarse nystagmus. Gaze to the opposite side evokes the same findings. Despite loss of adduction on attempted lateral gaze, convergence often remains intact. Damage to the medial longitudinal fasciculus unilaterally causes loss of adduction of the eye on the side of the lesion and nystagmus of the contralateral (abducting) eye. The eye that fails to adduct with gaze to one side can adduct with convergence, a finding demonstrating that the loss of adduction results from a supranuclear abnormality (i.e., an abnormality of neural structures at a higher level than the lower motoneuron nuclei). Unilateral internuclear ophthalmoplegia occurs usually with vascular disease of the brain stem, but it can also result from multiple sclerosis or, rarely, a tumor (glioma).

Lesions of the dorsolateral pons impair the function of the ipsilateral fifth and seventh nerves and evoke nystagmus and limb ataxia. Loss of pain and temperature sensation on the opposite side of the body occurs with inclusion of the spinothalamic tract in the lesion. Lesions in this location usually result from **occlusion of the anterior inferior cerebellar artery.** Deafness on the same side can result from secondary thrombosis of the internal auditory artery, which branches off the anterior inferior cerebellar artery.

Cerebellopontine Angle

Acoustic neuromas are slowly growing tumors that arise from Schwann cells in the sheath of nerve VIII close to the brain stem. As they expand in size, the tumor exerts pressure on the lateral region of the caudal part of the pons near the cerebellopontine angle (Fig. 13–2, lesion 2). The initial symptom consists of progressive unilateral deafness, which results from increasing damage to the eighth nerve, thereby interfering with nerve condition. Clinical testing at an early stage reveals decreased hearing on the side of the tumor, spontaneous horizontal nystagmus, and absent responses to natural labyrinthine (vestibular) stimulation on the affected side. Spontaneous horizontal nystagmus results from imbalanced input to the central nervous system from the vestibular apparatus on each side of the head. Natural labyrinthine stimulation can be evoked by caloric or rotational stimuli. In the normal subject, irrigating the external auditory canal with cold or warm water evokes nystagmus, a finding indicating intact labyrinthine function. Rotation of the patient in a special chair can also be used to evoke nystagmus. Damage to nerve VIII from an acoustic neuroma prevents nystagmus from appearing with these types of natural stimulation. Later in the course of the disease, cerebellar ataxia appears on the side of the lesion because of compression of the cerebellar peduncles. If the tumor becomes extremely large, damage to the spinal tract and nucleus of nerve V can occur, thus abolishing the corneal reflex and causing diminished pain and temperature sensibility in the face on the side of the lesion. A peripheral type of facial paralysis, also affecting the side of the lesion, can result from damage to the fibers of nerve VII. If they are detected in time, acoustic neuromas and other cerebellopontine angle tumors such as meningiomas usually can be removed surgically, and neurologic function can be fully restored.

Middle Region

A large lesion in the basal part of the right side of the middle pons can affect the right corticospinal tract and the emerging fibers of the right trigem-

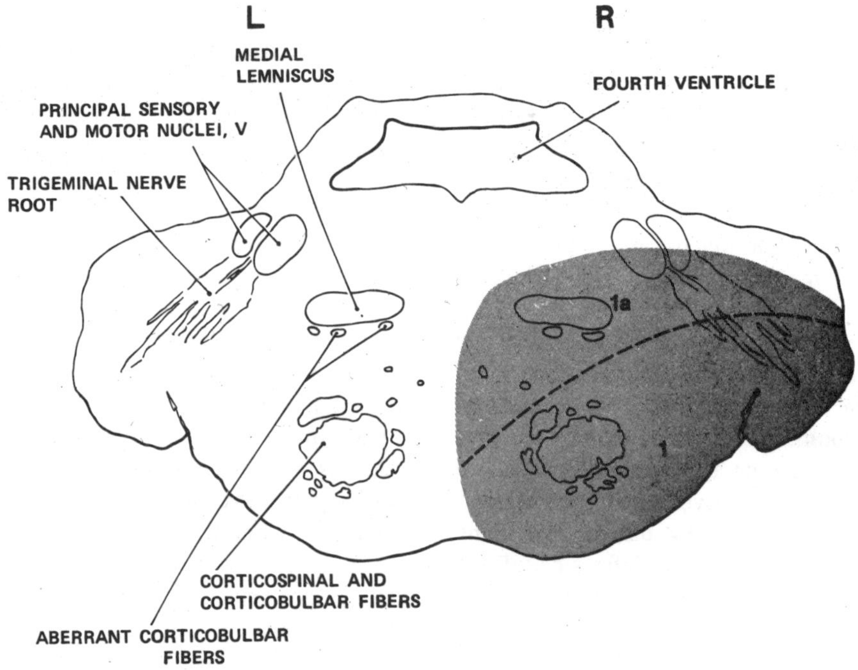

■ **FIGURE 13-3.** A cross section of the middle region of the pons. The *shaded areas* indicate the positions of the lesions. **(1)** A lesion affecting the right corticospinal tract and the emerging fibers of the right trigeminal nerve. **(1a)** An extension of this lesion involves the medial lemniscus and the aberrant corticobulbar tract. Compare with Figure 10–11.

inal nerve to produce ipsilateral fifth nerve palsy and contralateral hemiplegia (Fig. 13–3, lesion 1). Involvement of the motor fibers of nerve V leads to paralysis of the muscles of the right side of the jaw and causes the jaw to deviate to the right with opening of the mouth. Damage to the sensory fibers of nerve V causes anesthesia of the right side of the face and mouth, with loss of the corneal reflex when the right eye is stimulated. In the patient with an acute lesion, the hemiplegic limbs are hypotonic, and with chronic lesions, the limbs become hypertonic with hyperreflexia and an extensor plantar response.

A lesion in the same region that extends farther dorsally enters the pontine tegmentum and destroys the medial lemniscus. This results in losses of position sense, vibration sense, and tactile discrimination on the left side of the body. Extension of the lesion to the spinothalamic tract causes loss of pain and temperature on the contralateral side of the body. A lesion in this location also interrupts the few aberrant **uncrossed** fibers of the corticobulbar and corticotectal tracts that have separated from the corticospinal tracts and in this region lie near the medial lemniscus (Fig. 13–3, lesion 1a). In addition to the left limbs, the superficial muscles of the lower part of the left side of the face become paretic. Lesions of the middle part of the pons also destroy the tectal projections to the paramedian pontine reticular formation before they cross and thus interrupt the pathway from the right frontal lobe that produces voluntary turning of the eyes to the left. This results in paralysis of left lateral gaze and deviation of the eyes tonically to the right. Direct injury of the paramedian pontine reticular formation causes paralysis of conjugate ocular deviation to the side of the lesion and tonic deviation of the eyes to the opposite side. When hemiplegia accompanies these symptoms, the affected limbs are on the side opposite the lesion. Thus, the patient "looks toward the hemiplegia."

Lesions of the Midbrain

Medial Basal Part (Weber's Syndrome)

A lesion of the right crus cerebri, or cerebral peduncle, and of the right oculomotor nerve usually produces left hemiplegia with involvement of the face, arm, and leg combined with complete ptosis and external strabismus of the right eye. The external strabismus results from the unopposed action of nerve VI, and eye closure (i.e., ptosis) on the right results from paralysis of the levator palpebrae muscle. Additional findings include loss of the ability to raise the right upper eyelid, dilatation of the right pupil, loss of adduction of the eye beyond the midline, and loss of upward and downward movement of the eye (Fig. 13–4, lesion 1). The right pupil becomes dilated because of interruption of the parasympathetic fibers in nerve III. The combination of unilateral oculomotor palsy and contralateral hemiplegia is termed **Weber's syndrome.** In some cases, the corticobulbar tract may not be affected because many of its fibers diverge from the corticospinal tract at this level and shift to a more dorsal position as they continue downward. If the lesion extends dorsally, however, it may include most of these fibers and may cause weakness of the face. Weber's syndrome usually results from **vascular occlusion** or an **aneurysm** (an abnormally dilated portion) of the basilar artery.

Tegmentum (Benedikt's Syndrome)

A lesion of the tegmentum of the midbrain affects the fibers of the oculomotor nerve, medial lemniscus, red nucleus, and fibers of the superior cerebellar peduncle, which pass around the red nucleus in this area (Fig. 13–4, lesion 2). A lesion on the left side causes loss of function of the left oculomotor nerve and results in paralysis of movement of the left eye with ptosis and pupillary dilatation. Tonically abducted, the eye can be adducted only to the midposition, and it cannot move in the vertical direction. Because the left medial lemniscus and trigemionthalamic fibers have joined the left spinothalamic tract at this level, the right side of the body, including the face, loses tactile, muscle, joint, vibratory, pain, and temperature sensation from injury to the ascending sensory tracts. Involvement of the red nucleus and the superior cerebellar peduncle,

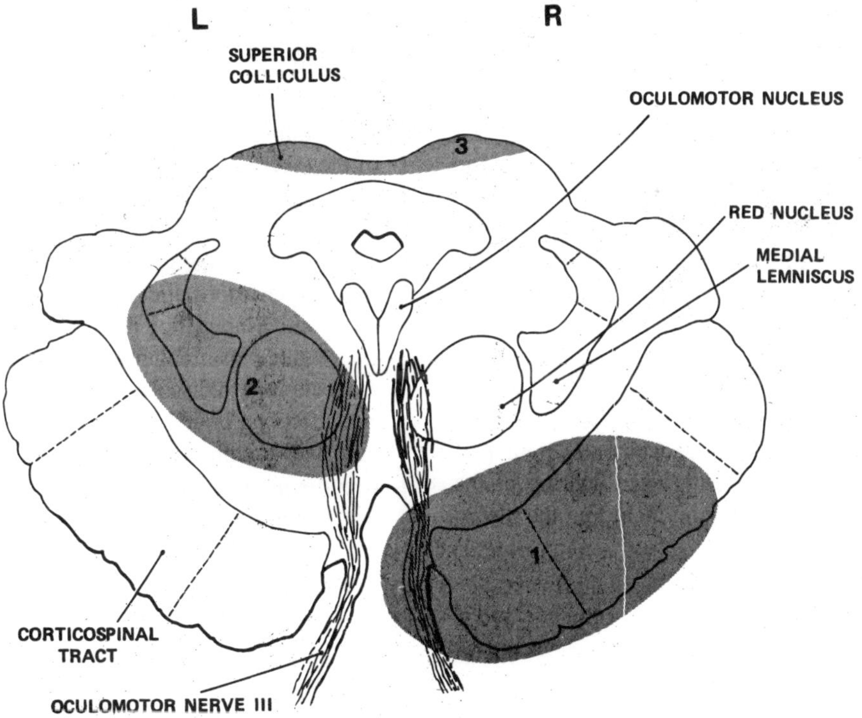

■ **FIGURE 13–4.** A cross section of the midbrain. The *shaded areas* indicate the positions of lesions. **(1)** A lesion of the right crus cerebri, or cerebral peduncle, and the oculomotor nerve. Dorsal extension of this lesion will involve the aberrant corticobulbar pathway. **(2)** A lesion of the tegmentum of the midbrain that affects the oculomotor nerve, the medial lemniscus, the red nucleus, and fibers of the superior cerebellar peduncle. **(3)** A lesion involving the superior colliculi. Compare with Figure 10–13.

which contains efferent fibers from the right cerebellar hemisphere, produces ataxia and involuntary (choreic) movements of the right arm and leg. The corticobulbar and corticospinal tracts remain unaffected; hence hemiplegia does not occur. The combination of third nerve palsy with contralateral loss of sensation, ataxia, and involuntary movements is termed **Benedikt's syndrome.**

Mesencephalic Tectum (Parinaud's Syndrome)

Injury in the vicinity of the superior colliculi (Fig. 13–4, lesion 3) causes paralysis of conjugate upward gaze, a disorder termed **Parinaud's syndrome.** The loss of upward gaze may be accompanied by pupillary abnormalities. The pupils may be fixed and unreactive to any stimulus, or they may react to near fixation but not to light. Paralysis of convergence can occur as well. This disorder often results from **tumors of the pineal gland** that compress the tectal and pretectal regions of the mesencephalon.

Brain Stem Lesions Causing Coma and "Locked-In" Syndrome

Bilateral lesions that damage substantial amounts of reticular formation in the upper pons and midbrain lead to **coma,** which is a state of unresponsiveness. Bilateral lesions of the ventral pons, usually caused by occlusion of the basilar artery, can completely interrupt the corticobulbar and corticospinal tracts. As a result, the patient becomes totally paralyzed and unable to speak but remains fully awake. Usually, the patient can open the eyelids and can make slight vertical eye movements. Retention of these movements results from sparing of the dorsal parts of the midbrain, including the rostral interstitial nucleus of the medial longitudinal fasciculus and its projections to the posterior commissure and the interstitial nucleus of Cajal. Communication can be established by asking the patient to move the eyes in response to a command. This establishes that the patient is completely immobile, or "locked in," but is not in a coma. The **locked-in syndrome** can also result from **central pontine myelinolysis,** a disorder seen in the late stages of chronic alcoholism and in several different severe chronic diseases. The disorder frequently occurs in such patients who come to emergency rooms with severe dehydration. Treatment with very rapid fluid and electrolyte replacement leads to central pontine myelinolysis.

Case Follow-up

The patient described at the beginning of this chapter had an ischemic infarction of the right crus cerebri, or cerebral peduncle, that damaged the descending corticobulbar fibers (weakness of the left lower face) and corticospinal fibers (weakness of the left arm and leg). The infarction also damaged the right nerve III (ptosis of the right eyelid with loss of the ability to elevate the lid, external strabismus of the right eye, loss of adduction of the eye beyond the midline, loss of upward and downward movement of the eye, and a dilated pupil). This constitutes Weber's syndrome. A computed tomography scan revealed no hemorrhage, and the patient was within the 3-hour time limit; hence treatment with tissue plasminogen activator was initiated in an attempt to dissolve the vascular occlusion affecting branches of the basilar artery. The attempt was successful in restoring strength in the left limbs and partial recovery of oculomotor function.

14

Hearing

Case Study

A 35-year-old woman gradually becomes aware of difficulty in hearing people who speak softly if they are on her right side. She also has a problem hearing on the telephone with the right ear and begins using her left ear instead. She consults her physician, who finds on examination that she cannot hear a softly whispered voice or the ticking of a watch with the right ear but can hear them with the left. The physician then places the base of a vibrating 256-Hz tuning fork on the middle of her forehead and asks whether the resulting sound seems louder in either ear. She hears the sound louder in the left than in the right ear. The physician then places the base of the vibrating tuning fork on her right mastoid process and asks her to indicate when the sound disappears, and at that point the physician asks whether she can still hear the vibrating tines when they are held in air close to her right ear. The physician performs the same maneuver with the left ear. On both sides, she can still hear the vibrating tuning fork in air after she can no longer hear it on bone. The physician then examines the eardrums, finds them to be intact, and irrigates each external auditory canal with cold water in succession. Nystagmus results from irrigating the left canal, not the right. From these findings, the physician formulates a localization and diagnosis and requests an imaging study.

What can be concluded from the test results? Can you localize the lesion responsible for this woman's symptoms? Can you develop a diagnosis? What imaging study would you request?

Ear

The eighth cranial nerve contains two divisions: vestibular and cochlear. Both consist of special somatic afferent systems, but each has such distinctive functions and anatomic relations that they can be considered separate cranial nerves. The vestibular division is discussed in Chapter 15.

Sound consists of sinusoidal waves—alternating condensations and rarefactions—of air molecules. The frequency of the waves, measured in **hertz (Hz),** determines the **pitch** of the sound. The amplitude of each wave, measured in **decibels (dB),** relates to the loudness of the sound. The human ear can detect sound frequencies from about 20 to 20,000 Hz and loudness from about 1 to 120 dB.

External Ear and Middle Ear

The auditory apparatus consists of three components: the external, middle, and inner ear. These components occupy three spaces in the skull, separated solely by membranes (Fig. 14–1A and B). The external ear, or auricle, leads to the **external auditory meatus,** which the **tympanic membrane** separates from the cavity of the middle ear. A chain of three ossicles—**malleus, incus,** and **stapes**—spans the middle ear (Fig. 14–1B). The first of the ossicles, the malleus, attaches to the tympanic membrane, and the last, the stapes, attaches to the **oval window** through a ligamentous membrane on its footplate. The **oval window** separates the air-filled middle ear cavity from the fluid-filled inner ear cavity.

Sound mediated by air strikes the tympanic membrane and induces motions in this membrane that the ossicles convey to the oval window. The

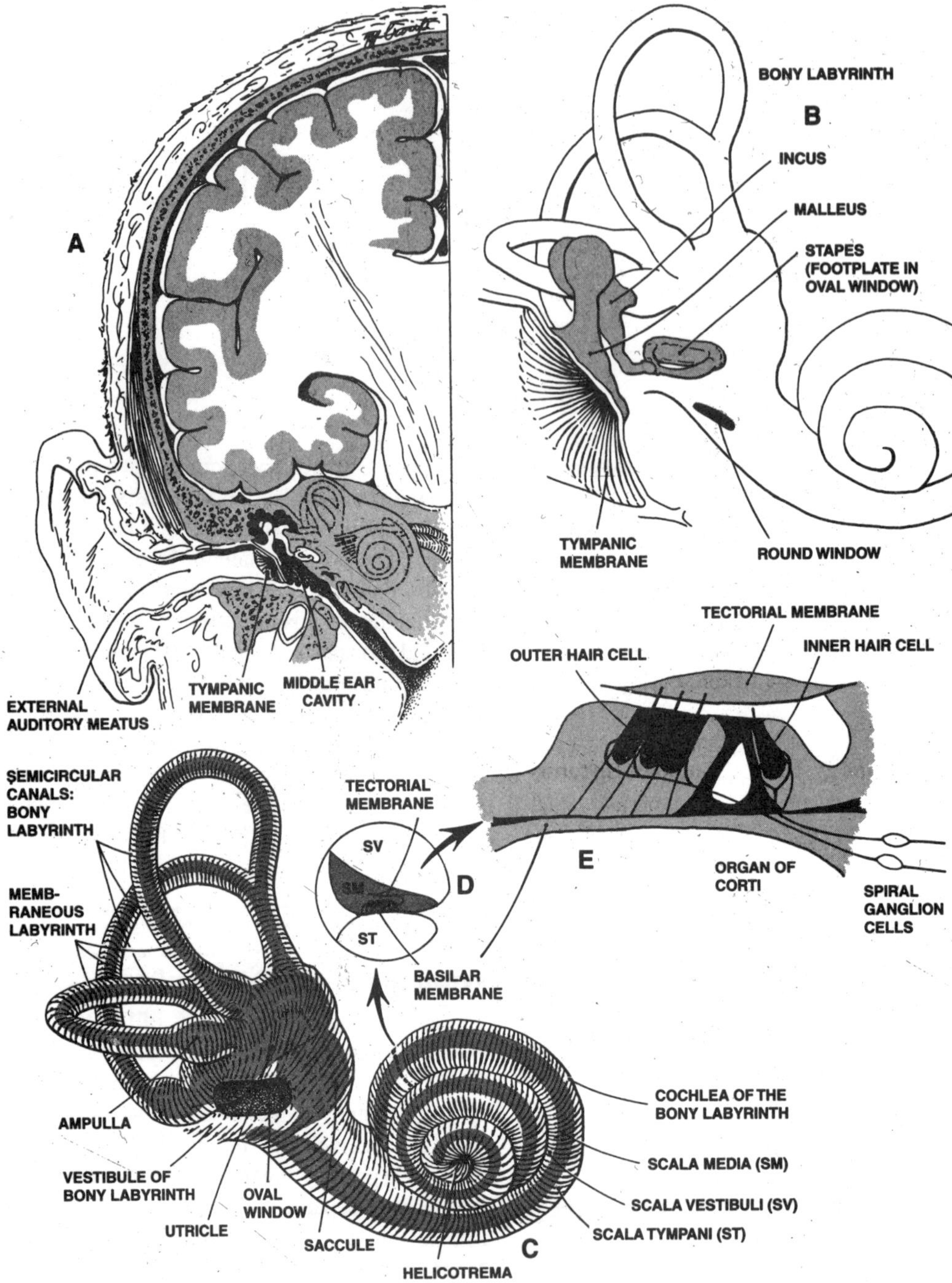

■ **FIGURE 14-1.** The ear. **(A)** The location of the three parts of the ear (external, middle, and inner) in relation to the skull and the brain. **(B)** The relationships among the eardrum (tympanic membrane) and the three bones (ossicles) in the middle ear that connect the eardrum to the inner ear. **(C)** The bony labyrinth and the membranous labyrinth within it (shown in *color*) form the inner ear. **(D)** A cross section through the bony and membranous labyrinths of the cochlea shows the location of the basilar membrane and tectorial membrane of the organ of Corti. **(E)** The organ of Corti rests on the basilar membrane. The stereocilia of the outer hair cells are embedded in the tectorial membrane; those of the inner hair cells (IHC) are not.

chain of three ossicles in the middle ear serves as an amplifier as well as an impedance-matching device that decreases the amount of energy lost by the sound waves in going from air to the fluid **(perilymph)** behind the oval window.

Inner Ear

The oval window provides an opening into the **vestibule** portion of the inner ear, which contains perilymph (Fig. 14–1C). The vestibule consists of a chamber that is continuous on one side with the **cochlea** and on the other side with the **semicircular canals.** The cochlea, a perilymph-containing tube, resembles a snail shell about 3.5 cm long wrapped around itself in 2.5 turns. The perilymph-containing semicircular canals are discussed further in Chapter 15. These three connected chambers within the temporal bone of the skull make up the **bony labyrinth.** A **membranous labyrinth** lies within the bony labyrinth and contains another fluid, the **endolymph.** The membranous labyrinth has a shape similar to that of the bony labyrinth, except in the vestibule.

Cochlea

In the cochlear part of the bony labyrinth, a conical central bony core, the **modiolus,** forms the axis of the cochlear turns. The **spiral lamina,** a ridge of bone turning around the modiolus, projects into the cochlear space. The spiral lamina partially divides the cochlear cavity into two perilymphatic chambers: the **scala vestibuli** and the **scala tympani.** The **scala media,** or **cochlear duct,** forms the membranous labyrinth within the cochlea. The cochlear duct stretches across the cochlea from the spiral lamina to the opposite wall of the cochlea and completes the separation of the scala vestibuli from the scala tympani. The **organ of Corti,** which contains sensory epithelium, or hair cells, forms a ribbon that stretches along the length of the cochlear duct and rests on the **basilar membrane** (Fig. 14–1D) as it spirals around the turns of the cochlea.

The piston action of the footplate of the stapes at the oval window produces an instantaneous pressure wave in the perilymph of the **scala vestibuli.** This pressure wave travels to the **helicotrema,** the apical connection between the scala vestibuli and scala tympani, within microseconds. The pressure wave in the perilymph of the scala vestibuli sets up a traveling wave on the basilar membrane. The basilar membrane is narrower at the base of the cochlea (near the vestibule) than at the apex (near the helicotrema). Hence the mechanical properties of the basilar membrane vary gradually from base to apex. As a result, the pressure wave produced by a sound of a specific frequency (i.e., pitch) causes the basilar membrane to vibrate maximally at a particular point along its length. This vibration maximally activates the hair cells of the organ of Corti located at that point.

Organ of Corti

The organ of Corti (Fig. 14–1E) contains two types of receptors: inner hair cells and outer hair cells. The **inner hair cells** function as auditory receptor cells. The base of each inner hair cell forms an indirect attachment to the basilar membrane. The apex of each cell bears **stereocilia,** which extend above the surface of the cell. The tips of the stereocilia lie just below the **tectorial membrane,** which forms an attachment to the wall of the cochlear duct separately from the attachment of the basilar membrane to the bony spiral lamina.

When sound waves enter the cochlea, the basilar and tectorial membranes move independently of each other, and the stereocilia touch the tectorial membrane and receive shearing forces. The resultant bending of the stereocilia opens ionic channels and causes changes of potential in the hair cell membrane. Synapses at the base of each hair cell activate the closely applied dendritic processes of the spiral ganglion cells. As many as 10 spiral ganglion cells innervate each inner hair cell, and each of these ganglion cells innervates only one inner hair cell. Thus, each inner hair cell can send information about its activity into the brain along 10 separate channels. These channels consist of the bipolar cells of the **spiral ganglion,** with cell bodies located within the modiolus of the cochlea and axons that form the cochlear division of the eighth nerve.

The **outer hair cells,** which contain **stereocilia** embedded in the tectorial membrane, possess contractile properties. This permits them to control the sensory response properties of the organ of Corti by regulating the apposition of the tectorial membrane to the inner hair cells. A system of efferent nerve fibers from the superior olivary complex of the pons, the olivocochlear bundle, accomplishes this important function (see later).

The organ of Corti serves as an **audiofrequency analyzer.** It is tonotopically organized so the highest tones (in pitch and frequency) maximally stimulate the hair cells in the most basal portion of the cochlea, which contains the narrowest segment of basilar membrane. The tones of lowest pitch maximally stimulate hair cells in the most apical portion of the cochlea, which contains the widest segment of basilar membrane. Tones or sounds of intermediate pitch stimulate the hair cells on the intermediate portion of the basilar membrane.

The inner hair cells and the spiral ganglion cells with which they synapse show frequency-dependent responses to sound. Each ganglion cell posseses a characteristic **tuning curve,** which is the relationship between the amplitude of sound needed to induce a barely detectable neuronal discharge and the frequency of the sound stimulus.

The pressure waves set up in the scala vestibuli traverse the scala media, vibrate the basilar membrane, and induce pressure waves in the scala tympani. Movements of an elastic diaphragm covering the **round window** dampen the pressure waves in the scala tympani. The round window consists of a bony opening between the scala tympani and the middle ear (Fig. 14–1A and B). Thus, air filling the middle ear dissipates these pressure waves.

Central Auditory Pathways

The cochlear nerve enters the brain stem at the junction of the medulla and pons. As it attaches to the brain stem, the nerve clings to the lateral side of the inferior cerebellar peduncle and enters the **posterior (dorsal) and anterior (ventral) cochlear nuclei.** Each entering nerve fiber bifurcates and connects synaptically with neurons in both cochlear nuclei. These nuclei contain tonotopically organized neurons. Three projections—the dorsal, intermediate and ventral acoustic striae—relay information from the cochlear nuclei to other structures centrally and rostrally. The **dorsal acoustic stria** originates in the dorsal cochlear nucleus, passes over the inferior cerebellar peduncle, and crosses to join the contralateral **lateral lemniscus** (Fig. 14–2). The two other striae arise from the ventral cochlear nucleus. The **intermediate acoustic stria** takes a course similar to that of the dorsal stria. The **ventral acoustic stria** takes a different route, by passing anterior to the inferior cerebellar peduncle to terminate in the **ipsilateral and contralateral nuclei** of the **trapezoid body** and **superior olivary nuclei** (Fig. 14–2; see also Fig. 10–10). These nuclei, in turn, project fibers into the ipsilateral and contralateral lateral lemnisci.

Fibers ascending from the dorsal and ventral cochlear nuclei through the dorsal and intermediate striae project to the contralateral inferior colliculus (although some of them synapse on relay neurons in the nuclei of the lateral lemniscus). These projections constitute the **monaural central auditory pathway,** which carries information about the frequency of auditory signals. The fibers of the ventral acoustic stria, in contrast, form a bilaterally ascending **binaural pathway** that includes synapses in the trapezoid body, superior olivary complex, and nuclei of the lateral lemniscus. This specialized pathway can analyze the location of origin, or direction, of auditory stimuli. The binaural pathway also ends in the **inferior colliculus,** which sends its axons to the **medial geniculate nucleus (body)** through the **brachium of the inferior colliculus.**

The medial geniculate nuclei (or bodies) serve as special sensory nuclei of the thalamus and constitute the final sensory relay stations of the hearing pathway. The efferent connection of the medial geniculate body to the temporal lobe forms the **auditory radiation,** which projects to the **transverse temporal gyri (gyri of Heschl)** and to the adjacent **planum temporale,** located on the dorsal surface of the superior temporal convolution and partly buried in the lateral fissure. Located within the transverse temporal gyri and the anterior part of the planum temporale, **Brodmann's areas 41 and 42** serve as the **primary and secondary auditory areas** of the cortex.

Processing in the Auditory Cortex

Sound can be heard when auditory impulses arrive at area 41; however, discriminations requiring a response to changes in the **temporal patterns** of sounds depend on neuronal processing in areas 41 and 42, particularly in the adjacent planum temporale (including part of area 22). Evaluation of combinations of different frequencies in a temporal sequence begins in the cochlear nuclei and continues through the inferior collic-

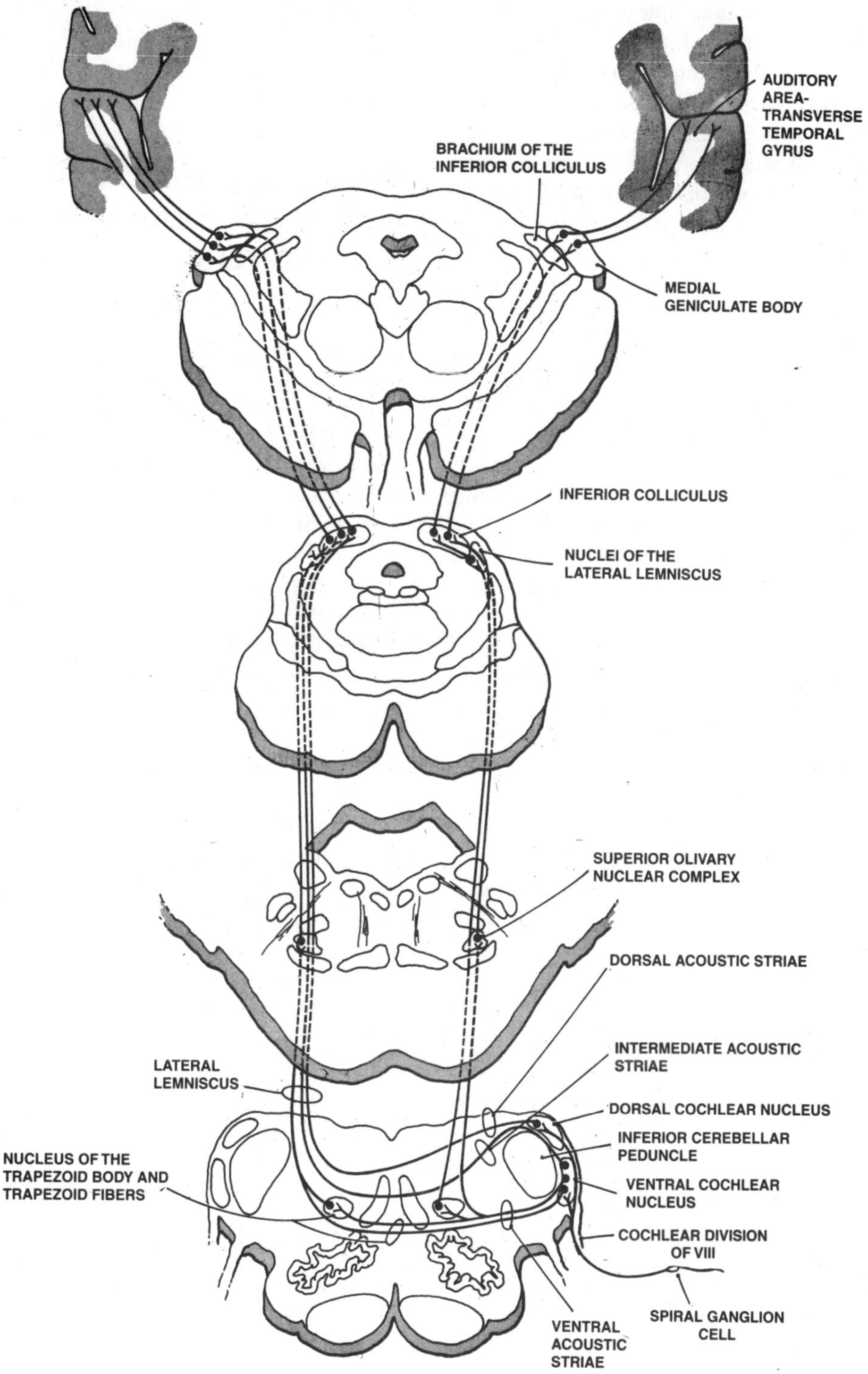

■ **FIGURE 14–2.** The auditory pathways. Axons of neurons in the cochlear nuclei actually cross the midline as they ascend, so they enter the lateral lemniscus at the level of the pontomedullary junction. For diagrammatic convenience, they are shown crossing completely in the medulla.

ulus, medial geniculate nucleus, and primary auditory cortex. A **tonotopic organization** has been demonstrated for all these central auditory nuclei, although **decoding the patterns of complex sounds** such as language requires the functioning of the primary, secondary, and surrounding association cortices. Information processing about the location of a sound begins in the superior olive and inferior colliculus, but the **ability to localize sound precisely** in space requires processing at all levels up to and including the auditory association areas in the superior temporal gyrus and the posterior parietal cortex.

A descending pathway beginning in the auditory cortex parallels the ascending sensory system and provides feedback that modulates sensory processing at all levels of the system, including the cochlea itself. From the region of the superior olivary complex, neurons projecting into the **olivocochlear bundle** travel by way of the eighth nerve and terminate directly on hair cells of the organ of Corti, where they regulate impulses originating in the cochlea. The efferent fibers of the auditory pathway, including the olivocochlear bundle, may be responsible for the phenomenon of selective auditory attention.

Bilateral Representation of the Cochlea in Each Temporal Lobe

As illustrated in Figure 14–2, above the level at which the cochlear nerve enters the brain stem, the hearing pathway consists of crossed and uncrossed fibers, most of which are crossed. Opportunity for auditory information to be redistributed in both crossed and uncrossed fashion exists at many levels of the brain stem. Fibers cross from one side to the other between the nuclei of the superior olive, trapezoid body, lateral lemnisci, and inferior colliculi. (These commissural connections are not illustrated in Figure 14–2.) Each lateral lemniscus therefore conducts stimuli from both ears. A lesion of the right lateral lemniscus, or of the right anterior transverse temporal gyrus, stops some impulses from both ears but does not interfere with other impulses from both ears projecting to the cortex of the left hemisphere. Therefore, deafness in one ear usually signifies damage to the acoustic (cochlear) nerve, the cochlea, or the sound-conducting apparatus of the middle ear on that side. The hair cells of the cochlea can be damaged bilaterally by toxic effects of some drugs, notably the aminoglycosides (antibiotics such as gentamicin and tobramycin) and salicylates (analgesics such as aspirin).

Diagnosing Hearing Deficits from Nerve Damage and from Conductive Defects

Air conduction or bone conduction can convey sound. **Air conduction** mediates sound when the source of the sound arises some distance from the ear and air transmits the sound waves to the tympanic membrane. **Bone conduction** mediates sound when the source of the sound, a vibrating body, maintains contact with the skull or bones of the body and these bones transmit sound waves to the ear. Injury to the sensory components of the inner ear or to the fibers of the eighth nerve commonly produces **hearing loss (sensorineural deafness)** and **tinnitus** (i.e., ringing or roaring in the ear). Disease affecting the auditory conducting mechanisms in the middle ear may also cause hearing loss and tinnitus, a condition termed **conductive deafness.**

Examination with a tuning fork can assist in distinguishing sensorineural deafness from conductive deafness. A 512-Hz or a 256-Hz tuning fork should be used. In the **Weber test,** the physician applies the base of a vibrating fork to the forehead in the midline and asks the patient whether the sound seems loudest in the midline or in one ear. In persons with normal hearing, the sound seems loudest in the midline. In patients with conductive deafness in one ear, the sound seems louder in the affected ear. This occurs because, in conductive deafness, an abnormality in middle ear structures reduces sound perception by air conduction, whereas perception by bone conduction becomes relatively enhanced as a result of the inability of that ear to perceive ambient noise in the environment by air conduction. In patients with sensorineural deafness in one ear, the sound seems louder in the other (normal) ear. This occurs because bone conduction of sound remains as ineffective in stimulating the damaged nerve as air conduction.

The **Rinne test** compares the patient's ability to hear a vibrating tuning fork by bone conduction and by air conduction. The physician places the base of a vibrating 512-Hz or 256-Hz tuning fork over one mastoid process of the skull and asks the patient to indicate when the sound can no longer be heard. At this point, the physician removes the tuning fork from the mastoid process and holds the tines of the still vibrating tuning fork in front of the ear. A person with normal hearing continues to hear by air conduction after bone conduction ceases. In conductive deafness, bone conduction functions better than air conduction; hence the patient cannot hear the vibrations in air. In sensorineural deafness, both are diminished, but air conduction remains better than bone conduction.

Audiometers provide refined testing of hearing because pure tones can be used at controlled intensities. Sound generators for both air and bone conduction are available, and the results of these tests in each ear can be graphed for both air conduction and bone conduction. Conductive deafness generally consists of impairment in the perception of pure tones during air conduction as compared with bone conduction. Sensorineural deafness generally consists of equal impairment in the perception of pure tones during air conduction and bone conduction. Most forms of conductive deafness affect the low frequencies to the greatest degree, whereas sensorineural deafness tends to affect the high frequencies.

Auditory evoked potentials, also known as **brain stem auditory evoked potentials,** can be recorded from electrodes applied to the scalp. The stimulus consists of a recurrent series of clicks, and the potentials can be amplified and then summated by a computer. A succession of structures in the auditory pathway from the auditory nerve to the auditory cortex generates the individual components of the auditory evoked potential. Auditory evoked potentials assist clinicians in determining the site of a disease process in the auditory pathway. Brain tumors, stroke, and multiple sclerosis are among the diseases that can alter the auditory evoked potential.

Sensorineural deafness commonly occurs with Ménière's disease (discussed in Chapter 15), trauma, drug damage, infection, aging, and occlusion of the internal auditory artery. Conductive deafness may result from wax in the external auditory canal, otitis media, and diseases that impair the capacity of the ossicles to function properly, such as otosclerosis.

Auditory Reflexes

Auditory reflexes consist of involuntary responses to sound that are mediated by branches from the main auditory pathway. **Audiomotor reflexes** consist of contractions of the tensor tympani and stapedius muscles in response to sound. The trigeminal and facial nerves innervate these muscles, respectively, and their contraction diminishes vibrations of the middle ear ossicles. Other reflex pathways synapse in the reticular formation to evoke autonomic responses. Among several pathways mediating auditory reflexes, fibers projecting from the inferior colliculus to the superior colliculus and fibers projecting from this site downward provide auditory input to the spinal cord by way of the **tectospinal tract.** These fibers terminate on lower motoneurons in the brain stem and cervical spinal cord and supply the oculomotor system and muscles of the head and neck that respond to sound. The **general acoustic muscle reflex** consists of a generalized startle reflex or jerking of the body in response to a loud, sudden sound. The **auditory-palpebral reflex** consists of a blink of the eyelids in response to a loud noise. The **auditory-oculogyric reflex,** an orienting response, involves deviation of the eyes in the direction of a sound. The **cochleopupillary reflex** consists of dilatation of the pupils (or constriction followed by dilatation) in response to a loud noise.

Case Follow-up

The patient described at the beginning of this chapter had decreased hearing in the right ear as shown by her presenting complaints and by tests demonstrating decreased perception of a whispered voice and a ticking watch. Hearing in the right ear was decreased when it was tested through bone conduction, as shown by the Weber test. Nevertheless, air conduction exceeded bone conduction in the right ear, as shown by the Rinne test. These findings indicate a sensorineural hearing loss from a disorder affecting the auditory component of the right eighth nerve. Testing vestibular function by irrigating the canals with cold water demonstrated dysfunction of the vestibular component of the eighth nerve. These findings suggest the diagnosis of a disorder slowly impairing the function of the right eighth nerve outside the brain stem. A magnetic resonance imaging study demonstrated an acoustic neuroma affecting the right eighth nerve in the cerebellopontine angle. Surgical removal of the tumor produced an excellent result, including preservation of hearing and recovery of vestibular function.

15

Vestibular System

Case Study

A 42-year-old woman experiences a sense of fullness in her right ear for several hours, followed by a sudden decrease of hearing in the ear, accompanied by a loud roaring sound. Within an hour, she develops a sensation of spinning of the room that requires that she lie down to avoid falling. Intense nausea ensues, and she becomes pale and breaks out in a cold sweat. These symptoms last for about 2 hours, and then the spinning sensation slowly diminishes, her hearing returns to normal, and the roaring sound disappears. About 1 year later, she has an identical episode and seeks medical help during the episode. Examination at the peak of her symptoms reveals constant lateral beating movements of her eyes (nystagmus), a low-frequency sensorineural hearing loss in the right ear, pallor, and sweating, but no other abnormality.

Where in the nervous system is the disorder responsible for this woman's symptoms? What causes it? Can she be treated?

The vestibular system consists of receptors located in the inner ear on both sides of the head, peripheral nerve fibers of the vestibular division of the eighth cranial nerve, and central connections that analyze information about the position and movement of the head in space. The vestibular system has the following functions: it maintains body balance; it coordinates eye, head, and body movements; and it permits the eyes to remain fixed on a point in space as the head moves. Commissural connections between the vestibular nuclei of the two sides mediate these reflex functions along with vestibulocerebellar, vestibulospinal, and vestibulo-ocular pathways. In addition, a thalamocortical pathway to the parietal lobe serves the conscious sense of head position and acceleration.

Vestibular Portion of the Inner Ear

The **inner ear,** or **labyrinth,** consists of a bony labyrinth and a membranous labyrinth. The **bony labyrinth** consists of a series of interconnected cavities in the petrous portion of the temporal bone. Inside the bony labyrinth lies the **membranous labyrinth,** a system of tubes and sacs of fine membranes. The vestibular membranous labyrinth contains five compartments: the utricle and saccule and three semicircular canals.

A fluid called **perilymph** fills the space between the bony labyrinth and the membranous labyrinth. **Endolymph** fills the membranous labyrinth. The endolymph in the vestibular membranous labyrinth communicates through a small channel with that in the cochlear duct. Similarly, the perilymphatic space of the vestibular part of the bony labyrinth is continuous with the perilymphatic spaces of the cochlea: the scala vestibuli and scala tympani.

The peripheral receptors of the vestibular system, the **vestibular hair cells,** reside in specialized receptor areas within the membranous labyrinth. These receptors serve both dynamic and static functions. The dynamic functions detect both linear (translational) and angular (rotational) motion of the head in space, whereas the static functions allow detection of the position (tilt) of the head. The control of posture, locomotion, and eye movements requires all components of vestibular function.

The labyrinth on each side of the body provides a baseline tonic discharge that constantly influences vestibular pathways to the ocular motor nuclei and the spinal cord. Responses of the labyrinthine receptors to natural stimulation can either increase or decrease this tonic discharge.

Utricle and Saccule

Within the vestibule of the bony labyrinth, the membranous labyrinth contains two swellings: the **utricle** and the **saccule** (see Fig. 14–1C). The floor of the utricle houses a specialized receptor region, the **macula.** The macula contains hair cells that synapse on the distal branches of vestibular ganglion cells. The apical surface of each hair cell bears numerous **stereocilia** and, on one side of the stereocilia, a single **kinocilium.** These "hairs" extend upward into an overlying gelatinous substance containing **otoconia,** which consist of calcium carbonate crystals.

When the head is in the erect position, the macula of the utricle lies in the horizontal plane, so the gelatinous matrix with its otoconia rests directly on the hair cells. If the head tilts or accelerates in the horizontal plane, the inertia of the otoconia causes the gelatinous matrix to lag behind the movement of the skull and thereby bends the hairs of the receptor cells. This movement changes the membrane potential of the receptor cells. When the force on a hair cell bends the stereocilia toward the kinocilium, the cell becomes depolarized; when the stereocilia bend away from the kinocilium, the cell becomes hyperpolarized. This results in a corresponding increase or decrease of activity at the synapses between the hair cells and the peripheral processes of the vestibular ganglion cells.

The macula of the utricle responds to changes in head position with respect to gravity or tilt and to earth-horizontal linear acceleration. The arrangement of hair cells in the macula creates a response to acceleration in any direction. The position of the kinocilium on only one side and the differential responses of the membrane potential to movement of the stereocilia with respect to the kinocilium cause each hair cell to be functionally polarized. In addition, the arrangement of the hair cells with respect to one another induces functional polarization of the macula itself. The hair cells are arrayed across the surface of the macula in curved rows. A specialized strip through the middle, called the **striola,** defines the site of change in orientation of the hair cells. Each hair cell is oriented with the kinocilium toward the striola. Thus, the hair cells on either side of the striola are organized as mirror images, and horizontal acceleration depolarizes one sector of the macula regardless of the direction of movement.

The saccule contains a macula of similar structure, but it is oriented vertically, approximately in a parasagittal plane. Thus, linear acceleration in the vertical direction stimulates the macula. This occurs in response to gravity or against gravity, as when we accelerate or decelerate in an elevator.

Semicircular Canals

The three semicircular canals—anterior (superior), lateral (horizontal), and posterior—are arranged in three planes that lie roughly at right angles to one another (see Fig. 14–1). The orientation of the canals is such that the horizontal canals on each side of the head lie in one plane, the right anterior and left posterior canals occupy the second plane, and the right posterior and left anterior canals are in the third plane.

The membranous labyrinth of each semicircular canal contains one enlarged end called the **ampulla** (see Fig. 14–1). Within the ampulla resides the **ampullary crest (crista ampullaris),** a ridge that bears hair cells like those of the maculae. A gelatinous capsule termed the **cupula** covers the ampullary crest and extends upward to the roof of the ampulla. This gelatinous matrix has the same specific gravity as the endolymph and therefore cannot sense the effects of gravity, but when the head undergoes angular acceleration or rotation, the viscous endolymph in the semicircular ducts lags behind as a result of inertia and pushes on the cupula.

Distortion of the cupula during angular acceleration evokes a receptor potential in the hair cells on the ampullary crest, and this alters the level of activity in the vestibular fibers of the eighth nerve with which the hair cells synapse. The afferent nerve fibers from each crista ampullaris respond with an increase in impulse frequency to rotation in one direction and with a decrease in impulse frequency to rotation in the opposite direction. These increases and decreases modify a baseline tonic level of vestibular activity that balances input from the two ears. Damage to the inner ear or vestibular nerve on one side causes an imbalance that can produce nausea, vertigo, postural imbalance, and abnormal eye movements.

Vestibular Nerve and Its Central Connections

The afferent fibers of the vestibular nerve have cell bodies in the **vestibular ganglion (of Scarpa).** Axons of bipolar cells of the vestibular ganglion pass through the internal auditory canal and reach the upper medulla in company with the cochlear nerve. The fibers of the vestibular nerve bifurcate into ascending and descending branches

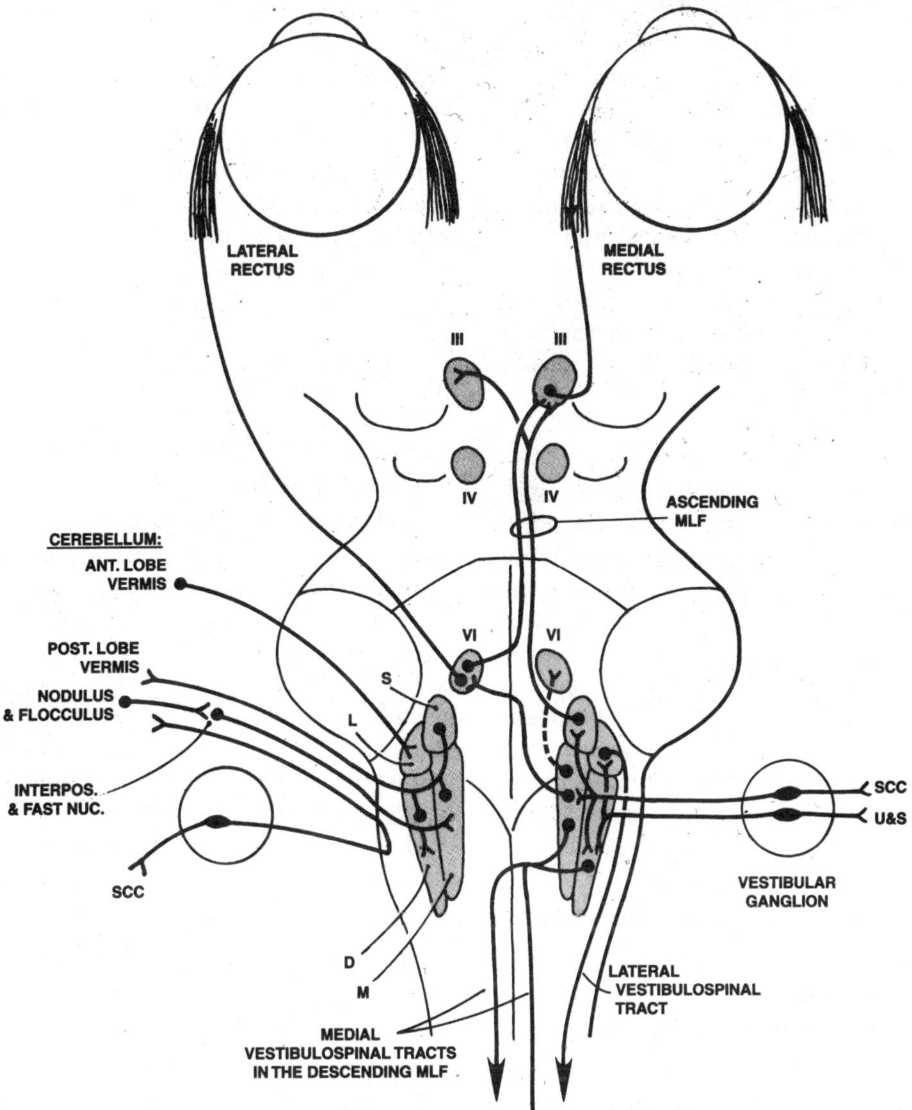

■ **FIGURE 15–1.** Selected connections of the vestibular ganglion cells and vestibular nuclei. The connections illustrated on the *right* and *left* have been separated only for clarity. All connections shown exist on both sides. Some of the connections of the vestibular nuclei with the oculomotor system and spinal cord are shown on the *right;* vestibular connections with the cerebellum are on the *left.* The *dashed line* indicates inhibitory connections that participate in vestibulo-ocular reflexes (see text). D = descending vestibular nucleus; FAST. NUC. = fastigial nucleus of the cerebellum; INTERPOS. = interpositus nucleus of the cerebellum; L = lateral vestibular nucleus; M = medial vestibular nucleus; MLF = medial longitudinal fasciculus; SCC = semicircular canals; S = superior vestibular nucleus; U&S = utricle and saccule; III = oculomotor nucleus; IV = trochlear nucleus; VI = abducens nucleus.

and terminate in the **vestibular nuclei,** which lie clustered in the lateral part of the floor of the fourth ventricle (Fig. 15–1). The four vestibular nuclei are the lateral vestibular nucleus, the medial vestibular nucleus, the superior vestibular nucleus, and the descending vestibular nucleus (also called the spinal or inferior nucleus).

The **cristae ampullares** of the semicircular canals provide input over vestibular afferents primarily to the central region of the vestibular nuclear complex, at the boundaries between the superior, medial, and descending vestibular nuclei. In contrast, the maculae of the utricle and saccule project vestibular afferents predominantly to the lateral and descending vestibular nuclei in this central core. The more peripheral neurons of these four nuclei make interconnections among the four nuclei and commissural connections with the contralateral vestibular nuclei, through which the balance of inputs from the two sides of the head can be analyzed.

In addition, some ascending branches of vestibular nerve fibers from the semicircular canals continue through the vestibular nuclei to end in the **nodulus of the cerebellum** (Fig. 15–1), although this projection may be small in humans. The vestibular nuclei project to the cerebellum and the reticular formation of the brain stem, to vestibulospinal pathways essential for postural reflexes and coordinated locomotion, to ascending pathways that regulate eye movements, and to thalamocortical pathways that mediate the conscious sense of position and movement of the head.

Vestibulocerebellar Connections

As mentioned earlier, some primary fibers of the vestibular nerve pass directly to the cerebellum and end in the cortex of the flocculonodular lobe. Other vestibular fibers to the flocculonodular lobe cortex and to the caudal part of the posterior lobe vermis arise from the superior, medial, and descending nuclei. In return, these cerebellar cortical areas influence the superior, medial, and descending vestibular nuclei by connections through two deep cerebellar nuclei, the **fastigial nucleus** and the **nucleus interpositus,** and by direct projections from the cerebellar cortex (not shown in Fig. 15–1).

The fastigial nucleus projects both crossed and uncrossed fibers that terminate widely in the vestibular nuclei and in the reticular formation of the pons and medulla. As they pass from the cerebellum, some of these fibers loop around the superior cerebellar peduncle to form the **uncinate fasciculus (hook bundle).** Other fastigiobulbar fibers, which remain uncrossed, pass from the cerebellum on the medial side of the inferior cerebellar peduncle and constitute a portion of the peduncle termed the **juxtarestiform body.**

The anterior lobe of the cerebellum strongly influences the lateral vestibular nucleus. The lateral nucleus sends major projections to the vermis of the anterior lobe and receives direct projections from Purkinje cells in the anterior lobe cortex.

Vestibulospinal Tracts

Lateral and Medial Vestibulospinal Tracts

Two major projections into the spinal cord arise from the vestibular nuclei. The uncrossed **lateral vestibulospinal tract** comes from the lateral vestibular nucleus. The **medial vestibulospinal tract,** which has both crossed and uncrossed axons, comes chiefly from the medial vestibular nucleus, with some fibers contributed by the descending (spinal) nucleus. The lateral vestibulospinal tract extends ipsilaterally from the cervical to the lumbosacral level of the spinal cord. The medial vestibulospinal tract, joining the descending portion of the medial longitudinal fasciculus (MLF), extends bilaterally, only through the cervical segments of the spinal cord. Both tracts terminate along their course almost exclusively on interneurons in laminae VII and VIII, which, in turn, synapse on alpha and gamma lower motoneurons in lamina IX. (See Chapter 8.) Both vestibulospinal tracts strongly facilitate motoneurons innervating antigravity muscles. These effects assist the local myotatic (muscle stretch) reflexes and reinforce the tonus of the extensor muscles of the trunk and limbs, to produce enough extra force to support the body against gravity and to maintain an upright posture. In addition, some projections in the medial vestibulospinal tract end on motoneurons of the neck that control **gaze** (coordinated movements of the neck and eyes).

Contributions of the Vestibulospinal System to Decerebrate Rigidity

An animal with a brain stem transection at the midbrain level develops a condition termed **decerebrate rigidity.** This condition is characterized by marked rigidity of the extensor muscles of all limbs as well as the trunk and neck. In humans, decerebrate rigidity consists of extension of all the limbs, with the arms adducted and internally rotated at the shoulders. Decerebrate rigidity results from a marked tonic enhancement of activity descending from the brain stem through the vestibulospinal and reticulospinal tracts, which strongly augment muscle tone, particularly in extensor muscles. Normally, a balance of inhibiting and facilitating activity descending from the cerebral hemispheres to the level of the spinal cord influences muscle tone. Removal of the influence of the cerebral hemispheres by transection at the upper levels of the brain stem allows activity in the vestibulospinal and reticulospinal tracts to occur without control. Decerebrate rigidity results principally from a marked tonic facilitation of gamma motoneuron activity in the spinal cord. This increases the firing rate of muscle spindle afferents and thereby, in reflex fashion, increases the firing of alpha motoneurons to extensor muscles. Transection of the dorsal roots abolishes decerebrate rigidity because this interrupts the gamma motoneuron influence on the muscle spindle afferent reflex arc. Central nervous system lesions that interrupt the descending vestibular and reticular pathways also abolish decerebrate rigidity, a finding indicating that these nuclei provide the driving force maintaining this state.

Vestibulo-ocular Systems

The vestibular system controls reflexive conjugate eye movements that compensate for brief head movements in any direction. Stimulation of the vestibular receptors evokes eye movements of equal magnitude in the direction opposite to the head, to keep the retina focused on the same visual field. This is a **vestibulo-ocular reflex.** The vestibular nuclei (particularly the medial nucleus) and their connections with the cerebellum influence the pathways used for smooth-pursuit eye movements. (See Chapter 19.)

Vestibulo-ocular Pathways

Fibers from the superior and medial vestibular nuclei and from the ventromedial part of the lateral nucleus project rostrally in the MLF. Collectively, these projections are both crossed and uncrossed. Most of them ascend in the MLF, but some also use alternate routes. They synapse primarily in the abducens (VI), trochlear (IV), and oculomotor (III) nuclei. Figure 15–1 illustrates only two examples of the numerous connections that make up this system. Those from the medial vestibular nucleus to the abducens nuclei in Figure 15–1 belong to the pathway that mediates horizontal eye movements in response to stimulation of the horizontal semicircular canals (see later). The ascending projections from the superior vestibular nucleus to the oculomotor nuclei in Figure 15–1 represent connections from the superior vestibular nucleus that control vertical eye movements in response to stimulation of the anterior and posterior canals.

Other fibers from the MLF project to several small nuclear groups in the vicinity of the oculomotor nuclear complex and the pretectal area that participate in vertical eye movements. (See Chapter 19.) They include the interstitial nucleus of Cajal and the rostral interstitial nucleus of the MLF. In return, the interstitial nucleus of Cajal sends descending fibers through the MLF to the vestibular nuclei and the spinal cord.

Vestibulo-ocular Reflexes

Vestibulo-ocular reflexes enable the eyes to remain fixed on stationary objects while the head and body move. Turning the head slightly to the right causes a slight flow of endolymph in the horizontal semicircular canals. The flow moves to the left because the inertia of the fluid causes it to lag behind the movement of the head. This flow of endolymph increases neural activity in the hair cells of the ampulla in the right horizontal canal and decreases activity in the left. This excites the vestibular nuclei on the right through the vestibular ganglion cells. Axons from the right medial vestibular nucleus cross the midline to excite the left abducens nuclear complex and induce contraction of the left lateral rectus muscle (Fig. 15–1). Simultaneously, projections from the right medial vestibular nucleus inhibit the ipsilateral abducens nucleus (Fig. 15–1, dashed line). From a separate group of cells in the left abducens complex, axons cross the midline and ascend through the MLF to the right oculomotor nucleus. These axons activate oculomotor neurons to the right medial rectus muscle. As a result, the eyes turn the proper distance to the left to compensate for the head movement to the right and keep the field of vision unchanged. (Additional information about eye movements is found in Chapter 19.)

Nystagmus

Persistent stimulation of hair cells in the ampulla of a semicircular canal causes the eyes to move slowly to one side until they reach the physical limit and then jerk quickly to the opposite side. These movements occur repetitively in rapid succession and produce tremor-like oscillations of the eyes known as **nystagmus.** Nystagmus consists of a normal reflex response to rotation or to unilateral (unbalanced) stimulation of one of the semicircular canals (see the later discussion of caloric tests). By convention, the direction of nystagmus refers to the direction of the fast component, although this is opposite to the movement induced by stimulation from the semicircular canal. The finding that vestibular stimulation evokes nystagmus provides a basis for clinical tests of vestibular function.

Clinical Testing to Elicit Nystagmus

A **rotation test** of vestibular function can be performed by turning the patient in a revolving chair with the head tilted forward 30 degrees to bring the horizontal canals parallel with the floor. After 10 or 12 turns, movement stops abruptly. During rotation, endolymph moves in the direction opposite to the movement of the head, but with stopping, momentum causes the endolymph to reverse direction and to flow in the direction in which the head had been turning, even though the head has become stationary. The induced nystagmus, called **postrotatory nystagmus,** lasts about 30 seconds in neurologically normal persons. When rotation is to the left, on cessation of movement, endolymph flows to the left, and the slow component of the nystagmus moves to the left. Because the quick component moves to the right, it is called "nystagmus to the right." With a special chair designed to rotate the patient's head in the plane of the horizontal semicircular canals, the vestibulo-ocular reflex can be evaluated quantitatively in response to physiologic rotation at various different test frequencies.

Caloric, or thermal, tests of nystagmus permit the vestibular system of each side to be tested separately. Usually, the examiner places the patient either prone with the head tilted forward about 30 degrees or seated with the head tilted backward about 60 degrees. Either of these positions brings the horizontal semicircular canal into the vertical plane. The examiner then irrigates the patient's external auditory canal with either cold or warm water. This maneuver lowers or raises the temperature of the endolymph on the side of the semicircular canal closest to the middle ear and causes a convection current to develop in the endolymph. The convection current causes deviation of the ampullary crest, which stimulates the hair cells and leads to nystagmus. With warm water irrigation in the right ear, the convection current moves superiorly, causing endolymph to flow toward the ampulla, similar to the effects of head acceleration to the right in the horizontal position. Thus, the nystagmus includes a slow component to the left and a quick component to the right. Irrigation with cold water causes the current to be reversed, and the nystagmus consists of a slow component to the right and a quick component to the left. The caloric tests of nystagmus can be recorded graphically by placing recording electrodes on the patient's face near the eyes and using appropriate amplification and recording equipment.

Spontaneous Nystagmus Is a Pathologic Condition

Loss of the tonic labyrinthine discharge on one side unbalances the stream of impulses from the two sides and leads to spontaneous nystagmus and vertigo. Unbalanced discharge can occur with destruction of the vestibular receptors, section of the vestibular nerve, or damage to the vestibular nuclei. Spontaneous nystagmus reflect neurologic dysfunction. Tonic deviation of the eyes to one side, along with nystagmus and vertigo, occurs after unilateral damage to the vestibular nuclei or their connections, but tonic ocular deviation does not occur after destruction of the vestibular receptors or section of the vestibular nerve. For example, severing the right vestibular nerve unbalances the influence of the remaining left vestibular apparatus and causes nystagmus with the fast component to the left.

Because most peripheral vestibular lesions destroy activity in the nerve rather than stimulating it, the fast component of the nystagmus usually beats away from the diseased ear. The compensatory influences of voluntary and visual reflex circuits overcome these effects in a few weeks.

Although horizontal nystagmus is the most common type, vertical or rotatory forms of spontaneous nystagmus also occur. Spontaneous nystagmus results not only from lesions of the vestibular system, but also from lesions of the brain stem and cerebellum. Nystagmus can also result from chronic visual impairment and from certain toxic substances. **Vertical nystagmus** is usually associated with central lesions, whereas **horizontal and rotatory nystagmus** often results from peripheral lesions affecting the labyrinth or the vestibular nerve.

Vestibulothalamocortical Pathway

Projections from the vestibular nuclei to the ventral lateral and ventral posterior nuclei of the thalamus provide conscious awareness of the position and movements of the head. From these thalamic nuclei, vestibular information projects to several separate areas associated with the somatosensory cortex, including primary somatosensory areas 2V, which receives primarily joint sensations, and 3a, which receives information from muscle spindles. Other cortical areas that have been implicated in vestibular function include posterior areas of the parietal lobe dorsally (in area 7) and in the posterior part of the superior temporal gyrus at its junction with the parietal and insular cortices. This last area is important in vestibulo-ocular functions.

Sensory Aspects of Vestibular Stimulation

Stimulation of the vestibulothalamocortical pathway causes a sense of motion. This occurs irrespective of the source of the stimulation, whether by motion of the entire body, by artificial means such as caloric test for nystagmus, or as a result of disease. **Vertigo** consists of a sense of whirling. The affected person may feel rotational movements of the body or may perceive external objects as spinning about the body. **Motion sickness** during travel by air or sea is a familiar manifestation of prolonged and excessive stimulation of the vestibular apparatus. The symptom of **dizziness** may refer to a sensation of vertigo, but more commonly it describes feelings of giddiness, faintness, light-headedness, or visual disturbances of various types. Careful questioning of the person complaining of dizziness usually allows the clinician to determine whether the patient has true vertigo or some other symptom. The distinction can be extremely important in diagnosis. Ménière's disease is a condition characterized by sudden attacks of severe vertigo, usually associated with nausea, vomiting, and prostration and usually lasting a few days at a time. Fluctuating but progressive unilateral deafness and tinnitus frequently accompany the attacks of vertigo. The disease results from the progressive accumulation of endolymphatic fluid in the labyrinth **(endolymphatic hydrops).**

Case Follow-up

The patient described at the beginning of this chapter has a vestibular and cochlear disorder affecting the right ear, as shown by the nystagmus and hearing loss. Her symptoms are typical of **Ménière's syndrome,** which can result from many causes, including congenital inner ear malformations, inflammatory disease, physical trauma, allergic disorders, autoimmune diseases, and vascular disorders, including diabetes mellitus and hypertension (high blood pressure). When none of these causes can be identified, the disorder is of unknown cause and is labeled **Ménière's disease.** As noted earlier, Ménière's disease is characterized pathologically by dilatation and ballooning of the membranous labyrinth, including the scala media of the cochlea and the saccule, utricle, and semicircular canals. Treatment is with medications to reduce the severity of the acute attack. About 20% of patients do not respond to medication, and for them surgical section of the vestibular nerve can be highly effective. Alternatively, killing the hair cells by administration of an aminoglycoside such as streptomycin may alleviate adverse symptoms. Fortunately, the patient described here had Ménière's disease, but the disorder arrested spontaneously, and she has had no attacks over an observation period of 10 years.

16

Cerebellum

Case Study

A 50-year-old man complaining of difficulty with walking, with frequent falls of 2 days' duration, comes to an emergency room. He gives a history of chronic alcoholism extending over 20 years. He frequently takes no food for several days in a row owing to constant alcohol intake with resulting anorexia. An alcoholic binge and several days without food precipitated his difficulty with walking. On examination, he walks with a wide-based, irregular gait, he has difficulty in turning around without falling, and he is poorly coordinated on tests requiring rapid leg movements. His speech, eye movements, and arm movements are normal.

Which part of his nervous system is affected? What has caused his symptoms? Can his disorder be treated?

Overview of Cerebellar Function

The **cerebellum,** along with other central nervous system structures, participates in the execution of a wide variety of movements. It maintains the fine control and coordination of both simple and complex movements. It is essential for the following: coordinating posture and balance in walking and running; executing sequential movements in eating, dressing, and writing; producing rapidly alternating repetitive movements and smooth-pursuit movements; and controlling certain properties of movements, including trajectory, velocity, and acceleration. Voluntary movements can proceed without the cerebellum, but such movements lack precision and appear clumsy and disorganized. Evidence suggests that the cerebellum participates not only in motor processes, but also in certain specific cognitive functions. Cerebellar damage has been implicated in disturbances of executive functioning, spatial cognition, aspects of personality, and linguistic performance.

Cerebellar Anatomy

The cerebellum consists of a bilaterally symmetrical structure situated in the posterior cranial fossa attached to the medulla, pons, and midbrain by three pairs of **cerebellar peduncles.** These peduncles lie at the sides of the fourth ventricle on the ventral aspect of the cerebellum. The **tentorium cerebelli,** a transverse fold of the dura mater, stretches horizontally over the superior surface of the cerebellum and separates it from the overlying occipital lobes of the cerebrum.

Numerous parallel folds known as **folia** corrugate the surface of the cerebellum. A layer of gray matter, the **cerebellar cortex,** covers the surface and encloses an internal core of white matter. Four pairs of **deep cerebellar nuclei** lie buried within the cerebellum. From medial to lateral, these include the **fastigial, globose, emboliform,** and **dentate nuclei.** Commonly grouped together, the globose and emboliform nuclei are termed the **interposed nuclei.**

Primary Subdivisions

Cerebellar Lobes Are Transversely Divided Subdivisions

The cerebellum includes a midline structure called the **vermis** and two large lateral masses known as the **cerebellar hemispheres** (Fig. 16–1). Together, the vermis and hemispheres can be divided transversely into three lobes:

1. The **flocculonodular lobe** includes the paired flocculi, which consist of small appendages in the posterior inferior region, and the nodulus, which lies in the inferior part of the vermis (Fig. 16–1B). The posterolateral fissure separates the flocculonodular lobe from the posterior lobe. Also termed the **archicerebellum,** the flocculo-

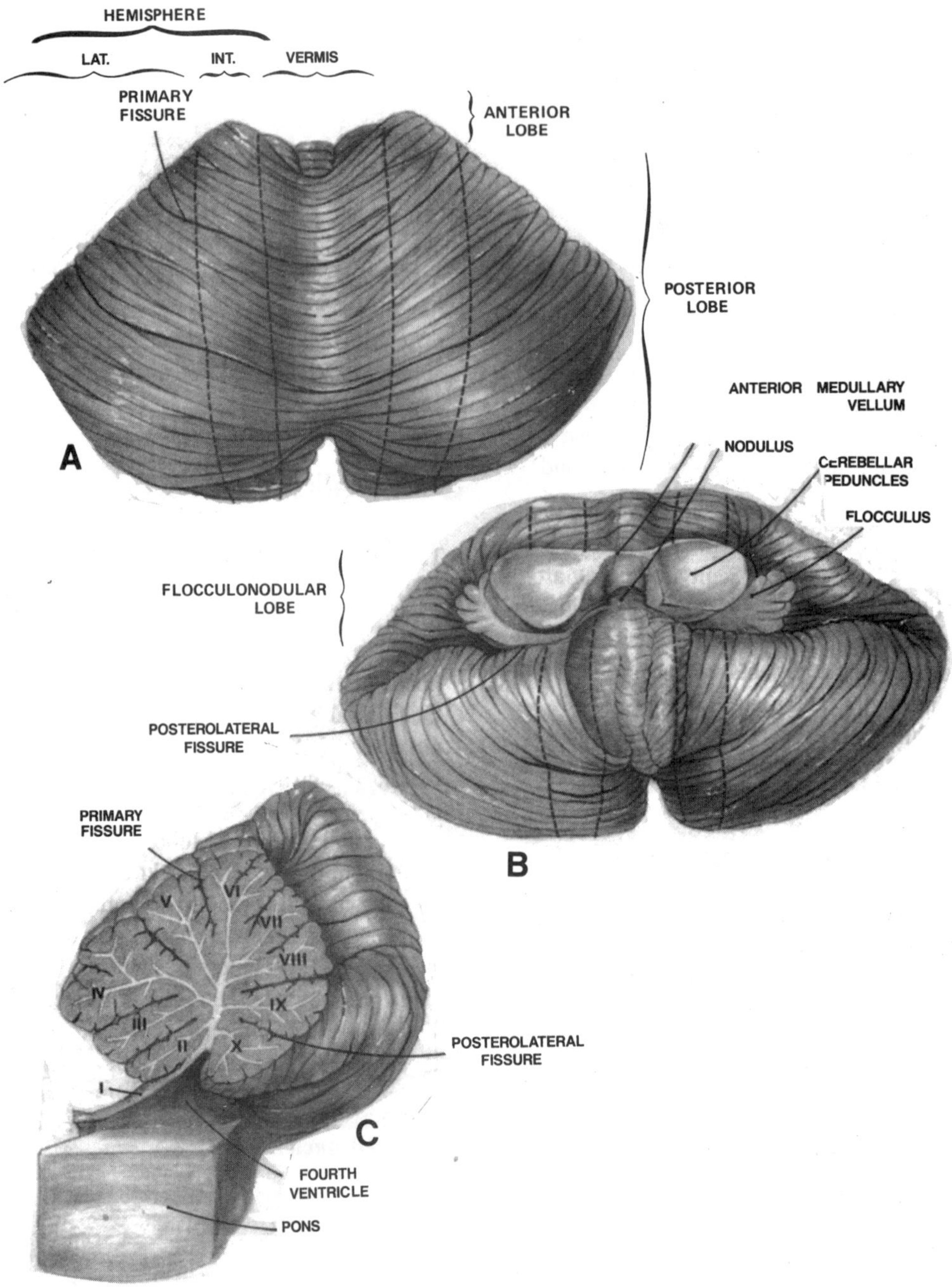

■ **FIGURE 16–1.** The human cerebellum seen from the dorsal **(A)** and ventral **(B)** surfaces and from the medial surface after a midline section through the vermis **(C).** The primary fissure divides the anterior and posterior lobes. The posterolateral fissure divides the posterior lobe from the flocculonodular lobe. Roman numerals identify the vermal structures.

nodular lobe constitutes the oldest part of the structure phylogenetically.
2. Modest in size, the **anterior lobe** lies anterior to the **primary fissure** (Fig. 16–1A). This lobe corresponds approximately to the **paleocerebellum,** the second oldest part of the cerebellum phylogenetically.
3. The largest part of the cerebellum, the **posterior lobe** lies between the other two lobes and contains the major portions of the cerebellar hemispheres. The newest part of the structure phylogenetically, the posterior lobe is also termed the **neocerebellum.** The lowest lying components of the cerebellar hemispheres, the **cerebellar tonsils,** lie immediately above the foramen magnum. When a disease process such as a tumor or hemorrhage in the cerebellum increases pressure in the posterior fossa, the cerebellar tonsils can herniate downward into the foramen magnum and can compress the medulla. This threatens survival because compression of the medulla leads to dysfunction of reticular formation neurons in the brain stem that control blood pressure and respirations.

The flocculonodular lobe receives many projections from the vestibular nuclei. The anterior lobe, particularly its vermal portion, receives input from the spinocerebellar and trigeminocerebellar pathways. The flocculonodular and anterior lobes are the predominant regions of the cerebellum in phylogenetically older vertebrates. Greatly expanded in mammals that have developed an extensive cerebral cortex, the posterior lobe receives projections from the cerebral hemispheres. The foregoing description of transverse divisions is based on the embryonic development of 10 rostrocaudally arranged lobules (numbered I to X on the vermis in Fig. 16–1C).

Cerebellar Zones Divide the Cerebellum into Sagittal Subdivisions

A more clinically useful method of describing the cerebellum comes from the **longitudinal sagittal zonal patterns.** This classification subdivides each half of the cerebellum into three longitudinal strips arranged mediolaterally that include the cerebellar cortex, underlying white matter, and the deep cerebellar nuclei, structures with anatomic linkage and functional integration. These strips include the following:

1. The vermal region with the fastigial nuclei.
2. The paravermal region or the intermediate zone of the hemisphere with the interposed nuclei.
3. The lateral hemisphere region with the dentate nuclei.

See Figure 16–1A and B.

Cerebellar Cortex

Cell Layers

The cerebellar cortex consists of the following three cell layers (Fig. 16–2):

1. The outermost **molecular layer** contains two types of neurons (**stellate cells** and **basket cells**), dendrites of Purkinje and Golgi type II cells, and axons (T-shaped **parallel fibers**) of granule cells.
2. The middle **Purkinje cell layer** contains the cell bodies of Purkinje cells. These very large, flasklike neurons have enormous dendritic arborizations extending upward into the molecular layer. This dendritic arborization is unusual in that it is confined to one plane—the sagittal plane of the cerebellum. As a consequence of this arrangement, Purkinje cell dendrites spread out in a plane perpendicular to the course of the millions of parallel fibers. These fibers run along the length of the folium and make thousands of synaptic contacts with the dendrites of each Purkinje cell (Fig. 16–2). Purkinje cells constitute the sole projection neurons of the cerebellar cortex. Their long axons synapse either on deep cerebellar nuclei or vestibular nuclei. Within the cerebellar cortex, collaterals of Purkinje cell axons make synaptic contact with Golgi cells, other Purkinje cells, basket cells, and stellate cells.
3. The innermost **granular layer** contains massive numbers of **granule** cells (neurons), **Golgi type II cells** (neurons), and **glomeruli** (synaptic complexes that contain axons of incoming mossy fibers, axons and dendrites of Golgi type II cells, and dendrites of granule cells). Glial cell processes encase each glomerulus.

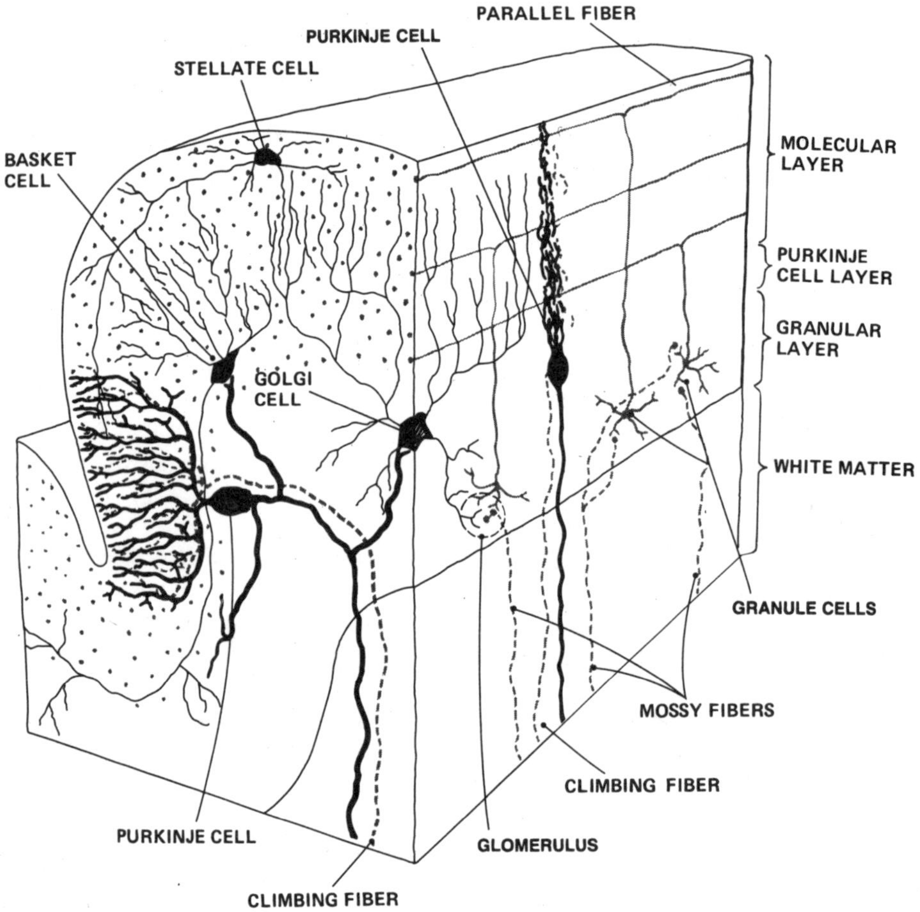

■ **FIGURE 16–2.** A piece of the cerebellar cortex. The smaller cut surface (*left side of the diagram*) represents the sagittal plane of the cerebellum, perpendicular to the length of the folium. This is the plane in which Purkinje cell dendrites arborize. At right angles to this surface, the larger cut surface (*right side*) represents the mediolateral plane of the cerebellum along the length of one folium.

Synaptic Organization

The cerebellar cortex has a simple synaptic organization. The output cells of the cortex, Purkinje cells, all inhibit neurons of the underlying deep cerebellar nuclei. Two types of excitatory inputs reach the Purkinje cells: mossy fibers and climbing fibers. Three sets of inhibitory fibers reach Purkinje cells, the three aminergic fiber systems: noradrenergic, dopaminergic, and serotonergic (not shown in Fig. 16–2). The cerebellar cortex contains two types of inhibitory interneurons and one type of excitatory interneuron. Most excitatory afferents to the cerebellar cortex send collateral projections to the deep cerebellar nuclei. Some afferents, notably those in the dorsal spinocerebellar and cuneocerebellar pathways, project mainly or exclusively to the cerebellar cortex. The afferents to the cortex terminate either in the granule cell layer (in the glomeruli) as mossy fibers or, in the molecular layer, on the dendrites of Purkinje cells as climbing fibers.

Mossy fiber afferents enter the cerebellum from the spinal cord, pontine nuclei, vestibular ganglia and nuclei, trigeminal nuclei, and reticular formation nuclei. Mossy fibers use glutamate as a neurotransmitter, except those derived from the pedunculopontine nucleus and some of the vestibular nuclei, which use acetylcholine. Granule cells, on which mossy fibers synapse, use glutamate as a neurotransmitter at their parallel fiber synapses with Purkinje cells and with interneurons: basket cells, stellate cells, and Golgi cells. These interneurons, in turn, release gamma-aminobutyric acid (GABA) and evoke inhibitory effects. **Climbing fiber afferents** originate exclusively in the inferior olive. Climbing fibers release glutamate or aspartate to excite the Purkinje cell dendrites on which they synapse.

Purkinje cells release GABA and thereby inhibit the deep cerebellar nuclei. These nuclei provide the origin of the efferent fibers from the cerebellum to the inferior olive, reticular formation, vestibular nuclei, red nucleus, and thalamus. All these projections release glutamate, except those to the inferior olive, which use GABA.

Patterns of Excitation

Both mossy fiber and climbing fiber inputs produce excitatory effects in both the deep cerebellar nuclei and the cortex. Mossy fiber input excites Purkinje cells indirectly by activating granule cells and their axons, the parallel fibers. Mossy fiber excitation of Purkinje cells evokes **simple spikes,** which consist of a single action potential. Climbing fiber input excites Purkinje cells directly and evokes **complex spikes,** which consist of an action potential followed by a long-lasting depolarization with multiple small wavelets. Granule cells, through their axonal processes (parallel fibers), excite Purkinje cells, basket cells, stellate cells, and Golgi type II cells. In turn, basket cells and stellate cells inhibit Purkinje and Golgi type II cells. The Golgi type II cells inhibit granule cells. Finally, Purkinje cells, the only route for all information exiting from the cerebellar cortex, inhibit the deep cerebellar and vestibular nuclei. Consequently, of all the neurons whose cells reside within the cerebellar cortex, only the granule cell causes excitation.

Aminergic Afferents

In addition to the mossy fiber and climbing fiber inputs, aminergic afferent projections reach all three layers of the cerebellar cortex. These projections are thought to be inhibitory. **Noradrenergic fibers** arise in the locus ceruleus, enter the cerebellum through the superior cerebellar peduncle, and make synaptic contact with cerebellar nuclei, Purkinje cells, and the interneurons of the cerebellar cortex. **Dopaminergic fibers** originating in the substantia nigra and the ventral mesencephalic tegmentum ascend to the interposed and dentate nuclei and to the Purkinje cell and granule cell layers of the cerebellar cortex. **Serotonergic fibers** project from the raphe nuclei of the brain stem to all parts of the cerebellar nuclei and cortex and terminate in both the granule cell and molecular layers.

Summary of Information Processing

Afferent input from essentially all sources reaches both the deep cerebellar nuclei and the cerebellar cortex and leads to an increase in excitability of the deep nuclei and the Purkinje cells of the cerebellar cortex. The Purkinje cells provide strong inhibitory control over neurons of the deep nuclei. The inhibitory control of Purkinje cells over the excitability of the deep cerebellar nuclei is a key aspect of cerebellar function. Through information received from afferents and interactions between the cerebellar cortex and the deep nuclei, the cerebellum monitors ongoing movements and triggers new or modified movements. The cerebellum can ensure that the speed and accuracy of movements are adequate for each task the motor system undertakes.

During ongoing motor tasks, the mossy fiber inputs furnish an excitatory "main-line" pathway providing drive for neurons in the deep cerebellar nuclei. The mossy fiber input to the cerebellar cortex constitutes a "side path" consisting of a mossy fiber–granule cell–parallel fiber–Purkinje cell circuit with related interneurons. This inhibitory cerebellar cortical side path controls the discharge of neurons in the deep cerebellar nuclei.

The climbing fiber input to the cerebellar cortex has a conditioning effect on the activity of Purkinje cells. Climbing fiber activity can adjust the flow of information through Purkinje cells by strengthening or weakening the influence of various synapses in the cerebellar cortical pathways converging on the Purkinje cells. Moreover, climbing fiber activity is thought to influence motor learning by inducing plastic changes in the synaptic activity of Purkinje cells.

Peduncles

The large numbers of fibers entering and leaving the cerebellum form the three pairs of **cerebellar**

peduncles. The peduncles attach the cerebellum to the brain stem and connect it with other parts of the nervous system.

The **inferior cerebellar peduncle (restiform body)** consists chiefly of afferent fibers. Its fibers enter the cerebellum from at least six sources:

1. The vestibular nerve and nuclei.
2. The inferior olivary nuclei.
3. The dorsal spinocerebellar tract.
4. Some of the fibers from the rostral spinocerebellar tract.
5. The cuneocerebellar tract from the accessory cuneate nuclei in the medulla.
6. Reticulocerebellar fibers.

The first three of these are illustrated in Figure 16–3. The inferior peduncle contains a single efferent pathway, the **fastigiobulbar tract** (also called the **juxtarestiform body;** see Chapter 15), which projects to the vestibular nuclei and completes a vestibular circuit through the cerebellum.

The **middle cerebellar peduncle** (brachium

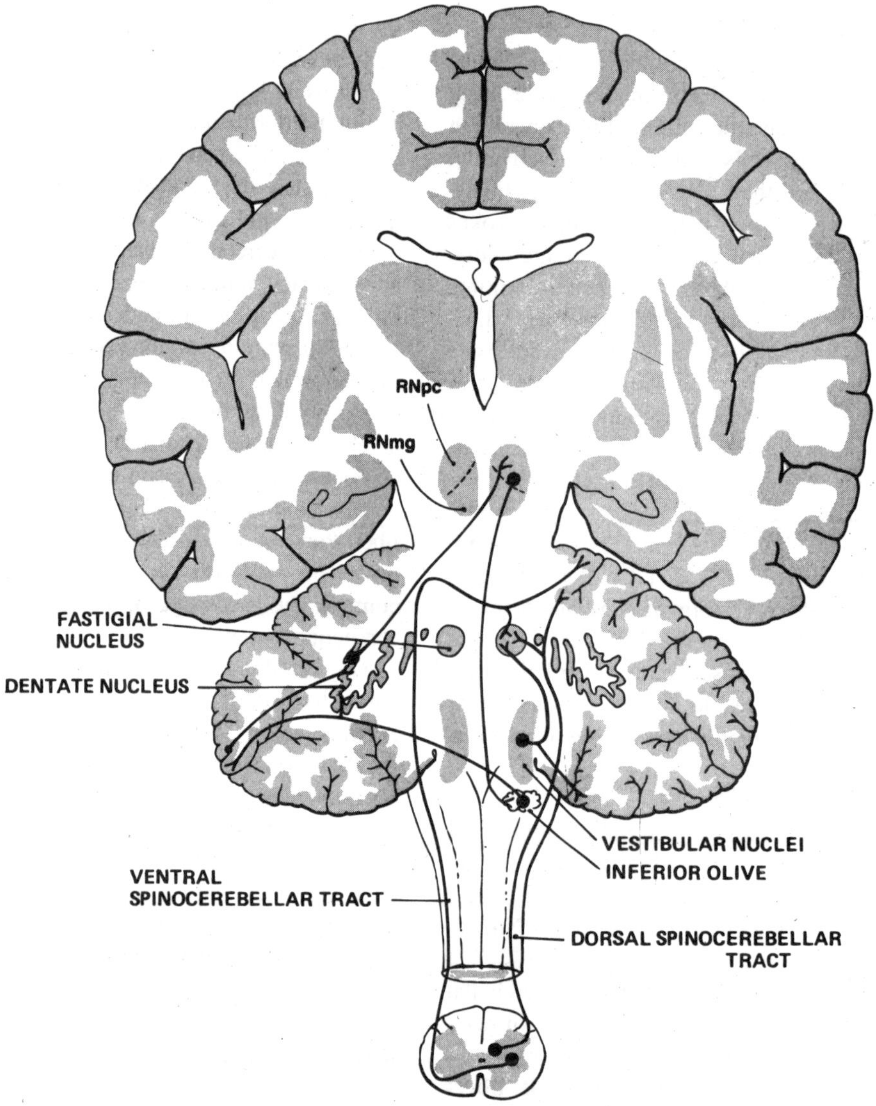

■ **FIGURE 16–3.** Inputs to the fastigial nucleus and cerebellar cortex from the spinal cord and vestibular nuclei and inputs to the dentate nucleus and cerebellar cortex from the inferior olive.

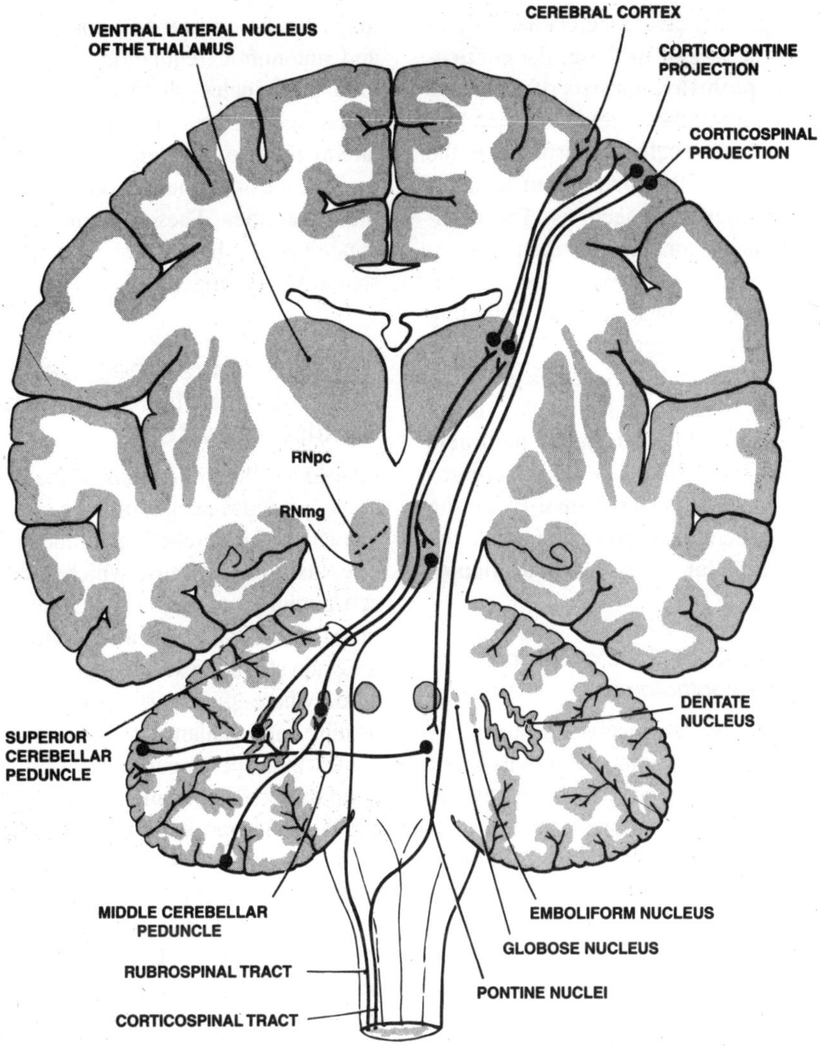

■ **FIGURE 16–4.** Connections of the dentate nucleus and interposed (emboliform and globose) nuclei.

pontis) consists almost entirely of crossed afferent fibers from the contralateral pontine nuclei in the gray substance of the basal pons (pontocerebellar or transverse pontine fibers). The major projections to these pontine nuclei originate within the cerebral cortex (Fig. 16–4).

The **superior cerebellar peduncle** (brachium conjunctivum) consists principally of efferent projections from the cerebellum. Rubral, thalamic, and reticular projections arise from the dentate and interposed (globose and emboliform) nuclei (Fig. 16–4). Some of the fastigiobulbar tract fibers run with the superior peduncle for a short distance before they enter the inferior cerebellar peduncle. The superior cerebellar peduncle also contains afferent projections from the ventral spinocerebellar tract (see Figs. 7–1 and 16–3), a portion of the rostral spinocerebellar tract, and trigeminocerebellar projections.

Major Circuits

Afferents to the Cerebellar Cortex

From the Cerebral Cortex

The cerebellar cortex and the deep cerebellar nuclei receive a constant stream of information originating in multiple sites. Neuronal activity emanating from the cerebral cortex reaches these structures through three cerebrocerebellar projection pathways. The largest of these, the **corticopontocerebellar pathway,** consists of a crossed path connecting most of the cortex of one cerebral hemisphere with the cerebellar hemisphere on the opposite side by way of the **corticopontine tract** and the **pontocerebellar** projections. The corticopontine projections contain information from primary motor and sensory areas of the cerebral cortex, and also from associative areas, including prefrontal and parietal regions, and from the primary visual cortex and, to some degree, the auditory cortex. These pontocerebellar fibers ascend through the **middle cerebellar peduncle** (see Figs. 10–10 and 16–4). The other cerebrocerebellar pathways originate primarily in the motor areas of the cerebral cortex and include the **cerebro-olivocerebellar** and **cerebroreticulocerebellar** pathways.

From the Spinal Cord, Special Sensory Systems, and Hypothalamus

The cerebellar cortex also receives a stream of information from the skin, joints, and muscles of the limbs and trunk of the body mediated by the three spinocerebellar tracts (dorsal, ventral, and rostral) and the cuneocerebellar tract. Most other sensory modalities, including the auditory, vestibular, and visual senses, also reach the cerebellum. Finally, the cerebellum receives direct connections from neurons in the hypothalamus. All this information enters a vast pool of cerebellar cortical neurons, in which integration takes place.

Afferents from Different Central Nervous System Areas Distribute to Cerebellar Zones with Different Functions

In general, the vermal and intermediate zones of the anterior lobe and the caudal part of the posterior lobe receive afferent input primarily from the spinal cord; the flocculonodular lobe receives a major projection from the vestibular system; and the cerebellar hemispheres receive their major input from the cerebral cortex. This distribution provides the basis of a general functional pattern. The vermal and intermediate zones of the anterior and caudal posterior lobes function primarily in the control of posture and locomotion. Evidence suggests that this region may also be concerned with affective processes and autonomic regulation. The flocculonodular lobe participates chiefly in vestibular function (balance, posture, and eye movements). The lateral zones of the cerebellar hemispheres focus on the control of finely coordinated movements of the extremities. These regions also appear to be concerned with executive functioning, visual-spatial processing, and language production.

Efferents of the Deep Cerebellar Nuclei Distribute to Different Functional Systems

Examining the projections of the deep cerebellar nuclei provides insight into the efferent pathways by which the cerebellum influences movement. The **fastigial nucleus,** which receives Purkinje cell output from the vermal zone, sends efferent fibers to the **reticular and vestibular nuclei** of the brain stem. These nuclei project into the spinal cord, where they participate in the control of posture and balance. Projections from these nuclei into the upper brain stem assist in the regulation of conjugate eye movements.

Many neurons of the **interposed nuclei** receive input from Purkinje cells in the vermal and paravermal (intermediate) zones and send projections through the superior cerebellar peduncle to the **magnocellular division of the red nucleus** on the contralateral side. The magnocellular division gives rise to axons of the rubrospinal tract (see Figs. 9–2 and 16–4), which crosses the midline and descends into the spinal cord. Hence this pathway originates in the interposed nuclei and terminates in the spinal cord on the same side of the body. The rubrospinal tract contributes to locomotion and coordinated movements of the extremities.

The lateral zone of the cerebellar cortex, which consists primarily of the lateral part of the posterior lobe, sends Purkinje cell axon into the **dentate and the interposed nuclei.** These nuclei project through the superior cerebellar peduncle to the contralateral red nucleus and the ventral lateral and intralaminar nuclei of the thalamus.

Fibers from the dentate nucleus terminate in the **parvocellular division of the red nucleus,** which gives rise to the rubro-olivary tract. These fibers descend ipsilaterally through the brain stem in the central tegmental tract to terminate in the inferior olivary complex and thereby provide a feedback

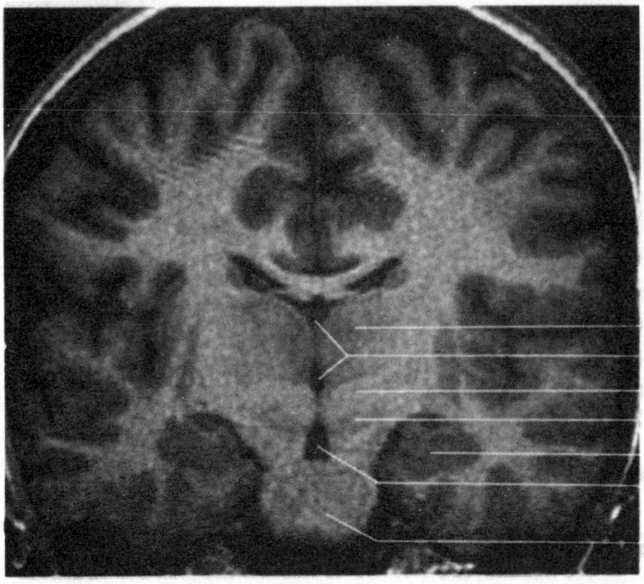

■ **FIGURE 16–5.** A magnetic resonance imaging (T1-weighted sequence) scan in the coronal plane through the brain of a neurologically normal adult showing the thalamus and the base of the midbrain and pons. The red nucleus appears like the white matter because of the capsule of heavily myelinated dentato-rubrothalamic fibers that surround it.

loop to the dentate nucleus and lateral zone of the cerebellar cortex (Figs. 16–3 and 16–5).

Thalamocortical fibers from the **ventral lateral thalamic nucleus** relay impulses to the motor regions of the ipsilateral frontal lobe. Through the pathway to the frontal lobe, the thalamocortical projections make synaptic contact with cortical efferent fibers that pass through the pyramidal tract and project to the contralateral side of the spinal cord through the corticospinal pathway. Hence this pathway arises in the dentate and interposed nuclei and terminates in the spinal cord on the same side of the body (Fig. 16–4). Through its connection with the corticospinal pathway, this part of the cerebellar circuitry exerts an important influence on finely coordinated, learned movement of the distal limb musculature. The projections through the **intralaminar nuclei** reach the posterior parietal, superior temporal, prefrontal, cingulate, and parahippocampal regions of the cerebral cortex. Evidence indicates that these projections influence multiple cognitive processes. Cerebellar connections with the prefrontal cortex participate in executive functioning, with the parietal lobe in visuospatial processing, with the frontal lobe in linguistic activity, and with the cingulate and parahippocampal region in affective and motivational phenomena.

Integration of the Cerebellum and Cerebral Cortex in Movement and Cognition

The intent to perform a movement originates in the motor association areas of the cerebral cortex, including the supplementary motor cortex. These areas act in cooperation with the lateral portions of the cerebellar hemispheres and dentate nuclei during the early phases of movement planning. The result is a command to move, which involves the dentate nuclei, followed by neurons in area 4 of the cerebral cortex. The intermediate parts of the cerebellar hemispheres, including the interpositus nuclei, receive information about the progress of the ongoing movement by inputs from collaterals of pyramidal tract fibers mediated by way of the pontine nuclei and also from peripheral receptors in the body parts being moved.

As indicated earlier, the connections of the cerebellum with thalamocortical projections to the prefrontal cerebral cortex suggest that the cerebellum influences cognitive processing. Presumably, the nervous system uses these connections in some kinds of processing, such as planning ahead. The cerebellum may learn a motor program and may quickly link elements within the program to a new situation so these elements can be used quickly and automatically.

Clinical Signs of Cerebellar Dysfunction

From the clinical perspective, the cerebellum consists of a series of two sagittal zones on each side. The clinical signs of cerebellar dysfunction can be separated into those resulting from disease of the midline zone of the cerebellum and those resulting from disease of the lateral portions.

Clinical Signs of Midline Zone Dysfunction

The midline zone of the cerebellum consists of the anterior and posterior parts of the vermis, the flocculonodular lobe, and the fastigial nuclei. Disease of these regions produces the following signs and symptoms:

1. **Disorders of stance and gait.** The patient usually stands on a broad base, with the feet several inches apart. There may be a severe truncal tremor. The patient cannot walk in tandem, placing the heel of one foot directly in front of the toes of the other foot. With disease of the midline zone, the gait disturbance usually occurs without ataxia of the movements of individual limbs.
2. **Titubation.** This consists of a rhythmic tremor of the body or head occurring several times per second.
3. **Rotated or tilted postures of the head.** The head may be maintained rotated or tilted to the left or the right. The side of the deviation does not usually indicate the site of the cerebellar disease.
4. **Ocular motor disorders.** Certain disturbances of ocular function result from cerebellar disease, the most prominent of which is **spontaneous nystagmus** (i.e., not resulting from physiologic vestibular stimulation). This consists of rhythmic oscillatory movements of one or both eyes occurring with the eyes gazing straight ahead or with ocular deviation.
5. **Affective disturbances.** These were described recently and consist of flattening or blunting of emotional expression, as well as disinhibited or inappropriate behavior.

Clinical Signs of Lateral (Hemispheric) Zone Dysfunction

For clinical purposes, the lateral cerebellar zone consists of the cerebellar hemisphere and the dentate and interposed nuclei of each side. Disease of this region produces the following signs and symptoms:

1. **Decomposition of movement.** The patient performs various components of a motor act in a jerky and irregular manner, rather than in a smooth sequence. Evidence indicates that decomposition of movement is a voluntary, adopted strategy that compensates for the inability to make complex movements accurately. The person with a cerebellar disorder learns to make movements more accurate by moving one joint at a time in a serial manner.
2. **Disturbances of stance and gait.** The patient stands on a broad base and walks unsteadily, with a tendency to fall to the side, forward, or backward. Ataxia of individual movements of the limbs accompanies the gait disorder.
3. **Hypotonia.** This is a decrease in the resistance to passive manipulation of the limbs that appears in one or several limbs at the time of cerebellar injury. Hypotonia often decreases with time. It can be detected clinically by manipulating the limbs about the joints and not by palpating the muscles.
4. **Dysarthria.** In cerebellar disease, speech may be slow, slurred, and labored, but comprehension remains intact, and grammar does not suffer.
5. **Dysmetria.** This is a disturbance of the trajectory or placement of a body part during active movements. The limb may fall short of its goal in hypometria, or it may extend beyond its goal in hypermetria.
6. **Dysdiadochokinesis and dysrhythmokinesis.** Dysdiadochokinesis reflects the decomposition of movements in cerebellar disease, and it is demonstrated by testing alternating or fine repetitive movements. Dysrhythmokinesis is a disorder of the rhythm of rapidly alternating movements. It can be evoked by asking the patient to tap out a rhythm such as three rapid beats followed by one delayed beat. In cerebellar

disease, the rhythm of the movements becomes disturbed.

7. **Ataxia.** This term comprehensively describes the various problems with movement resulting chiefly from the combined effects of dysmetria and decomposition of movement. The patient makes errors in the sequence and speed of the components of each movement. A patient with an ataxia of gait veers from side to side and has difficulty in walking in a straight line.
8. **Tremor.** Cerebellar disease results in **static** and **kinetic tremors.** Static tremor can be demonstrated by asking the patient to extend the arms parallel to the floor with the hands open. A rhythmic oscillation generated at the shoulder appears. Having the patient place the heel of one foot on the knee of the opposite leg and run the heel down the shin evokes a kinetic tremor. Having the patient alternately touch the nose and then touch the examiner's finger, which is held at a full arm's length away from the patient, also evokes a kinetic tremor. These movements result in a side-to-side coarse tremor that is generated at the proximal joints (shoulder and hip).
9. **Impaired check and rebound.** These are related signs of cerebellar dysfunction. The examiner asks the patient to maintain the arms extended forward while the examiner taps the patient's wrist enough to displace the arm. Normally, the arm returns rapidly to the resting position, but with cerebellar disease, the limb becomes markedly displaced and repeatedly overshoots when returning to the original position.
10. **Ocular motor disorders.** Certain disorders of eye movement result from injury to the cerebellar hemispheres. The most common disorder is nystagmus.
11. **Disturbances of executive functioning.** These disturbances consist of deficient planning, set shifting, abstract reasoning, working memory, and decreased verbal fluency.
12. **Impaired spatial cognition.** This condition includes visuospatial disorganization and impaired visuospatial memory.
13. **Personality change.** Flattening or blunting of affect has been described, along with disinhibited or inappropriate behavior.
14. **Linguistic difficulties.** These difficulties include abnormalities in the rhythmic and intonational aspects of speech and language, or **dysprosody,** and nongrammatical construction and naming disorders (**anomia**).

Cerebellar defects gradually improve with time after sudden lesions such as traumatic injury or loss of blood supply (stroke). Improvement of motor function over time occurs partially because the patient learns compensatory strategies and partially because of the **plasticity** of the central nervous system (the capacity to form new connections or to use existing connections differently).

Somatotopic localization of separate body regions in the cerebellar cortex has been demonstrated in experimental animals. These studies have revealed an extremely complex representation of body parts. Despite the complexity of the organization of the cerebellum, however, clearly the right cerebellar hemisphere influences the right side of the body, and any symptoms occurring unilaterally should be found on the same side as the lesion in the cerebellum. This finding contrasts strikingly with cerebral lesions, which produce contralateral effects.

Diseases

Many neurologic diseases affect the cerebellum. The **spinocerebellar ataxias** consist of inherited disorders transmitted as dominant or recessive traits. The dominantly inherited spinocerebellar ataxias have been numbered successively as they are described, and thus far 16 of them have been identified (SCA1 through SCA16). Most of them result from expanded triplet (CAG) repeats. These diseases cause degeneration of the inferior olives, pons, cerebellum, and various other components of the nervous system, including the corticospinal tracts, basal ganglia, and peripheral nerves. The disorders usually present clinically with ataxia of gait, dysarthria, and incoordination of limb movements.

Friedreich's ataxia, a recessively inherited spinocerebellar ataxia, results from an expanded triplet (GAA) repeat that leads to degeneration of peripheral nerves, spinocerebellar pathways, dorsal columns, and corticospinal tracts in the spinal cord. The disease begins in childhood or early adolescence with ataxia of limb movements and gait, accompanied by the appearance of extensor plantar responses. As the disease progresses, patients develop scoliosis, pes cavus (high arches), limb weakness, and ataxia. The disease progresses to include paraparesis (i.e., severe weakness of the legs), with loss of the muscle stretch reflexes and position and vibration sense in the limbs.

Sporadic olivopontocerebellar atrophy is a progressive neurodegenerative disease of unknown cause. The disease results in the gradual loss of neurons of the inferior olives, pons, and cerebellar cortex and causes ataxia of gait, dysarthria, cerebellar tremors of the trunk and limbs, and incoordination of movements of all limbs. In some patients, sporadic olivopontocerebellar atrophy evolves into multiple system atrophy, which includes cerebellar ataxia with autonomic insufficiency and parkinsonian features.

Alcoholic cerebellar degeneration is a disease associated with severe chronic alcoholism with malnutrition. Degenerative changes appearing in the anterior and superior parts of the cerebellar vermis are associated with ataxia of gait but with preservation of speech and coordinated movements of the upper extremities.

Case Follow-up

The patient described at the beginning of this chapter had alcoholic cerebellar degeneration. He was treated with vitamin B_1 (thiamine), fluid replacement for dehydration, and a well-balanced, nutritious diet. His symptoms gradually improved, and he left hospital able to walk without difficulty. He entered Alcoholics Anonymous, and with help he was able to remain sober for many years, with no return of his neurologic disorder. Fortunately, he had received medical attention soon enough to prevent permanent damage to his cerebellum, and also to avoid the more dire symptoms of Wernicke-Korsakoff disease. This disease, which also results from malnutrition and occurs frequently as a complication of alcoholism, causes ataxia of gait, paresis of ocular movements, and loss of recent memory. If untreated, this disease leads to progressive coma and death, but if diagnosed and treated promptly, it can be reversed entirely. In addition to severe chronic alcoholism, Wernicke-Korsakoff disease can be found in people who have undergone gastric bypass procedures for obesity. Some of these people become progressively malnourished, and their stores of thiamine drop to critical levels, thus triggering the onset of Wernicke-Korsakoff disease.

SECTION 5

Forebrain

17

Basal Ganglia

Case Study

A 55-year-old man develops a feeling of stiffness and clumsiness of his left hand, and, when sitting still, he observes a tremor involving the wrist and fingers of this hand. About the same time, he also begins to scuff his left foot on the floor occasionally while walking. About 1 year later, the tremor has become constant, and he trips occasionally because of misplacement of the left foot. He consults a neurologist, who notes that the patient has a somewhat immobile face and that he blinks infrequently. The neurologist also finds a four- to six-cycle per second tremor of the left wrist and fingers, mild rigidity on passive manipulation of the left arm and leg, and slowness of fine finger movements of both hands.

Which part of this man's nervous system is responsible for these symptoms? What has caused these symptoms? Is this condition treatable?

Overview

The **basal ganglia** comprise a network of subcortical nuclei of the telencephalon, subthalamus, and midbrain that modulate motor and cognitive functions of the cerebral cortex. Whereas the cerebral cortex influences motor function directly through the corticospinal and corticobulbar pathways, the basal ganglia and the cerebellum influence lower motoneurons indirectly through modulation of the cerebral cortex and brainstem. Recurrent circuits accomplish cortical modulation through cortical–brain stem–cerebellar–thalamic–cortical and cortical–basal ganglia–thalamic–cortical loops. Although tightly integrated, these cerebellar and basal ganglia loops perform different functions; hence diseases affecting them produce distinctive neurologic deficits.

Both the cerebellum and the basal ganglia also project to the brain stem. In contrast to the major influence the cerebellum exerts over multiple descending brain stem pathways (rubrospinal, vestibulospinal, and reticulospinal), the basal ganglia make limited brain stem connections, and these principally involve the reticular formation and the superior colliculus. Compelling evidence indicates that the basal ganglia participate in cognitive functioning, but relatively little solid information has been acquired about this, particularly in comparison with the role of the basal ganglia in motor functioning.

Traditionally, clinicians have divided the motor system into two groups of circuits: the **pyra-**

midal system and the **extrapyramidal system.** The pyramidal system consists of the corticobulbar and corticospinal pathways. The extrapyramidal system includes all other projection pathways that influence motor control, including the basal ganglia and the projection pathways from brain stem to spinal cord (e.g., rubrospinal, reticulospinal, vestibulospinal, and tectospinal tracts). Physiologically, extrapyramidal neuronal circuits interact closely with those of the pyramidal system, and separating them must be viewed as artificial. Nevertheless, distinguishing disorders of the extrapyramidal system from those of the pyramidal system makes good clinical sense, because diseases affecting these two systems present with distinctive and separable clinical signs.

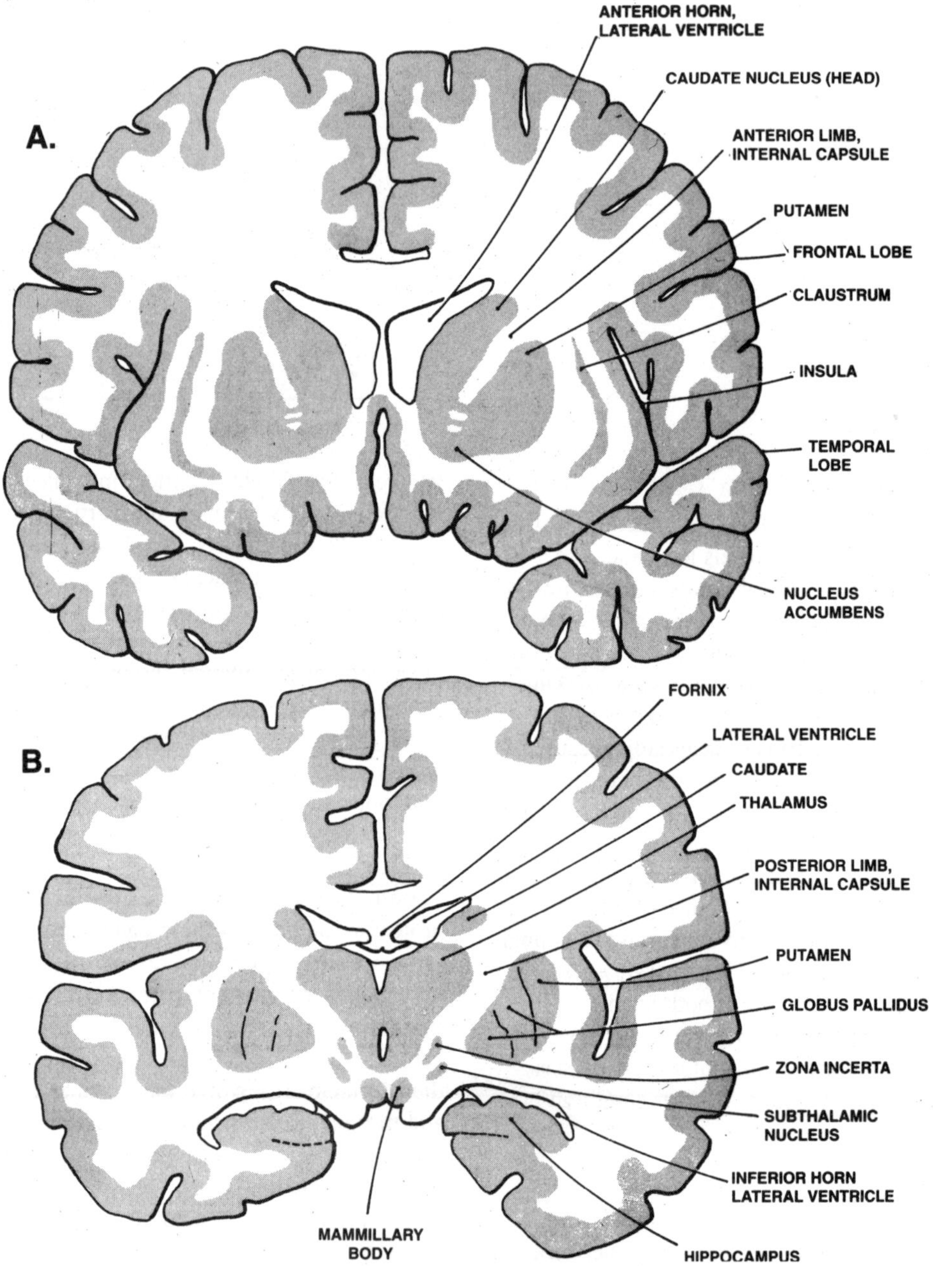

■ **FIGURE 17–1.** Two coronal sections through the cerebral hemispheres. **(A)** Section through the rostral part of the frontal lobe shows the relation of the caudate nucleus, putamen, and nucleus accumbens to the surrounding telencephalic structures. **(B)** Section through the caudal part of the frontal lobe shows the location of the lentiform nucleus lateral to, and the body of the caudate nucleus dorsal to, the diencephalon.

Components

The largest nuclei of the basal ganglia lie deep within the telencephalon and extend to the base of the cerebral hemisphere. These nuclei include the **dorsal striatum** (**caudate nucleus** and **putamen**), the **ventral striatum** (**nucleus accumbens** and **anterior perforated substance**), the **dorsal pallidum** (**globus pallidus**) and the **ventral pallidum.** Several other subcortical nuclei, the **subthalamic nucleus,** the **substantia nigra,** and the **ventral tegmental area,** reside at the interface between the diencephalon and midbrain. Intimately interconnected anatomically and functionally with the striatum and pallidum, these nuclei constitute part of the basal ganglia. Table 17–1 provides a guide to the terminology associated with the basal ganglia used in this book.

■ TABLE 17-1. BASAL GANGLIA NOMENCLATURE

Term	Components
Dorsal striatum	Caudate nucleus and putamen
Dorsal pallidum	Globus pallidus, pars externa, and pars interna
Lenticular (lentiform) nucleus	Putamen and globus pallidus
Ventral striatum	Nucleus accumbens and anterior perforated substance*
Ventral pallidum	
Substantia nigra	Pars compacta and pars reticulata
Ventral tegmental area	
Subthalamic nucleus	

* In most nonprimate mammals, the entire area equivalent to the anterior perforated space of the human brain receives direct projections from the olfactory bulb and is called the olfactory tubercle. In the human, olfactory projections are limited to the lateral part of this area, adjacent to the piriform cortex (see Fig. 22–1).

Dorsal Striatum and Pallidum

The **caudate nucleus** occupies a position in the floor of the lateral ventricle (Figs. 17–1B, 17–2, and 17–3). The bulge at the cephalic end of the caudate nucleus comprises the **head** (Figs. 17–1A and 17–2). The **body** passes backward, dorsolateral to the thalamus (Figs. 17–1B and 17–3), and tapers gradually to form the **tail,** which curves ventrally, follows the inferior horn of the lateral ventricle into the temporal lobe, and ends near the amygdala.

The putamen and globus pallidus together form the **lenticular,** or **lentiform, nucleus** (Figs. 17–1B and 17–3), a thumb-sized mass wedged against the lateral side of the internal capsule. Fibers of the internal capsule separate the lenticular nucleus from the caudate nucleus, except in the cephalic part, where cell bridges through the anterior limb of the internal capsule fuse the caudate nucleus and putamen together.

The **putamen** constitutes the lateral portion of the lenticular nucleus and presents the same

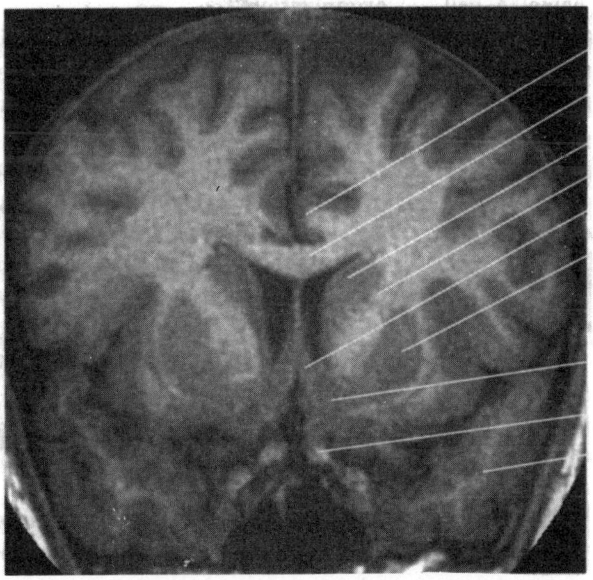

■ **FIGURE 17-2.** A T1-weighted (spoiled gradient echo) magnetic resonance image. This coronal sequence, from a neurologically normal adult, shows the dorsal striatum (caudate and putamen) and the ventral striatum (nucleus accumbens and anterior perforated substance) in the frontal lobe of the cerebral hemisphere. Compare with Figure 17–1A.

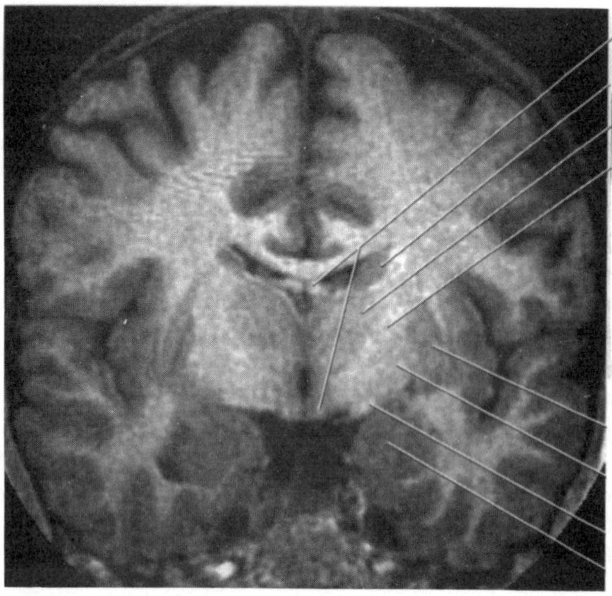

■ **FIGURE 17–3.** A T1-weighted (spoiled gradient echo) magnetic resonance image. This coronal sequence, from a neurologically normal adult, shows the dorsal striatum (caudate and putamen) and the globus pallidus of the basal ganglia. Compare with Figure 17–1B.

histologic appearance as the caudate nucleus, with numerous, densely packed, small neurons. The **globus pallidus,** in the medial region of the lenticular nucleus, contains sparsely distributed large cells traversed by many myelinated fibers. These fiber bundles account for the pale appearance of the globus pallidus in the fresh state, a characteristic that determined its name. A cell-sparse lamina separates the globus pallidus from the putamen, and a similar lamina divides the globus pallidus into two parts: the **globus pallidus pars externa** and the **globus pallidus pars interna.**

Connections of the Dorsal Striatum and Pallidum with the Cerebral Cortex

The striatum receives the major inputs to the basal ganglia. The cerebral cortex, thalamus, and substantia nigra provide these afferents.

The Dorsal Striatum (Putamen and Caudate) Receives Excitatory Input from the Isocortex

Axons project to the dorsal striatum from neurons in all areas of the isocortex, but most heavily from the frontal and parietal lobes. The primary motor (area 4), premotor (lateral area 6), supplementary motor (medial area 6), and somatosensory (areas 3, 1, and 2) cortices project preferentially to the putamen (Fig. 17–4). In contrast, the frontal eye fields and association areas of the frontal and parietal lobes project heavily onto the caudate nucleus. These projections have a **topographic organization.**

The neurons projecting from isocortex to striatum provide strong **excitation,** using **glutamate** as their neurotransmitter. Stimulation of cerebral cortical neurons evokes in striatal neurons sequences of excitatory postsynaptic potentials followed by inhibitory postsynaptic potentials. The excitatory postsynaptic potentials result from the actions of excitatory glutamatergic cortical efferents and the inhibitory postsynaptic potentials from gamma-aminobutyric acid (GABA)–ergic interneurons in the striatum.

The Dorsal Striatum Inhibits the Substantia Nigra Reticulata and the Globus Pallidus

Groups of neurons in the striatum project to the substantia nigra pars reticulata and to the external and internal segments of the globus pallidus. These projections continue the **topographic organization** initiated in the isocortex to the dorsal striatum, from the striatum to the globus pallidus–

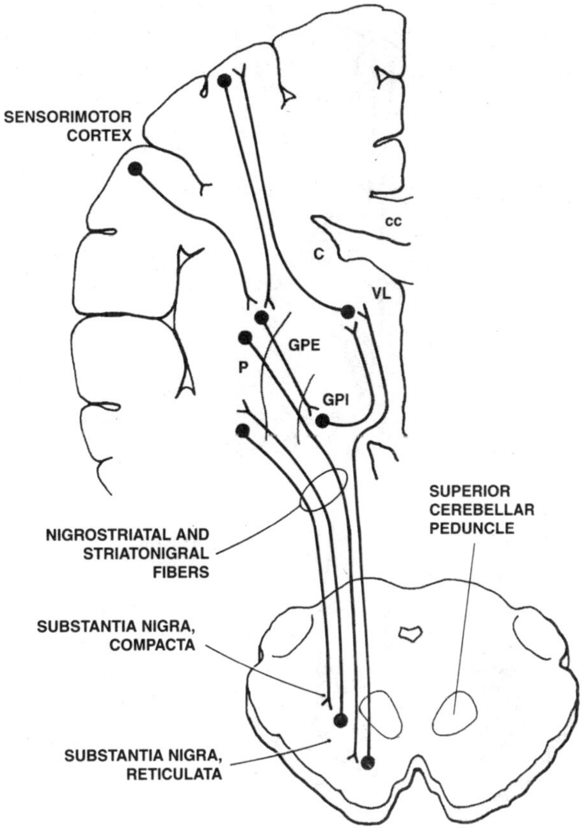

■ **FIGURE 17–4.** The direct loop through the putamen and the connections of the striatum with the substantia nigra pars compacta. The striatonigral fibers represented in this diagram arise in the putamen. However, most striatonigral fibers arise from the caudate. C = caudate nucleus; cc = corpus callosum; GPe = globus pallidus pars externa; GPi = globus pallidus pars interna; P = putamen; VL = ventral lateral nucleus of the thalamus.

substantia nigra reticulata, and from these nuclei to the thalamus.

Neurons projecting from the striatum to the external segment of the pallidum provide **inhibition** using the neurotransmitters **GABA** and **enkephalin.** Projections from the striatum to the internal segment of the pallidum and the substantial nigra also provide inhibition, but they use the neurotransmitters **GABA** and **substance P.** Many of the interneurons within the striatum provoke **excitation** using the neurotransmitter **acetylcholine.**

The Substantia Nigra and Globus Pallidus Influence the Thalamus

A major outflow of efferent fibers from the basal ganglia comes from the internal segment of the globus pallidus and the substantia nigra pars reticulata. Both these areas develop in the caudal ventral diencephalon region called the **subthalamus.** As development proceeds, the fibers of the internal capsule pass between them and thus separate them in the mature brain, but their connections and functions nevertheless develop in synchrony. Efferents from these nuclei stream across and ventral to the internal capsule, around the zona incerta and into the **thalamic fasciculus** (Fig. 17–5), where fibers traveling from the cerebellar nuclei to the thalamus join them. The fibers from the globus pallidus interna and the substantia nigra reticulata synapse in the **intralaminar** nuclei (including the centromedian) and in the **ventral lateral, ventral anterior,** and **mediodorsal** nuclei of the thalamus. Axons from cells of the intralaminar nuclei provide feedback to the striatum (not shown in Fig. 17–5), whereas those of the ventral lateral, ventral anterior, and mediodorsal nuclei complete the ''basal ganglia loop'' by projecting to frontal lobe cortex (Fig. 20–4).

The Direct Loop Disinhibits (Excites) Thalamocortical Projections to the Cortex

Figure 17–4 illustrates an example of this simple circuit, called the **direct loop,** in which excitatory glutamatergic fibers from several functionally related areas of the isocortex converge on a particular region of the dorsal striatum (the putamen in this illustration). GABAergic neurons

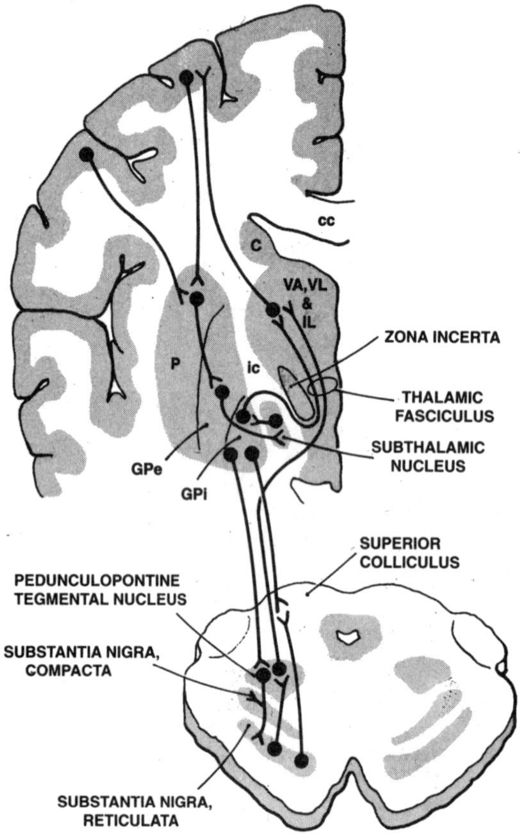

■ **FIGURE 17–5.** The indirect loop through the subthalamic nucleus; also represented are the efferents from the globus pallidus interna and substantia nigra pars reticulata to the superior colliculus and midbrain tegmentum. C = caudate nucleus; GPe = globus pallidus pars externa; GPi = globus pallidus pars interna; ic = internal capsule; IL = intralaminar nuclei of the thalamus; P = putamen; VA = ventral anterior nucleus of the thalamus; VL = ventral lateral nucleus of the thalamus.

in this striatal region, in turn, project to and inhibit neurons in discrete areas of the globus pallidus interna and the substantia nigra reticulata. These areas then provide GABAergic projections to inhibit discrete targets in the thalamus.

Striatal inhibition of GABAergic pallidothalamic and nigrothalamic projections removes the inhibiting effects of these projections on thalamocortical glutamatergic cells. The term **disinhibition,** meaning inhibition of an inhibiting projection, describes this effect. The disinhibition of thalamic neurons leads to excitation of a discrete target within the broader area of cerebral cortex at the origin of the loop. **Through the direct loop, then, information from several functionally related cortical areas funnels through one sector of the basal ganglia and results in recurrent excitation of one of these cortical regions.**

The direct loop schematically represented in Figure 17–4 flows through the putamen. This loop originates in the sensorimotor cortex, which includes the primary motor, primary somatosensory, premotor, and supplementary motor cortices. All these areas contribute input to the putamen, but the outflow of this direct loop reaches only specific parts of the ventral lateral nucleus of the thalamus and, through this nucleus, projects primarily to the supplementary motor area in Brodmann's area 6.

Basal Ganglia Loops Modulate Function in Different Regions of the Cerebral Cortex

Five distinct basal ganglia loops, four through the dorsal striatum and one through the ventral striatum, can be distinguished by the functions of the cortical areas they modulate. The cortical targets of the four loops through the dorsal striatum include the **supplementary motor area,** the **dorsolateral prefrontal cortex,** the **frontal eye fields,** and the **lateral orbitofrontal cortex.** By inference, these loops can be described as **motor, cognitive/executive, oculomotor,** and **emotional/social,** respectively.

Although anatomically and functionally distinctive, these loops remain integrated pathways, not segregated or isolated. Each loop flows through its own preferred subdivisions of the striatum (e.g., putamen, head of caudate nucleus, or body of caudate nucleus), globus pallidus interna–substantia nigra reticulata, and thalamus (ventral lateral, ventral anterior, and/or mediodorsal nuclei). At each level (especially cortical and thalamic levels), intrinsic interconnections between their separate target zones interdigitate the loops.

An Indirect Loop Inhibits Thalamocortical Neurons

Each of the basal ganglia loops includes both direct loop and **indirect loop** fibers. The indirect loop can be viewed as a side arm of the direct loop, through which the subthalamic nucleus influences the outflow of the globus pallidus interna (Figs. 17–5 and 17–6). Striatal efferents reach the **external segment of the globus pallidus,** and after synaptic articulation, pallidal efferents cross the posterior limb of the internal capsule to reach the **subthalamic nucleus.** Neurons of the subthalamic nucleus project **excitatory glutamatergic** fibers back to both parts of the globus pallidus, but primarily to the internal segment and to the substantia nigra reticulata, where they excite GABAergic projections to the thalamus and thereby inhibit the thalamus. The subthalamic nucleus also receives direct input from the cerebral cortex. **The net result of activation of this indirect loop is to decrease thalamocortical activation.**

Dopaminergic Nigrostriatal Connections Modulate the Direct and Indirect Loops

The cells of the **substantia nigra compacta** produce **dopamine.** Their projections to the dorsal striatum enhance cerebral cortical activation through both the direct and the indirect loops. This results from differences in the types of striatal receptors that receive nigrostriatal dopaminergic input. Dopaminergic projections **excite** striatal cells of the direct (excitatory) loop

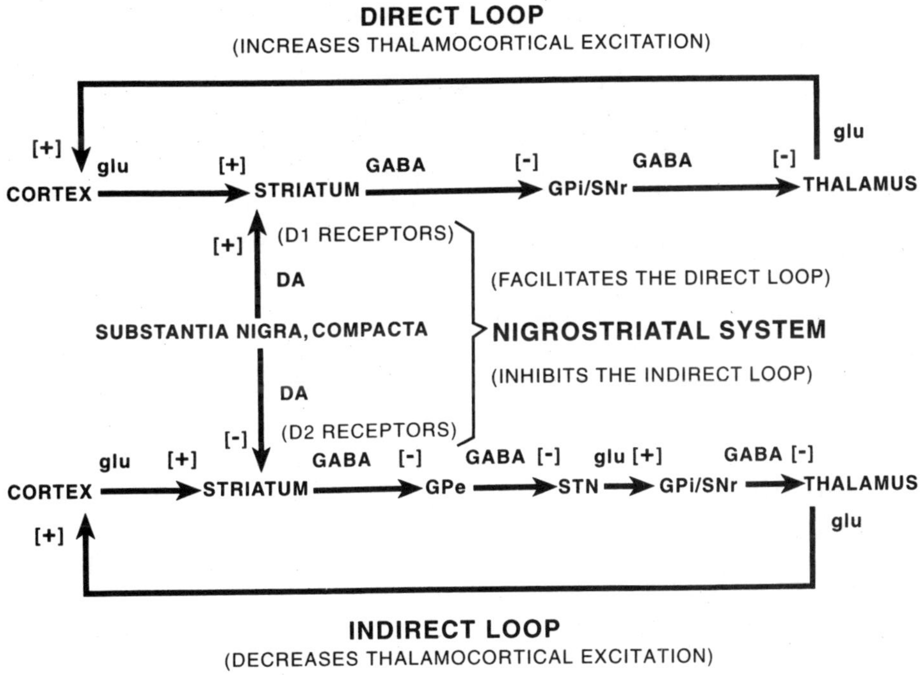

■ **FIGURE 17–6.** The nigrostriatal dopaminergic projections have opposite effects on the direct loop and the indirect loop of the basal ganglia, but the same net excitatory effect on thalamocortical projections. Dopamine facilitates the direct loop (which is an excitatory loop) by acting at D1 receptors on striatal cells that control this loop, whereas it inhibits the cells of the indirect loop (which is an inhibitory loop) through its action at D2 receptors. DA = dopamine; GABA = gamma-aminobutyric acid; glu = glutamate; GPe = globus pallidus pars externa; GPi = globus pallidus pars interna; SNr = substantia nigra pars reticulata; STN = subthalamic nucleus.

through D1 receptors on these cells, and they **inhibit** striatal cells of the indirect (inhibitory) loop through D2 receptors on these cells (Figs. 17–4 and 17–6).

Connections of the Pallidum with the Brain Stem

Important projections of the globus pallidus interna–substantia nigra reticulata descend into the midbrain, where they terminate in the superior colliculus and the pedunculopontine tegmental nucleus (Fig. 17–5). The projections of substantia nigra reticulata to the **superior colliculus** contribute to the regulation of saccadic eye movements. (See Chapter 19.)

The **pedunculopontine tegmental nucleus** belongs to a midbrain region that coordinates states of arousal with fundamental motor patterns. The nucleus contains **cholinergic neurons** that project to the brain stem reticular formation, where they influence eye movements and both trunk and limb musculature during rapid-eye-movement sleep and wakefulness. Pedunculopontine tegmental neurons also project rostrally to other cholinergic neurons at the base of the forebrain (in the basal nucleus of Meynert) that induce arousal by widespread activation of the cerebral cortex; and they influence sensory and motor processing through connections to the posterior and lateral parts of the thalamus. Pedunculopontine tegmental nucleus neurons also excite other parts of the basal ganglia, including the substantia nigra compacta (see Fig. 23–1).

Ventral Striatum and Pallidum

The circuitry of the dorsal striatum described earlier receives input from the motor, sensory, and association areas of the frontal, parietal, occipital, and lateral temporal lobes. These are all isocortical areas. The **allocortex,** or **limbic lobe,** and ventral areas of the temporal lobe project to the **ventral striatum,** which includes the **nucleus accumbens** and the **anterior perforated substance** (Fig. 17–1A). This constitutes the fifth of the five functionally defined basal ganglia loops, and by modulating the **limbic cortex,** it participates in motivational and visceral functions associated with emotion.

In general, the circuitry of the ventral striatum and pallidum parallels that of the dorsal. Like the dorsal striatum, the ventral striatum receives afferents from the intralaminar nuclei of the thalamus as well as from the cerebral cortex, and it projects to the substantia nigra reticulata, the globus pallidus, and the ventral extension of the globus pallidus, the **ventral pallidum.** Through direct and indirect loops, these pallidal regions control specific parts of the ventral anterior and mediodorsal nuclei of thalamus that modulate the anterior cingulate gyrus and medial orbitofrontal gyri (see Fig. 20–4). Both the ventral pallidum and the nucleus accumbens provide input into the pedunculopontine tegmental nucleus.

The ventral striatum also parallels the dorsal striatum in having reciprocal connections with a dopaminergic cell group in the midbrain, but in this circuit most of the dopaminergic neurons reside in the **ventral tegmental area,** a nuclear area medial to the substantia nigra compacta. In parallel with the nigrostriatal fibers, these ventral tegmental area neurons project back to the nucleus accumbens and anterior perforated substance. In addition, these neurons, along with some medial cells in the substantia nigra compacta, make projections that profoundly and directly affect the cerebral cortex, especially the frontal and limbic lobes. This is the **mesocortical dopaminergic system** (see Fig. 23–2).

The ventral striatum and pallidum modulate cerebral cortical areas that participate in motivation, mood, affect, and in social behaviors and visceral functions associated with emotional states. These structures also participate in behaviors associated with addiction to substances of abuse.

Function and Dysfunction

As described earlier in this chapter, the basal ganglia can be viewed as participants in a series of parallel pathways extending from cerebral cortex to basal ganglia, then to thalamus and back to the cerebral cortex. These pathways collect information from multiple forebrain structures, process this information through the basal ganglia, and move it back to the cerebral cortex. These pathways participate in the control of movements and in certain cognitive functions.

Physiologic Properties of Basal Ganglia Neurons

Recordings from neurons in the basal ganglia of experimental animals during various motor tasks reveal that the discharge of single cells in the neostriatum correlates directly with movements of the contralateral arm or leg. Neuronal activity related to movement usually occurs at the same time as the movement or even slightly after movement has occurred. Neuronal activity also has been related to learned cues and to behavioral context and motivation. These findings suggest that the basal ganglia monitor the progress of movements and participate in the sequencing and automatic execution of learned motor plans.

The Basal Ganglia Regulate Sequences of Movement and Influence Cognition

The movements influenced by the basal ganglia include those related to posture, automatic movements (e.g., swinging the arms while walking), and skilled volitional movements of the trunk and limbs, including eye movements. The basal ganglia also participate in cognition, a function that may be mediated through the circuits connecting these nuclei with the prefrontal cortex.

Diseases

Diseases of the basal ganglia in humans cause difficulty in initiating movements, disturbances in continuing or stopping ongoing movements, abnormalities of muscle tone (rigidity), and development of involuntary movements (tremor or chorea). These disorders can be divided into three functional categories: (1) parkinsonism; (2) hyperkinetic movement disorders, including ballism, chorea, and athetosis; and (3) dystonia. Parkinsonism results from degeneration of the substantia nigra or interference with dopaminergic neurotransmission in the striatum. The hyperkinetic movement disorders result from striatal or subthalamic dysfunction. Dystonia results from pallidal dysfunction but can occur with disorders of other component parts of the basal ganglia.

Parkinsonism

A common neurodegenerative disorder of undetermined cause, **Parkinson's disease,** or paralysis agitans, affects principally older people. The neuropathologic changes consist of degeneration (neuronal loss and depigmentation) in the substantia nigra and locus ceruleus with inclusions **(Lewy bodies)** in remaining neurons. The pathologic changes in the substantia nigra involve dopaminergic neurons that project to the striatum and thus lead to the depletion of dopamine in the caudate nucleus and putamen. The depletion of dopamine leads to complex changes in the activity of striatal projection neurons, with similar effects on thalamocortical projections over both the direct pathway and the indirect pathway. In the direct pathway, **decreased** nigrostriatal **excitation** of D1 receptors decreases the striatal inhibition of neurons in the internal segment of the globus pallidus and the substantia nigra reticulata. Consequently, the pallidothalamic and nigrothalamic inhibition of thalamocortical neurons becomes enhanced.

The end result is decreased cerebral cortical excitation over thalamocortical projection fibers. In the indirect pathway, **decreased** nigrostriatal **inhibition** of D2 receptors increases the striatal inhibition of neurons in the external segment of the globus pallidus. This decreases the inhibitory effects of external segment pallidal neurons on subthalamic nucleus neurons and thereby enhances the excitatory effects of subthalamic projections on the internal segment of the globus pallidus and the substantia nigra reticulata. Consequently, the pallidothalamic and nigrothalamic inhibition of thalamocortical neurons becomes enhanced. The end result is decreased cerebral cortical excitation over thalamocortical projection fibers.

Patients with Parkinson's disease develop **bradykinesia** (slowness of movement), rigidity, gait instability, and tremor, usually beginning first on one side of the body, then affecting the other. These symptoms improve markedly with administration of levodopa. The bradykinesia becomes apparent with difficulty in initiating and performing volitional movements of the most common type, including standing, walking, eating, and writing. The lines of the patient's face become smooth, the expression becomes fixed (the so-called masked face), and the facial expression gives little overt evidence of spontaneous emotional responses. The patient stands with the head and shoulders stooped and walks with short, shuffling steps. The arms remain at the sides with walking and do not automatically swing in rhythm with the legs, as they should. Although patients have difficulty in starting to take their first steps, once they are under way, the pace becomes more and more rapid, and patients have trouble stopping, even though they have reached their goal. This abnormality of walking has been termed a **festinating gait.**

Rigidity of the limbs (i.e., increased resistance to passive movement) can be found in most patients with Parkinson's disease and often consists of **cogwheel rigidity.** When the examiner passively flexes or extends one of the patient's extremities, an increased resistance occurs that suddenly gives way and then returns sequentially as the movement continues, in the manner of a cogwheel. The muscle stretch (deep tendon) reflexes usually are normal. The **tremor** of Parkinson's disease typically occurs when the patient sits at rest and consists of four- to six-cycle per second flexion and extension movements of the fingers and wrists, at times in the form of a ''pill-rolling'' movement.

Treatment of Parkinson's disease consists of the administration of medications that enhance striatal dopaminergic activity. These include a combination of levodopa and carbidopa, the latter to prevent hepatic inactivation of levodopa. Multiple other medications have been developed to overcome some of the side effects of this medication.

Surgical therapy, consisting of the placement of a lesion in the globus pallidus or ventrolateral nucleus of the thalamus, was used extensively in the past in treating the symptoms of Parkinson's disease. Discovery of the utility of levodopa caused the surgical approach to fall into disuse, but a resurgence of interest has resulted from the finding that patients become less responsive to levodopa and related medications over time. Moreover, dopaminergic medications cause marked involuntary movements (dyskinesias), which worsen with time, and titrating the level of drug sufficient to improve symptoms without inducing dyskinesias becomes increasingly difficult as the disease continues. Currently, surgical approaches include placing a lesion in the basal ganglia or thalamus and implanting stimulating electrodes in the subthalamic nucleus for chronic stimulation. High frequency stimulation of the subthalamic nucleus inhibits these neurons, thereby decreasing their excitation of the globus pallidus interna and substantia nigra reticulata. Both approaches have been shown to benefit the symptoms of Parkinson's disease in the late stages of the disorder. Implantation in the striatum of fetal tissue that produces dopamine has been attempted, but the results generally have been disappointing.

A severe form of parkinsonism has been described in young adults who have taken intravenous recreational drugs. Improper synthesis of a synthetic heroin-like compound results in the production of 1-methyl-4-phenyl-1,2,3,6-tetrahydropyridine. This drug causes severe degeneration of the dopaminergic neurons of the substantia nigra. Other neurodegenerative diseases can also cause parkinsonism, including progressive supranuclear palsy and multiple system atrophy. A form of parkinsonism has been described as the result of multiple small infarctions affecting the basal ganglia.

Hyperkinetic Movement Disorders

The **hyperkinetic movement** disorders include **ballism, chorea,** and **athetosis.** These disorders may share a pathophysiologic mechanism consisting of decreased activity of the subthalamic nucleus. Decreased subthalamic nucleus function can result from destruction of the structure, as when a small stroke affects this structure and causes **hemiballismus,** which is a series of flinging movements of the arm and leg of one side. Dysfunction of subthalamic nucleus neurons causes loss of subthalamic excitation on the internal segment of the globus pallidus and substantia nigra pars reticulata. The result is **disinhibition** of thalamocortical neurons that thereby excessively enhances their excitatory effects on the cerebral cortex.

A movement disorder that can result from disease of the basal ganglia, **chorea** consists of a rapid, irregular flow of motions, including ''piano-playing'' flexion and extension movements of the fingers, elevation and depression of the shoulders and hips, crossing and uncrossing of the legs, and grimacing movements of the face. **Sydenham's chorea** occurs in children as a complication of rheumatic fever, but the disease is self-limited, and recovery is complete. A disorder inherited as an autosomal dominant trait, **Huntington's disease** frequently presents in adult life with severe depression and progresses to include involuntary choreiform movements and progressive dementia. The disorder can begin in childhood, but it usually presents more in children with hypokinetic and dystonic movements than in those with choreic movements. The genetic locus responsible for the disease has been found, and the gene product, huntingtin, has been characterized. The neuropathologic features consist of marked degenerative changes in the basal ganglia, particularly in the caudate nucleus and putamen, which show profound destruction of striatal GABAergic neurons. This change leads to disinhibition of neurons in the external segment of the pallidum. These latter neurons excessively inhibit subthalamic neurons, thereby reducing excitatory drive to the internal segment of the globus pallidus and substantia nigra pars reticulata. The result of this is disinhibition of thalamocortical neurons.

Hemichorea consists of choreiform movements limited to one side of the body, usually resulting from a vascular lesion of the contralateral basal ganglia. The disorder usually occurs abruptly in middle age, and weakness of the affected limbs often accompanies the involuntary movements.

Athetosis consists of a movement disorder characterized by slow, writhing movements of a worm-like character involving the extremities, trunk, and neck. Athetosis frequently occurs in cerebral palsy and results from brain damage that occurred at birth as a result of hypoxia and ischemia. The pathologic changes involve the cerebral cortex and the basal ganglia. **Tics** consist of repetitive movements or vocalizations, usually of undetermined cause. The repetitive movements can be subtle or obvious, with repetitive blinking, twitching of the face, trunk, or limbs, clearing of the throat, and even word production. Tics likely result from disorders of the basal ganglia, and increased dopaminergic nigrostriatal activity may underlie this movement disorder. **Tourette's syndrome** consists of repetitive tics with vocalization, usually beginning in childhood and at times diminishing or disappearing with age.

Dystonia

The **dystonias** consist of postural and movement disorders frequently beginning in childhood and characterized by fixed or relatively fixed postures of the trunk and limbs. In some dystonias, a combination of athetosis and dystonia occurs simultaneously. One of the most common causes of dystonia is **cerebral palsy,** a disorder associated with prematurity and stemming from hypoxic or ischemic insults to the brain either in utero or in the perinatal period. Afflicted children frequently show delayed developmental milestones, with varying degrees of spasticity and rigidity, athetosis, and dystonia occurring with growth and development. Speech commonly becomes affected, but intellect can be entirely normal. Common forms of cerebral palsy include bilateral hemiplegic postures with spasticity (flexion of the upper limbs, extension of the lower limbs) and **double athetosis,** with moderately fixed postures in flexion of all limbs, along with abnormal involuntary movements of the athetotic type. Another dystonia, **dystonia musculorum deformans,** presents in childhood as a dominantly inherited disorder or as a sporadic disorder. Slowly progressive, the disorder can cause severe contortions of the limbs, with progressive difficulty in the use of the arms and legs that leads to complete immobility in severe cases. Dystonias can appear in adult life in either focal areas of the body or in more generalized forms. The most frequent focal form of dystonia is **spasmodic torticollis** or wryneck. Injection of botulinum toxin into dystonic muscles has proven highly effective in relieving the symptoms of many focal dystonias.

Case Follow-up

The patient described at the beginning of this chapter has a movement disorder resulting from disease of the basal ganglia. The history and findings are characteristic of Parkinson's disease. Because the symptoms were mild when the patient first received the diagnosis, the only treatments recommended were physical therapy and active exercise. Over the next 2 years, progressive involvement of the right limbs interfered with the patient's business activities, and the neurologist administered a combination of levodopa and carbidopa. This medication relieved the symptoms almost completely, and the patient was able to continue his business, leisure, and family-related activities. He continues to do well now, approximately 10 years after the diagnosis was made.

18

Vision

Case Study

A 25-year-old woman has a traffic accident when she passes through an intersection without noticing that an automobile on her right has already proceeded through the intersection. She frequently bumps into walls when rounding corners going to either the left or the right, and she finds that her golf game is deteriorating. She consults a neurologist, who finds an abnormality in her visual fields. Although she has preserved central vision, she cannot see even large moving objects in the temporal (outer) fields of both eyes.

What part of the nervous system has been affected? What has caused this problem? Can it be treated?

Overview of the Visual Pathways

For vision to occur, reflected rays of light from an object must reach the eye, pass through the **cornea** and **lens,** where refraction occurs, and form an image on the retina. The optical properties of the lens invert and reverse the projection of the visual field on the retina; hence the image forms upside down (inverted) and turned left for right (reversed). Thus, light entering the superior half of the visual field projects onto the inferior half of the retina, and light entering the inferior half of the visual field reaches the superior half of the retina. Similarly, light from the left half of the visual field projects onto the right (nasal) half of the left retina and right (temporal) half of the right retina (Fig. 18–1, colored lines), and this information passes along to the right cerebral hemisphere. The reverse occurs in the right half of the visual field. The organization of the entire visual path within the brain conforms to the peripheral optical system, so the right hemisphere receives inverted images of objects that lie to the left. The organization of other systems of the brain matches this apparent reversal and inversion of position. Thus, the motor areas of the frontal lobes and the somesthetic zones of the parietal lobes contain inverted and reversed representations of body parts.

Retina

Light Hyperpolarizes Rods and Cones

The human **retina** develops from the optic vesicles, which grow out of the prosencephalon. Thus, the retina forms as an extension of the central nervous system. It contains two types of photoreceptors: **rods** and **cones.** Cones mediate color vision and provide high visual acuity. Rods mediate light perception; they provide low visual acuity with good perception of contrasts and function chiefly in nocturnal vision. The retina has an overall ratio of rods to cones of 20 to 1, but the **fovea centralis** within the **macula,** a specialized region in the retina adapted for high visual acuity, contains only cones, whereas the periphery of the retina contains primarily rods.

Both rods and cones respond to light because they contain visual pigments that can trap photons of light. Rods contain a single type of pigment, **rhodopsin,** whereas three different types of cones contain three forms of the pigment **iodopsin.** Each type of iodopsin absorbs light maximally in a different part of the visible light spectrum (i.e., light of a different color). The absorption of light by the visual pigments in both rods and cones

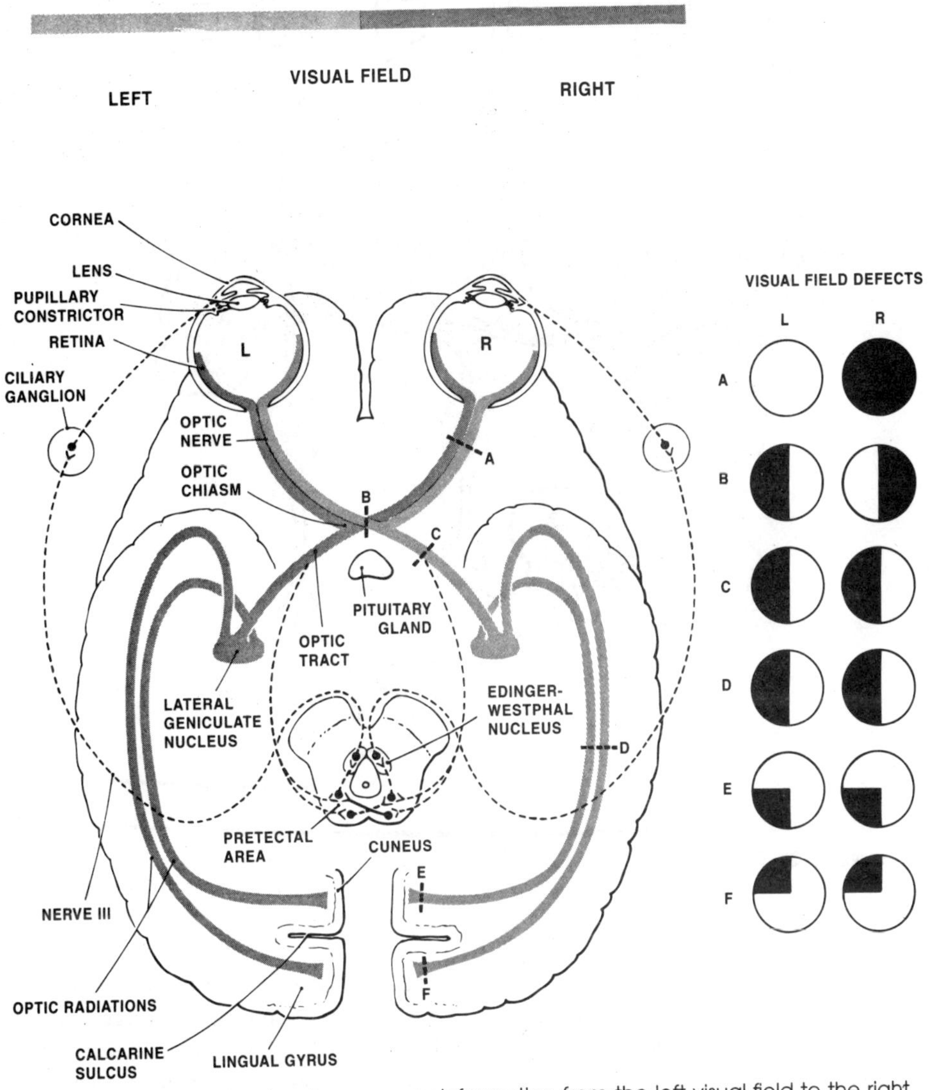

■ **FIGURE 18–1.** The visual pathways carry information from the left visual field to the right visual cortex *(colored lines)* and from the right visual field to the left visual cortex. Lesions (**A** through **F**) along the pathway from the eye to the visual cortex cause deficits in the visual fields shown as *black areas* on the corresponding visual field diagrams. The diagram also shows the pathway through the pretectum and cranial nerve III, which mediates reflex constriction of the pupil in response to light. This reflex pathway is described in Chapter 19.

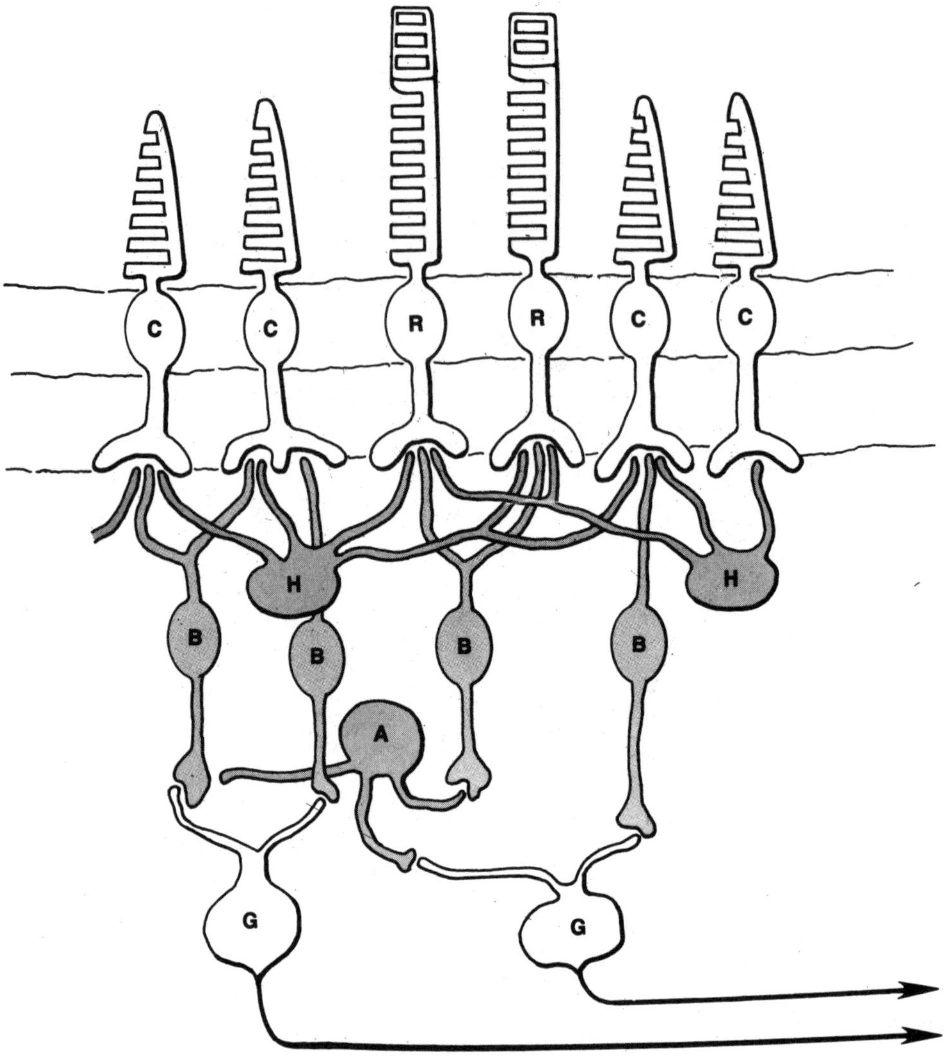

■ **FIGURE 18–2.** Six basic cell types form the circuitry of the retina. A = amacrine cell; B = bipolar cell; C = cone receptor cell; G = ganglion cell; H = horizontal cell; R = rod receptor cell.

isomerizes the pigment molecules. A cascade of chemical reactions initiated by this isomerization decreases the sodium conductance of the receptor cell membrane, which leads to a slow hyperpolarization, or a graded potential, across the cell. Most retinal cells transmit information by using graded potentials, in contrast to most other neurons of the central nervous system, which use action potentials to transfer information.

Rods and Cones Influence Retinal Ganglion Cells through Bipolar Cells

Figure 18–2 shows, in simplified form, the basic cell types in the retina and their interconnections. The activity of several **rods,** as many as 1500 in the peripheral retina, converges onto a single **bipolar cell,** which influences a **ganglion cell** through the **amacrine cell** interneurons. In contrast, individual **cones** connect singly and directly through bipolar cells to ganglion cells. These cells interact through both electrical and chemical synapses, where they generate graded potentials. Numerous neurotransmitters have been identified at the chemical synapses. The **receptor cells** and **bipolar cells** most likely use the excitatory amino acid glutamate at their chemical synapses as they transmit visual signals to ganglion cells. The intervening interneurons, the **horizontal cells** and amacrine cells, transmit signals in all directions equally well and apparently exert inhibitory actions by release of gamma-aminobutyric acid, although they also contain several other important neurotransmitter molecules, including dopamine, acetylcholine, and various neuropeptides.

Visual Pathways

Retinal Ganglion Cell Axons in the Optic Nerve Project to the Diencephalon and Midbrain

The functional circuits connecting rods and cones to **ganglion cells** process information about the color and contrast of images that fall on the retina. Thus, action potentials generated by ganglion cells provide highly processed information about visual images to the thalamus and brain stem. The axons of ganglion cells converge to form the **optic nerve head,** the first part of the **optic nerve.** Myelination occurs after the nerve exits from the eye (Fig. 18–1).

Optic nerve fibers from both eyes combine to form the **optic chiasm,** which lies superior to the anterior portion of the sella turcica of the sphenoid bone, immediately above the pituitary gland. A partial decussation (crossing) of fibers takes place in the chiasm. Fibers from the nasal halves of each retina cross; those from the temporal halves of each retina approach the chiasm, but leave it without crossing. At the level of the optic chiasm, a small number of ganglion cell axons terminate in the **suprachiasmatic nucleus of the hypothalamus,** where periods of ambient light and darkness entrain circadian rhythms.

Most axons, the crossed nasal and uncrossed temporal fibers, continue behind the chiasm as the **optic tracts.** The optic tracts terminate in the **lateral geniculate nuclei (LGNs) of the thalamus,** the **superior colliculus,** and the **pretectal area,** as well as on a series of nuclei along the optic tract that participate in optokinetic eye movements. (See Chapter 19.)

The Lateral Geniculate Nucleus Receives Retinotopically Organized Input

Large numbers of fibers in the optic tract terminate in the LGN. Each LGN receives inputs from the retina in an orderly **retinotopic pattern** representing the contralateral visual half-field. In other words, ganglion cells in adjacent areas of the retina project systematically on adjacent neurons in the LGN. Nevertheless, the LGN does not contain an equal reconstruction of all parts of the visual field; the central visual field, containing the fovea, has more extensive representation than the peripheral field, a feature that reflects the higher density of photoreceptors in the central field.

Each LGN contains six layers of neurons, and each layer receives input from one eye only. The optic tract fibers originating in the ipsilateral eye distribute only to layers 2, 3, and 5 of the six layers; those from the contralateral eye distribute to the remaining three layers—1, 4, and 6. Thus, LGN cells do not have binocular receptive fields.

The Superior Colliculus Uses Retinal Input to Influence the Visual Cortex, Cerebellum, and Oculomotor System

The **superior colliculus** receives direct, retinotopically organized input from the ipsilateral optic tract. It also has reciprocal connections with neurons in the visual cortex. The neurons in the superior colliculus receiving visual input project to motoneurons in the pons and spinal cord by way of the tectopontine and tectospinal tracts, respectively. The tectopontine projection relays visual information to the cerebellum and participates in the control of eye movements through the paramedian pontine reticular formation. (See Chapter 19.) The tectospinal tract mediates the reflex control of head and neck movements in response to visual inputs.

The Pretectal Area of the Midbrain Mediates Pupillary Reflexes

An important site for the mediation of pupillary reflexes, the **pretectal area,** resides just rostral to the superior colliculus, where the midbrain fuses with the thalamus. The pretectal area receives input from the optic tract (Fig. 18–1), and pretectal neurons project into the mesencephalon and reach the **Edinger-Westphal** nucleus, a component of the oculomotor complex bilaterally. Preganglionic parasympathetic neurons in the Edinger-Westphal nuclei project with the third nerve out of the brain stem to neurons in the **ciliary ganglion.** Ciliary postganglionic fibers project to the pupillary constrictor muscles and to the ciliary muscles, which control the shape of the

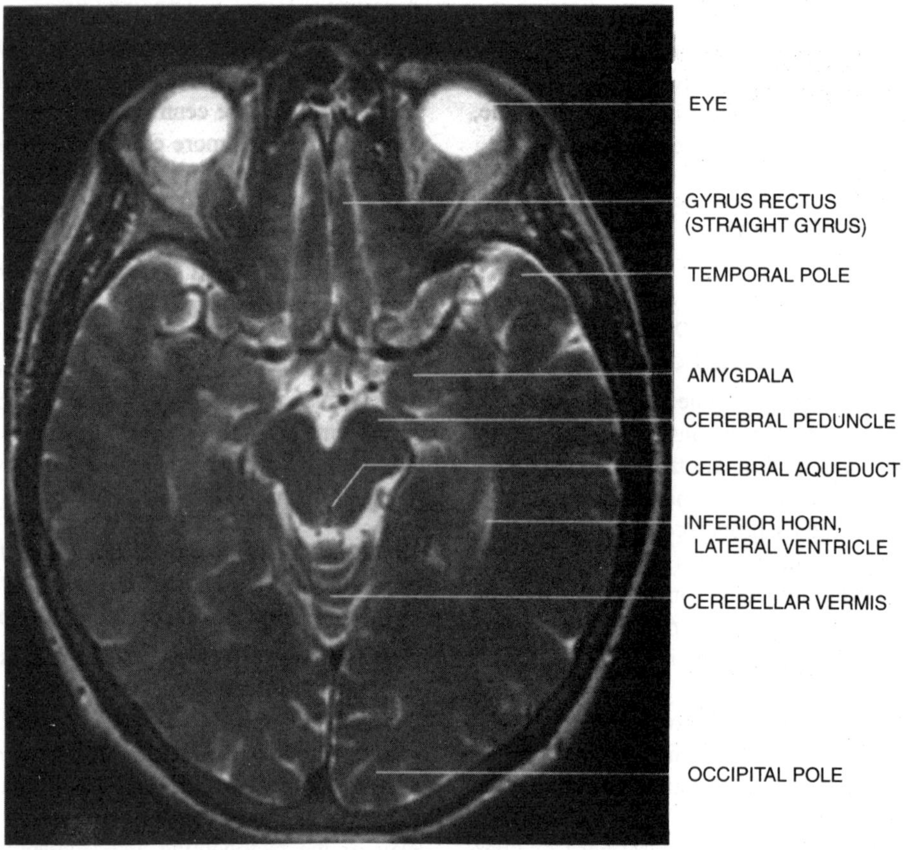

■ **FIGURE 18-3.** A T2-weighted magnetic resonance image in the axial plane from a neurologically normal adult illustrates the location of the optic radiations in the lateral wall of the lateral ventricle and the visual cortex on the medical surface of the occipital lobe.

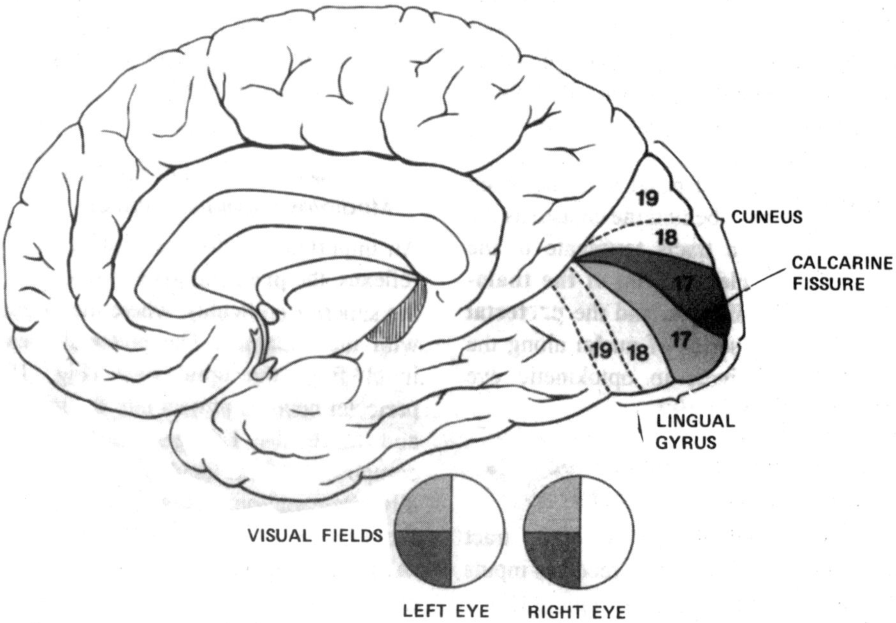

■ **FIGURE 18-4.** The visual cortex on the medial surface of the right occipital lobe. This brain area receives input from stimuli in the left half of the visual field of each eye.

lens. The reflexes mediated by the pretectal area are described in Chapter 19.

Optic Radiations and Visual Cortex

Neurons of the LGN give rise to fibers that form the **geniculocalcarine tract (optic radiations),** which projects to the primary visual cortex of the occipital lobes. The radiating fibers from the lateral part of each LGN course downward and forward initially. Then they bend backward in a sharp loop and form a flat band that passes through the temporal lobe in the lateral wall of the inferior horn of the lateral ventricle and sweep posteriorly to the occipital lobe. Fibers from the medial portion of the LGN travel adjacent to those from the lateral LGN, but they take a more direct, nonlooping course over the top of the inferior horn and then travel posteriorly to the occipital lobe. The location of the optic radiations along the lateral wall of the ventricle and the calcarine cortex can be seen in the magnetic resonance image shown in Figure 18–3.

The area of cortex that receives the optic radiations surrounds the **calcarine fissure** (sulcus) on the medial side of the **occipital lobe.** The **cuneus,** the gyrus above the calcarine fissure, receives visual impulses from the upper quadrant of the ipsilateral side of both retinas (this corresponds to the lower quadrant of the contralateral visual field). The **lingual gyrus,** below the calcarine fissure, receives impulses that arise from the lower quadrants of the retina (Fig. 18–4). The **primary visual cortex** or **V1** (Brodmann's area 17) is also called the **striate cortex** because histologic sections of the cortex reveal a horizontal stripe of white matter (the line of Gennari) within the gray matter. Created by the large number of myelinated fibers in layer IV of the cortex, this stripe can be seen with the naked eye.

Fibers from the LGN to the cortex maintain their **topographic** arrangement, so the receptive areas of cortex contain a retinal map. The information from the upper quadrant of the left half of the visual field projects onto the lower right quadrant of the retina. From there, the information passes to the lateral portion of the right LGN and then to the right visual cortex below the calcarine sulcus (Figs. 18–1 and 18–4). Information received in the central part of the quadrant (the fovea) projects to the posterior part of area 17, the occipital pole. Peripheral retinal information projects to the anterior part of area 17.

Areas 18 and 19, which surround area 17, participate in **visual perception** (i.e., visual sensory processing). Areas 18 and 19 also contribute to pathways for visually guided saccades, ocular pursuit movements, accommodation, and convergence through connections with the frontal lobes and the brain stem. Areas 18 and 19 together constitute the proximal **visual association areas,** a component of the unimodal visual association cortex.

Information Processing in the Visual Pathways

Receptive Field Characteristics of Ganglion Cells, Lateral Geniculate Nucleus Cells, and Visual Cortex

Retinal ganglion cells respond when light strikes the retina, and a spot of light focused on a specific, small area of the retina provides the most effective stimulus for these cells. Each ganglion cell has a **receptive field,** a specific area of the retina that maximally stimulates or inhibits the firing of that ganglion cell when stimulated with light. Two types of **ganglion cells** exist: **on-center** and **off-center.** On-center cells have a receptive field that is characterized by a central excitatory zone and an inhibitory surround. Shining a focused light beam in the center of the receptive field excites the cell, and shining a light beam in a doughnut-shaped area around the center of the field inhibits the cell. Off-center ganglion cells have reverse properties; light falling on the center of their receptive field inhibits them, and illumination of the surrounding area excites them. Diffuse light does not excite ganglion cells. Thus, ganglion cells respond chiefly to contrasts.

Like ganglion cells, neurons in the LGN respond to small spots of light and show on-center and off-center receptive fields. These neurons also show no response to diffuse illumination.

Striate cortex neurons have more complex behavior than LGN neurons. Small spots of light have minimal effects on neuronal discharge; optimal light for cortical cell excitation must have contrasting areas of light and dark with linear properties (i.e., consist of a short line, a bar, or some other configuration with a clear edge). These linear stimuli also must have a specific orientation in the visual field. For an individual striate neuron, for example, a vertical bar of light falling on a specific part of the retina may be ineffective, but an oblique bar of light falling on that same part of the retina at a particular angle to the vertical will maximally alter its neuronal discharge.

The visual cortex is organized functionally into narrow vertical columns of neurons running from the cortical surface to the white matter. Within each column, all the neurons respond to bars or slits of light in essentially identical receptive field locations and with the same orientation, but primarily from only one of the two eyes. These **ocular dominance columns** lie in a row so that, across the series of adjacent columns, the neurons respond successively to a shifting axis of rotation of the visual stimulus. Neurons in an adjacent row, or stripe, have matching receptive field properties but respond primarily to stimulation of the other eye. Neurons in the peristriate cortex (areas 18 and 19) also respond to edges of light, but these neurons require more complex stimuli for activation than most striate neurons.

Two Classes of Retinal Ganglion Cells Project Different Visual Information through Magnocellular and Parvocellular Streams to the Visual Cortex

Several separate streams of visual information flow from the retina to the LGN and then to the striate cortex. Two major streams have been named, based on the LGN neurons that process information in each. The **magnocellular stream** begins with large cells of the retinal ganglion cell layer (termed **Y-cells**) that project to the magnocellular layers (layers 1 and 2) of the LGN, which, in turn, course on to the striate cortex, where they terminate in a particular part of layer IV. From the striate cortex (V1), this stream projects through the visual association cortex to posterior temporal and dorsal parietal cortex. Most cortical neurons of the magnocellular stream respond to movement, orientation, and contrast, especially in dim illumination. They do not respond to color. Thus, the magnocellular stream processes information required for quickly locating a moving object in visual space.

The **parvocellular stream** begins with small cells of the retinal ganglion layer (termed **X-cells**) that project to the parvocellular layers of the LGN (layers 3 through 6). The parvocellular layers project information to the striate cortex about the color and shape of objects in bright illumination. The parvocellular stream from the LGN terminates in a different part of layer IV of the cortex and then projects to two functionally distinct types of cerebral cortical neurons: those responsive to shape and orientation and those responsive to color. This pathway for analysis of form and color continues through the visual association cortices to the inferior temporal cortex.

Effects of Lesions Interrupting the Visual Pathway

Testing the Visual Fields for Defects

The **visual fields** can be measured in detail by perimetry. The visual fields can also be examined for **scotomas** (small areas in the fields with diminished or absent vision) in the office or at the bedside using the **confrontation method.** This method requires that the patient and the examiner sit facing each other, initially with the patient's left eye covered and the examiner's right eye covered. The patient fixes gaze with the **right eye** on the examiner's **left eye.** Examination in this manner permits a comparison of the examiner's nasal and temporal fields with the patient's nasal and temporal fields. The examiner then introduces an object, usually a 3- or 4-mm white ball, from some point halfway between the examiner and the patient but beyond the normal periphery of vision. The examiner moves the object slowly toward the line of vision and notes the points at which the patient sees the object as compared with the point at which the examiner sees the object. After repeating the process multiple times through all four quadrants, the examiner estimates the extent of the patient's field of vision. The patient's blind spot can be mapped in this way and compared with the examiner's blind spot, and scotomas can be detected. The examiner depicts the information obtained from this examination by drawing the patient's visual fields on paper. By convention, examiners draw the visual fields from the patient's perspective. The examiner then follows the same procedure for testing the patient's left eye.

The confrontation method of testing the visual fields can also be used to screen the visual fields quickly for gross deficits. For this, the patient and the examiner sit facing each other, with the patient's left eye covered and the examiner's right eye covered. The patient fixes gaze with the right eye on the examiner's left eye. The examiner then moves an index finger quickly in each visual quadrant and asks the patient to tell the examiner when a movement occurs. The examiner can also ask the patient to count the number of fingers (usually one to three) that the examiner presents in each visual quadrant.

Lesions in Different Parts of the Pathway Can Produce Distinctive Visual Field Defects

Figure 18–1 depicts visual field deficits as patients with lesions in sites A to F would experience them. With partial damage to an optic nerve, the visual field may be contracted. Frequently, the visual field abnormality has an altitudinal pattern, which consists of a deficit occupying part or all of the nasal and temporal fields limited to the upper quadrants or the nasal and temporal fields limited to the two lower quadrants of vision. Injury of the portion of the optic nerve carrying fibers from the macular region results in partial or complete loss of vision at the center of the visual field; that is, the patient has a **central scotoma.** Visual acuity and color vision also may be affected. Injury of the portion of the optic nerve adjacent to the macular representation results in a **paracentral scotoma.** Complete destruction of one optic nerve produces complete blindness in the involved eye (Fig. 18–1, lesion A).

Lesions of the optic chiasm frequently result from compression inferiorly from a pituitary gland tumor (adenoma) or superiorly from a craniopharyngioma. The decussating fibers from the nasal retina of each eye, carrying information from the temporal fields, typically become affected first with loss of both temporal visual fields, known as **bitemporal hemianopia** (Fig. 18–1, lesion B). The term hemianopia refers to a visual field defect respecting the vertical midline (or meridian).

A lesion in the right optic tract that involves fibers from the nasal retina in the right eye and the temporal retina in the left eye causes a defect in the temporal field of the right eye and nasal field of the left eye (Fig. 18–1, lesion C). This defect, which affects the left visual fields of both eyes, is termed left **homonymous** (identical side) **hemianopia.** A lesion of the optic radiation usually results in homonymous hemianopia (Fig. 18–1, lesion D); however, a lesion in the anterior temporal lobe, where the fiber bundles are most separate, can cause a predominantly superior visual field defect.

Lesions that destroy the entire primary visual cortex of the right occipital lobe also cause left homonymous hemianopia. Visual acuity remains unaffected in the other hemifield, and if the visual field loss occurs slowly, the patient may not be aware of the hemianopia. **Macular sparing,** preservation of the central 5 to 10 degrees of vision in an otherwise blind hemifield, frequently occurs in patients with occipital lesions. The likely explanation is incomplete destruction of the extensive macular representation in the occipital cortex.

The cuneus receives visual input from the upper halves of the retina (lower visual field), and the lingual gyrus receives impulses from the lower halves of the retina (upper visual field) (Figs. 18–1 and 18–4). Thus, a lesion confined to the right lingual gyrus interrupts visual information from the lower part of the right half of each retina and corresponds to a visual field defect in the left superior quadrant of each eye, left superior quadrantanopia (Fig. 18–1, lesion F).

Restricted, or tunnel, visual fields can be found in people who have no organic disease. The constricted visual fields result from a **conversion reaction,** in which the affected person believes that the field deficits result from an organic cause and not from psychoneurosis. Tunnel vision can also occur in people who are malingering, in which case the affected person is falsifying the test results, usually in an attempt to receive some sort of financial reward. In both these disorders, although the affected people claim to have markedly constricted visual fields, they do not stumble over objects or search the visual environment to avoid stumbling, as do patients with severe organic visual loss. Visual field testing of people with conversion reactions and with malingering usually reveals inconsistent, frequently nonphysiologic patterns of visual loss.

Case Follow-up

The woman described at the beginning of this chapter had bitemporal hemianopia, which results from disease affecting the optic chiasm. An imaging study revealed a pituitary tumor compressing the optic chiasm. Neurosurgical removal of the tumor was accomplished with complete restoration of her visual fields. Initially, she needed supplemental hormonal treatment because of pituitary injury, but subsequently she was able to stop all medications and currently remains well. She is pleased that she has had no additional automobile accidents, and she is particularly happy that her golf game has improved to its previous level.

19

Optic Reflexes and Eye Movements

Case Study

A 25-year-old woman develops decreasing vision in the right eye over a 2-day period, accompanied by an aching pain in the right eye. By the second day, she can barely read using the right eye alone. She consults an ophthalmologist, who refers her to a neurologist. The neurologist finds markedly reduced visual acuity in the right eye with normal acuity in the left eye. The pupils are 4 mm in diameter on the right and 3 mm in diameter on the left. Shining a light into the right eye evokes only slight constriction of both the right pupil and the left pupil. Shining a light into the left eye evokes brisk constriction of both the left pupil and the right pupil. Examination of the optic fundus (the interior portion of the eye) with an ophthalmoscope reveals no abnormalities. There is no other abnormality on examination.

Where is the disease process responsible for these findings located? What kind of process could this be? Can this woman be treated to restore her vision?

Light Reflexes

Flashing light into the eye causes the normal pupil to constrict promptly, and removing the light causes the pupil to dilate. The rods and cones of the retina serve as the sensory receptors for this, the **direct light reflex.** The afferent pathway follows the course of the visual fibers through the retina, optic nerve, and optic tract almost to the lateral geniculate nuclei, but instead of entering this nucleus, the pupillary reflex fibers turn in the direction of the superior colliculus. They end in a region rostral to the superior colliculus known as the **pretectal area** (see Fig. 18–1). Interneurons located in this region send axons around the cerebral aqueduct to the **Edinger-Westphal nucleus,** a group of parasympathetic neurons in a rostral subdivision of the oculomotor nuclear complex. The efferent path begins with cells in the Edinger-Westphal nucleus whose **axons** leave the midbrain in the oculomotor nerve and end in the parasympathetic **ciliary ganglion.** Postganglionic fibers coming from the ganglion enter the eyeball and supply the sphincter muscle in the iris, which constricts the pupil when it contracts. Shining light into one eye evokes not only pupillary constriction of the ipsilateral eye, but also constriction of the pupil of the contralateral eye, the **consensual light reflex.** Crossing connections in the pathway at the level of the pretectum carry out this reflex (see Fig. 18–1).

Diseases that severely damage the retina or the optic nerve reduce the direct light reflex. Damage severe enough to cause complete blindness abolishes both the direct and the consensual light reflex. Lesions of the visual pathway located in the lateral geniculate nuclei, optic radiations, or visual cortex of one side, however, do not interfere with this reflex. Even in cortical blindness produced by complete destruction of the primary visual areas of both occipital lobes, the direct and consensual light reflexes remain preserved. The efferent path for the light reflex may be interrupted by damage to the oculomotor nuclear complex, the oculomotor nerve, the ciliary ganglion, or the iris sphincter muscle. Neither a direct light reflex nor a consensual light reflex can be obtained on the affected side when the efferent path for the light reflex has been interrupted.

The pupillary light reflexes can provide important diagnostic information. When light shined into one eye of a patient evokes a consensual response but no direct response, the afferent (receptive) limb of the reflex is intact but the efferent (effector) limb is defective in the eye tested. When light shined into one eye evokes no direct or consensual response, but light shined into the opposite eye evokes both a direct and a consensual response, the afferent limb of the reflex is impaired in the first eye tested. Usually, this results from a lesion in the retina or the optic nerve.

Reflexes Associated with the Near-Point Reaction

Directing the eyes to an object close to the face brings three different reflex responses into cooperative action.

1. **Convergence.** The medial rectus muscles contract to move both eyes toward the midline so the image in each eye remains focused on the fovea (the area of highest acuity within the macula). Without convergence, diplopia (i.e., double vision) occurs.
2. **Accommodation.** The lenses become thickened as a result of contraction of the **ciliary muscles.** This response maintains a sharply focused image on the foveas. Postganglionic parasympathetic neurons in the ciliary ganglia innervate the ciliary muscles, in addition to the pupillary sphincter.
3. **Pupillary constriction.** The pupils constrict as an optical aid to regulate the depth of focus. Pupillary responses to accommodation and convergence result from processes separate from the light reflex, because pupillary constriction occurs without change in illumination. Moreover, pupillary constriction accompanies accommodation even when prisms prevent convergence, and it accompanies convergence when plus lenses eliminate accommodation. The pathway mediating the pupillary response to accommodation and convergence passes through the optic nerve, optic tract, lateral geniculate nucleus, optic radiations, occipital cortex, corticotectal projections, superior colliculus, Edinger-Westphal nucleus, oculomotor nerve, and ciliary ganglion.

Changing gaze from a distant to a near object or following an object moving from a distance to near the face usually initiates all three reactions. The near reflex occurs involuntarily with a change in fixation or in following an object from far to near. Thus, the voluntary act of looking first at a distant target and then at a near target triggers the involuntary changes in accommodation, convergence, and pupil size. The reflex requires concentration on the task, because the reflex does not appear when a person in the process of changing gaze from distant to near fails to concentrate on the task or defocuses. In clinical examinations, the examiner provides the test stimulus for the near reaction. Although the usual stimulus for the near reaction is visual, proprioceptive pathways can provide input, so the reflex can be initiated by having a blind patient put a hand in front of the face and focus on the hand.

Disorders of Pupillary Function

Adie's Tonic Pupil

A benign condition, **Adie's tonic pupil** consists of a unilateral dilated pupil. It occurs most commonly between 20 and 50 years of age, with a predilection for women. Most people with Adie's pupil also have absent deep tendon reflexes. Over time, the pupil tends to become small and may mimic an Argyll Robertson pupil (discussed in the next section). Adie's tonic pupil shows no constriction or a segmental constriction to light, better constriction to a near target, and a pathologically slow redilation with a distant target. The pupil responds normally to drugs that cause **miosis** (constriction of the pupil) and **mydriasis** (dilation of the pupil). Adie's tonic pupil, however, constricts on instillation of 0.1% pilocarpine in the conjunctival sac, whereas the normal pupil does not respond to this drug. The response to pilocarpine reflects denervation supersensitivity.

Adie's tonic pupil results from a lesion of the parasympathetic postganglionic fibers of the ciliary ganglion or nerves. Viral infection probably causes the disorder, although orbital trauma or surgery may be implicated.

Argyll Robertson Pupil

The **Argyll Robertson pupil** consists of a small, irregular pupil that does not react to light but does react to accommodation. The pupil dilates in response to administration of atropine or cocaine unless iris atrophy has occurred. Initially described in association with central nervous system syphilis, the Argyll Robertson pupil currently results more commonly from other disorders, such as diabetes mellitus. The site of the lesion causing the altered responses of the Argyll Robertson pupil has not been established with certainty. The region of the gray matter around the cerebral aqueduct was thought to be responsible previously, but more recently, damage to the ciliary ganglion or the iris has been implicated.

Eye Movements

Five eye movement subsystems participate in placing a viewed object on the fovea, to permit the best visual resolution and to keep it there as the object or observer moves. These subsystems include the following:

1. **Saccades,** fast conjugate eye movements that place an object on the fovea.
2. **Pursuit,** slow conjugate eye movements that track a moving object and keep it on the fovea.
3. **Vergence,** converging or diverging the eyes to keep both foveas aligned to a target that moves closer or farther away.
4. **Vestibulo-ocular reflex,** which uses vestibular signals to move the eyes in an equal and opposite direction if the viewer's head moves.
5. **Optokinetics,** an adjunct to the vestibulo-ocular system in moving the eyes in response to motion of images across the retina during sustained head motion.

These subsystems have distinct functional characteristics and separate pathways through shared neural centers. Thus, although they overlap neuroanatomically, they can be both stimulated and injured separately.

Saccades

The **saccadic subsystem** places the fovea on a target rapidly and accurately and thus establishes fixation. This system can be assessed clinically by asking a patient to look alternately from one target to another within the visual field.

There are several types of saccades. Internally generated, **volitional saccades** direct the gaze to either a remembered location or a location where a target likely will appear. A nonvisual stimulus such as sound automatically triggers **reflexive saccades.** Internally generated, **volitional visually guided saccades** develop to view a specific target in the visual field. A new target appearing on the retina automatically triggers **reflexive visually guided saccades.**

The **frontal eye fields,** including parts of Brodmann's areas 6 and 8 in the precentral sulcus, initiate volitional and reflexive saccades. The **parietal eye fields** in the posterior parietal cortex mediate visually guided saccades of both volitional and reflexive types. Nevertheless, owing to interconnections between the frontal and parietal eye fields, each influences the other in initiating saccades.

For both visually guided and nonvisually guided saccades, neuronal activity from the cerebral cortex travels downward to the contralateral **paramedian pontine reticular formation (PPRF)** (Fig. 19–1). Impulse streams from the frontal eye field move directly to the PPRF, and impulses from the parietal eye fields synapse in the **superior colliculus** before moving to the PPRF. An important downward pathway from the frontal eye field to the caudate nucleus and adjacent putamen turns off the tonic inhibitory influence of the substantia nigra reticulata on the superior colliculus (Fig. 19–1).

Horizontal Saccades

For horizontal saccades (Fig. 19–1), PPRF burst cells send signals to the **abducens nucleus** of cranial nerve VI, where the pathway activates both abducens motor neurons and interneurons. Signals for horizontal saccades then proceed through abducens motor neurons to the lateral rectus muscle and by means of the abducens interneurons through the **medial longitudinal fasciculus** to the contralateral **oculomotor nucleus** of cranial nerve III (the medial rectus

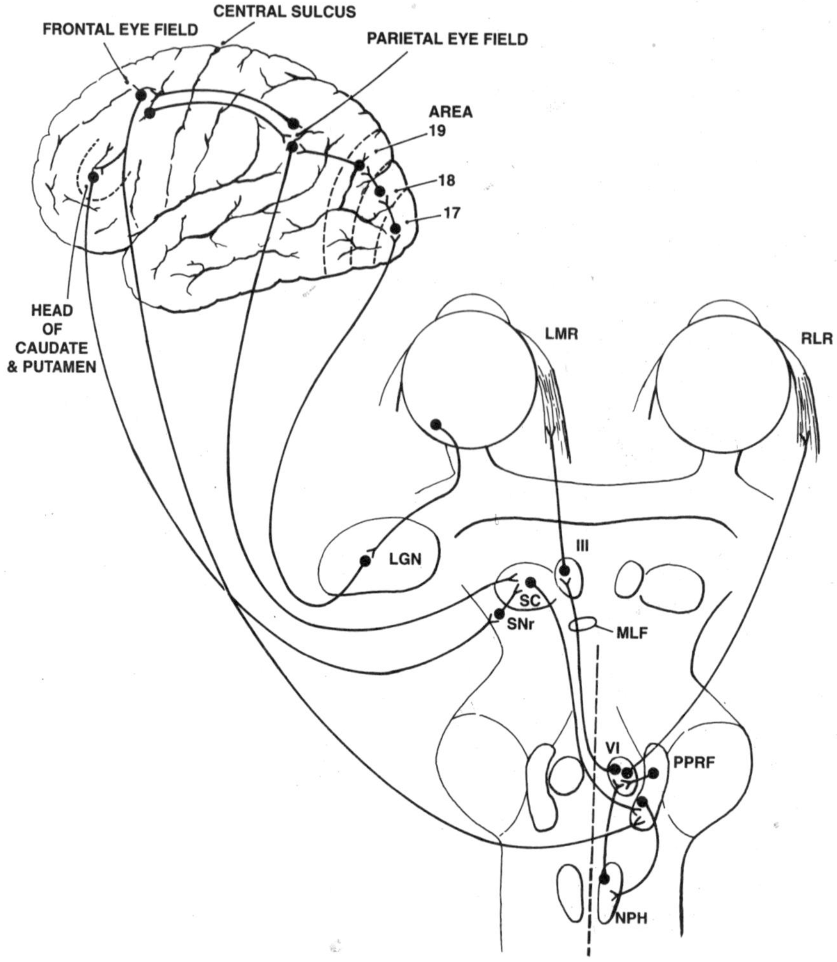

■ **FIGURE 19–1.** Pathways for visually guided and nonvisually guided saccadic eye movements. Only horizontal eye movements to the right, which are initiated in the left cerebral hemisphere, are illustrated. LGN = lateral geniculate nucleus; LMR = left medial rectus muscle; MLF = medial longitudinal fasciculus; NPH = nucleus prepositus hypoglossus; PPRF = paramedian pontine reticular formation; RLR = right lateral rectus muscle; SC = superior colliculus; SNr = substantia nigra pars reticulata; III = oculomotor nucleus; VI = abducens nucleus.

subnucleus). Input to the abducens nucleus from the **nucleus prepositus hypoglossi** (Fig. 19–1) supplies information about the current position of the head and eyes and holds the eyes on the target at the end of the saccade.

Vertical Saccades

The pathway for vertical saccades (not shown in Fig. 19–1) uses the same pathway to the PPRF, but impulses from the PPRF cells reach the motor neurons after an additional relay in the midbrain. This relay is in the rostral interstitial nucleus of the medial longitudinal fasciculus and the nearby interstitial nucleus of Cajal. These nuclei reside in the tegmentum of the rostral midbrain, just lateral to the oculomotor nucleus. These interstitial nuclei regulate vertical and torsional saccades through connections to the subnuclei of the oculomotor nucleus and to the trochlear nucleus.

Effect of Lesions of the Saccadic Pathway

Lesions of the saccadic pathway in humans cause saccades that are too small **(hypometric),** too slow, inaccurate **(dysmetric),** delayed in onset, or completely absent **(saccadic palsy).** Large, acute lesions of the cerebral hemisphere result in absent, small, or slow saccades in the direction contralateral to the side of the lesion. The eyes often deviate tonically toward the side of the lesion. The disorder occurs temporarily because other pathways can compensate. Lesions of the basal ganglia cause slow, small, long-latency saccades, or excessive saccades apparently unrelated to purposeful behavior **(saccadic intrusions).** Pontine lesions result in disturbances similar to those caused by cerebral lesions but affect eye movements toward the side of the lesion. Cerebellar lesions cause small, dysmetric saccades and difficulty in maintaining eccentric gaze.

Pursuit Movements

The **pursuit subsystem** maintains fixation on slowly moving targets. If it fails, saccades are needed to catch up with the target.

Pursuit Pathway

Visual inputs to the temporo-occipital junction initiate pursuit movements (Fig. 19–2). This area of the extrastriate cortex receives information about speed and direction of movement of a

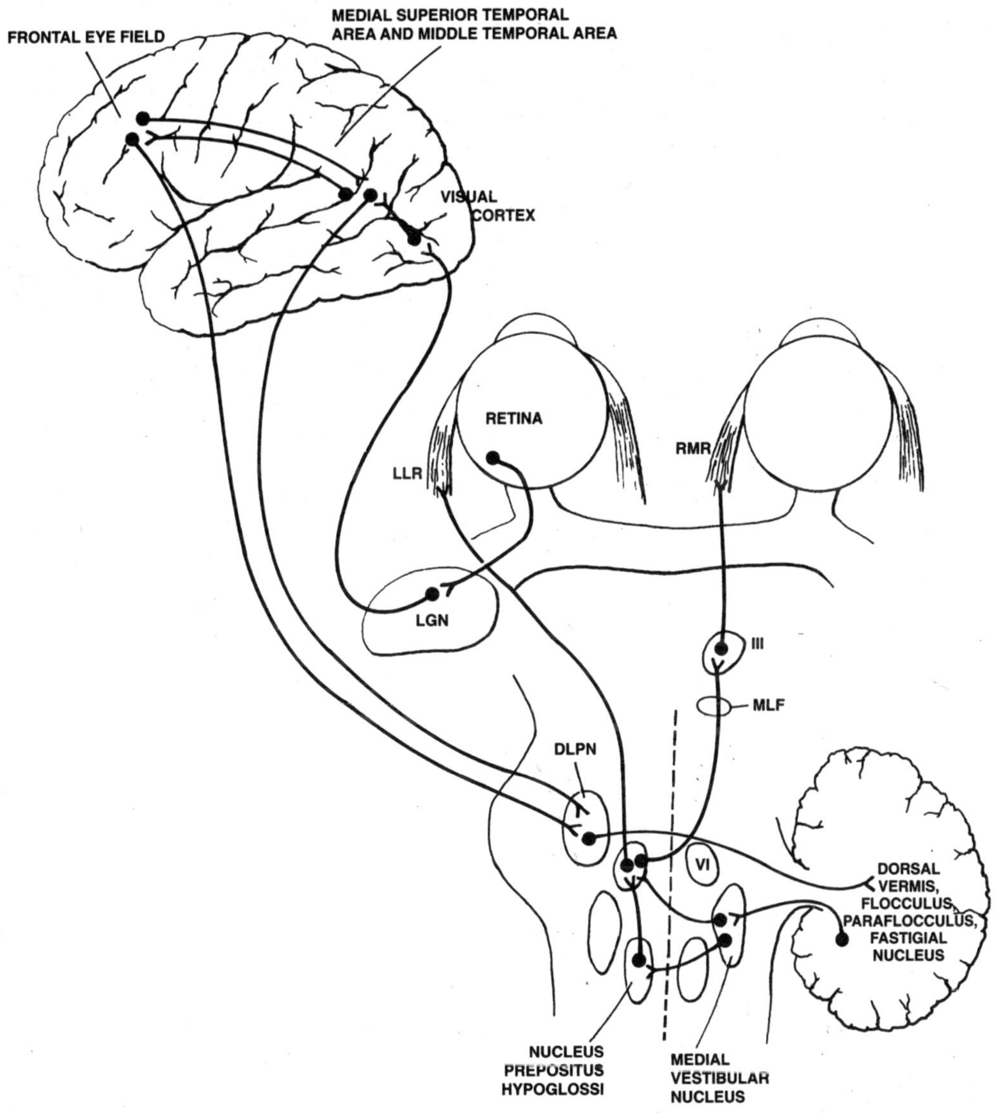

■ **FIGURE 19–2.** Pathways for horizontal pursuit movements of the eyes. DPLN = dorsolateral pontine nuclei; LGN = lateral geniculate nucleus; LLR = left lateral rectus muscle; MLF = medial longitudinal fasciculus; RMR = right medial rectus muscle; III = oculomotor nucleus; VI = abducens nucleus.

visual target from the **visual cortex** in areas 17, 18, and 19. From this **middle temporal cortex,** corticopontine fibers project to the ipsilateral **dorsolateral pontine nuclei.** The pathway for pursuit movements then leads to the **cerebellar vermis** and **flocculus,** the **vestibular nuclei,** especially the medial vestibular nucleus, and the **nucleus prepositus hypoglossi.** Finally, for horizontal pursuit movements, the medial vestibular nucleus excites the contralateral abducens nucleus to activate cranial nerve VI and the medial rectus subnucleus of cranial nerve III through the medial longitudinal fasciculus.

Lesions of the Pursuit Pathway

With a lesion of the pursuit pathway, movement of the object of interest off the fovea (**retinal slip**) leads to a saccade instead of a pursuit movement. This results in a series of small saccades as the patient follows a target, so-called saccadic pursuit.

Vestibulo-ocular Subsystem

Organization

The **vestibulo-ocular subsystem** prevents the image of interest from moving away from the fovea during head movements. This is called **image slip.** The pathway for the vestibulo-ocular subsystem begins with signals generated by the hair cell receptors in the **semicircular canals,** which travel to the **vestibular nuclei.** Each of the six semicircular canals controls a yoked pair of extraocular muscles that move the eyes approximately in the same plane as that of the canal. The three yoked pairs of muscles include the lateral rectus and medial rectus, the inferior oblique and superior rectus, and the inferior rectus and superior oblique.

The horizontal canals control movements in the horizontal plane, each canal exciting eye movements to the contralateral side of the head. Each anterior canal occupies the same plane as the opposite posterior canal; if the head undergoes angular acceleration that stimulates the anterior canal, the contralateral posterior canal will be inhibited, and vice versa. Stimulation of the anterior canal raises the eyes in the plane parallel to that canal. Stimulation of the anterior canal induces contraction of the contralateral inferior oblique and ipsilateral superior rectus muscles, and the eyes move upward. If angular acceleration occurs in the same plane but the opposite direction, the posterior canal of this same pair will be stimulated, and the eyes will be lowered. Stimulation of a posterior canal lowers the eyes in the plane of that canal by excitation of the contralateral inferior rectus and the ipsilateral superior oblique. To accomplish these actions, each semicircular canal articulates with neurons in the ipsilateral vestibular nuclei that excite one yoked pair of muscles and with other vestibular neurons that inhibit the antagonistic yoked pair.

Testing and Identifying Abnormalities

Clinicians assess the vestibulo-ocular subsystem by stimulating vestibular receptors with head movement, body rotation, or introduction of warm or cold water into the external auditory canal (caloric testing; see Chapter 15). The **head shaking acuity test** requires an alert patient with a full range of eye movements. The patient identifies the smallest line possible on a Snellen visual acuity card and then shakes the head quickly while reading the same line in reverse order. A **fall in acuity** indicates a deficient vestibulo-ocular subsystem. Another test of the vestibulo-ocular system, the **oculocephalic test,** or **doll's eye** or **doll's head** test, can be applied to awake or comatose patients. With the patient fixating on a target while awake, the examiner moves the patient's head horizontally and vertically. In patients with an intact vestibulo-ocular response, the eyes move in a direction opposite that of the head movement, and they maintain fixation on the target. A greater range of eye movements with the oculocephalic test than with voluntary movements indicates a gaze palsy rostral to the midbrain. This is termed a **supranuclear gaze palsy.** In the comatose patient, a normal oculocephalic response indicates an intact vestibulo-ocular pathway from the medulla to the midbrain and intact ocular motor nuclei and internuclear connections.

A prominent symptom of vestibulo-ocular reflex dysfunction, **oscillopsia,** consists of abnormal movement of the visual environment. After bilateral injury to the vestibulo-ocular pathways, the eyes cannot respond to head movements, and the patient complains of "bouncing" or "blurred" vision with movement. With complete destruction of the vestibulo-ocular pathways bilaterally, the patient cannot even correct for the tiny head movements associated with the carotid pulse. If the lesion interrupts only one vestibulo-ocular pathway, the vestibular system becomes unbalanced, and the patient develops a rhythmic oscillation of the eyes called **nystagmus.** The patient may report oscillopsia, vertigo, or dysequilibrium.

Vergence

The **vergence subsystem** converges or diverges the eyes to keep the image on the fovea as the object of interest moves closer or farther away. Clinicians assess this subsystem by having the patient focus on distant and near targets and determining whether the eyes diverge or converge. Activation of the vergence subsystem results from a blurred image or from an image falling on noncorresponding retinal areas. Signals in the posterior temporal, peristriate, and prefrontal cortex project to vergence cells in the mesencephalon and from there to cranial nerves III and VI. Usually affecting the diencephalon or mesencephalon, lesions of the vergence system in humans cause insufficient or excessive convergence or divergence and insufficient or excessive accommodation.

Optokinetic Movements

The **optokinetic subsystem** evokes eye movements in response to retinal slip during prolonged head movement at a constant velocity. The vestibulo-ocular subsystem produces compensatory eye movements initially in response to the acceleration of the head, but it fades away because the stimulation of the vestibular receptors ceases when the motion of the endolymph in the semicircular canals reaches equilibrium with the motion of the head. At this point, the continued retinal slip from movement of the visual field maintains the compensatory eye movements, which are optokinetic eye movements. For clinical examination, these movements can be induced by providing a constantly moving series of images (preferably one that fills the visual field) and asking the patient to focus on the images while observing the eyes for optokinetic nystagmus (see later).

A series of nuclei along the optic tract, the **nucleus of the optic tract,** and **nuclei of the accessory optic system** in the midbrain receive visual input directly from retinal ganglion cell axons and project to the cerebellum and the vestibular nuclei in the **direct optokinetic pathway.** The accessory optic system nuclei are also interconnected with the pursuit pathway by reciprocal connections with the temporo-occipital cortex (Fig. 19–2). This is the **indirect optokinetic pathway.**

A unilateral lesion in the optokinetic pathway results in decreased **optokinetic nystagmus,** elicited by moving a striped drum or tape in front of the patient. The normal response to a series of vertical stripes moving to the right is smooth pursuit to the right and then a saccade to the left when the eye reaches its limit of movement to the right in the orbit. In patients with a unilateral cerebral cortical lesion, optokinetic nystagmus does not occur when the target moves to the side of the lesion.

Case Follow-up

The woman described at the beginning of this chapter has a lesion affecting the right optic nerve behind the eye. This results in decreased visual acuity and a poor direct and consensual response to light shined into the right eye. The normal pupillary response of both eyes to light shined into the left eye demonstrates that the motor component of the pupillary response on the right side remains preserved. Additional history revealed that she had experienced a similar event in the left eye 2 years earlier. Her vision returned to normal after about 3 months. A magnetic resonance imaging study revealed multiple lesions in the white matter of her brain in addition to a lesion affecting the right optic nerve behind the globe and in front of the optic chiasm. A diagnosis of multiple sclerosis was made, and she was prescribed treatment with a beta-interferon medication. Her vision cleared completely in about 6 weeks, and 2 years later, she remains without symptoms.

20

Cerebral Cortex and Thalamocortical Connections

Case Study

A 55-year-old man suddenly develops weakness of his right arm and leg while at work. When he attempts to tell a coworker about his weakness, he can speak only slowly and can produce single words or brief phrases. He feels frustrated about his inability to communicate and frightened about the sudden weakness of his limbs. His coworker takes him immediately to hospital, where a neurologist sees him promptly. On examination, the man can speak only single words such as "weak" or short phrases such as "no pain head." Nevertheless, he understands complex language, as shown by his ability to carry out multiple tasks on command such as "touch your left index finger to your right ear, then close your eyes, then open your mouth." The lower right side of his face appears weak, and his right arm and leg have approximately 25% of the strength of his left arm and leg. Deep tendon reflexes on the right side are decreased compared with the left, and the right plantar response is extensor, the left flexor. Sensory testing with pinprick, light touch, cold, vibration sense, and position sense reveals no abnormalities.

Where in the nervous system does this patient have a lesion causing his speech difficulty and right-sided weakness? What would cause this? Is treatment available?

Cerebral Cortex

The human brain possesses the capacity to undertake a vast number of intellectual and cognitive functions. Performing these functions requires the circuits of the **cerebral cortex** to be engaged and to interact with other parts of the nervous system. The cerebral cortex participates in many aspects of memory storage and recall. It is necessary for the comprehension and execution of language and for certain special talents such as musical and mathematic abilities. It participates in processes responsible for attention, and it contributes to the perception and conscious processing of all sensations, as well as to the integration of sensory inputs from several modalities, providing recognition of individuals, objects, and places. The cortex is necessary for the planning and execution of complex motor activities such as fine digit, hand, and phonatory movements and for the planning of complex behavior.

The cerebral cortex is a mantle of gray matter on the surface of the cerebral hemispheres. With limited exceptions, the thalamus provides the input to the cortex, and corticothalamic projections uniformly reciprocate the thalamocortical connections. This chapter therefore includes an overview of the organization of the thalamus and some details of the thalamocortical relationships.

Cortical Cell Layers: The Basis for Structure and Function Relationships within and between Cortical Areas

Cells arranged in layers that follow the contours of the gyri and sulci densely populate the cerebral cortex. The cortex can be divided into regions based on differences in the number of cell layers. **Isocortex** contains six layers; **allocortex** has three; and **mesocortex,** which forms a zone between isocortex and allocortex, varies from three to six layers. The zone of mesocortex that borders isocortex contains five to six layers, and the mesocortex adjacent to allocortex has three to four. Corticoid, or cortex-like, regions have neurochemical features and neuronal connections characteristic of cortex, but **corticoid areas** contain no clearly discernible layering of cells.

Isocortex

The Six Cell Layers of Isocortex Differ in Cell Type and Connections

In the human brain, most of the cerebral cortex consists of isocortex. From the pial surface, the cell layers of isocortex have been named: **I, molecular; II, external granular; III, external pyramidal; IV, internal granular; V, internal pyramidal;** and **VI multiform** (or **fusiform**). These names refer to the size and shape of the cell types that predominate in each layer, and the cells' sizes and shapes, in turn, relate directly to their input and output connections. Very small cells (like grains of sand) fill the granular layers; the pyramidal layers contain large neurons with pyramidal shape; and the multiform layer consists of a variety of cell types, but mostly spindle-shaped (fusiform).

A radial pattern of fibers to and from the cortex, and fibers making connections between the layers of cells of the cortex, organizes the cortex into **vertical columns.** Afferent fibers to the cortex run radially toward the surface (i.e., along the length of the vertical columns). They distribute to the small stellate (star-shaped) cells, which can be found in all layers, but they constitute the predominant cell type in the granular layers (II and IV). Input from the thalamus projects primarily to layer IV. The stellate cells, which are interneurons, make short-axon connections within their vertical column to form a great variety of closed processing loops.

Efferent projections of pyramidal cells in many layers, especially those in layer III, coordinate neuronal processing in both adjacent and distant vertical columns of the cortex. These projections form interhemispheric connections through the **corpus callosum** and intrahemispheric **association fibers** that provide the backbone of functional cortical networks. The output of the columns to subcortical targets comes from the pyramidal cells of layer V. These cells project to the basal ganglia, brain stem and spinal cord, and to those thalamic nuclei that have only subcortical and diffuse cortical connections. Layer VI cells project back to the thalamic nuclei that provide input restricted to a specific cortical area.

Functional Regions of Isocortex Vary in the Relative Thickness of Their Cell Layers

The relative thickness of each of the six cortical layers, and the density of neuron cell bodies within each layer vary in different regions of the isocortex. Recognized early in the 20th century, these histologic differences were thought to reflect functional differences. At that time, Brodmann designated a total of 52 cytoarchitecturally different areas of the isocortex, many of which are now recognized as functionally distinct and can be identified by number as part of the standard anatomic nomenclature of the cortex (Figs. 20–1 and 20–2).

The term **homotypic isocortex** refers to isocortical areas that form the prototype pattern of six well-developed layers of cells, whereas the term **idiotypic isocortex** designates those with extreme variations from the homotypic pattern. The **primary motor area (MI)** and the **primary sensory areas** consist of idiotypic cortex. MI contains an enlarged layer V and reduced layers II to IV, whereas the primary visual, somatosensory, and auditory areas have thick layers II, III, and IV and a relatively thin layer V.

The **association areas** of the cortex consist of homotypic isocortex. **Unimodal association areas** surround (or lie adjacent to) the primary areas. In these areas, the cells process only one sensory modality (e.g., visual, auditory, or somatosensory association areas) or deal exclusively with programming movements (motor association cortex). Lesions of the unimodal sensory association areas lead to complex defects in sensory perception, with the elemental sensations remaining intact.

Heteromodal association areas receive input from multiple unimodal areas. Thus, heteromodal association neurons deal with integrated sensory or sensorimotor contingencies, or, in some cases, fire only in response to stimuli of motivational significance. The heteromodal association areas can be found in the prefrontal region, the posterior

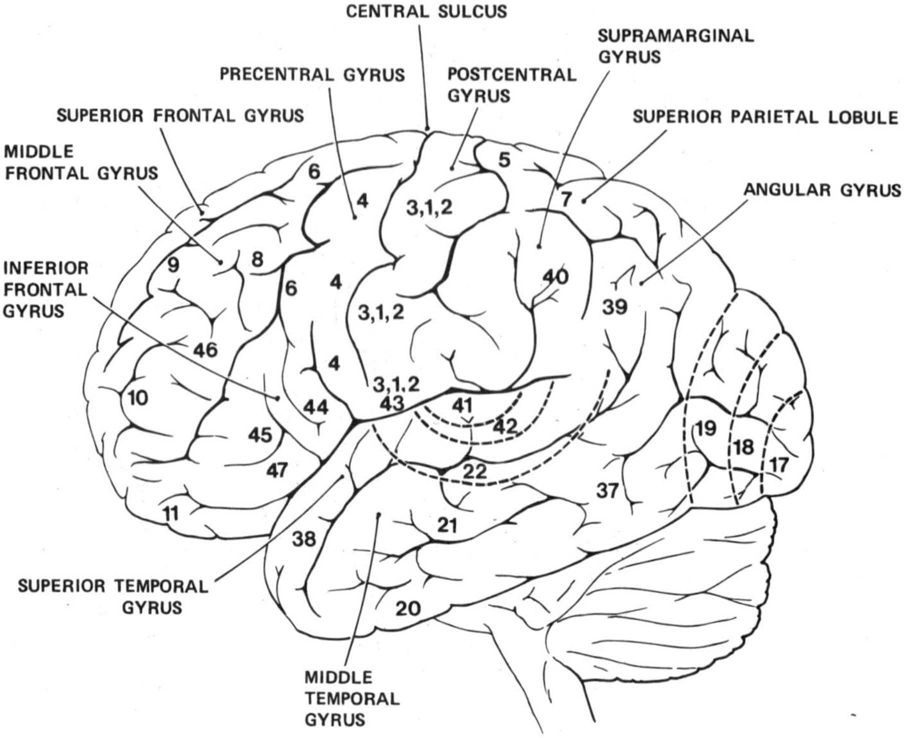

■ **FIGURE 20-1.** A lateral view of the surface of the brain, showing the numbered Brodmann's areas of the cerebral cortex.

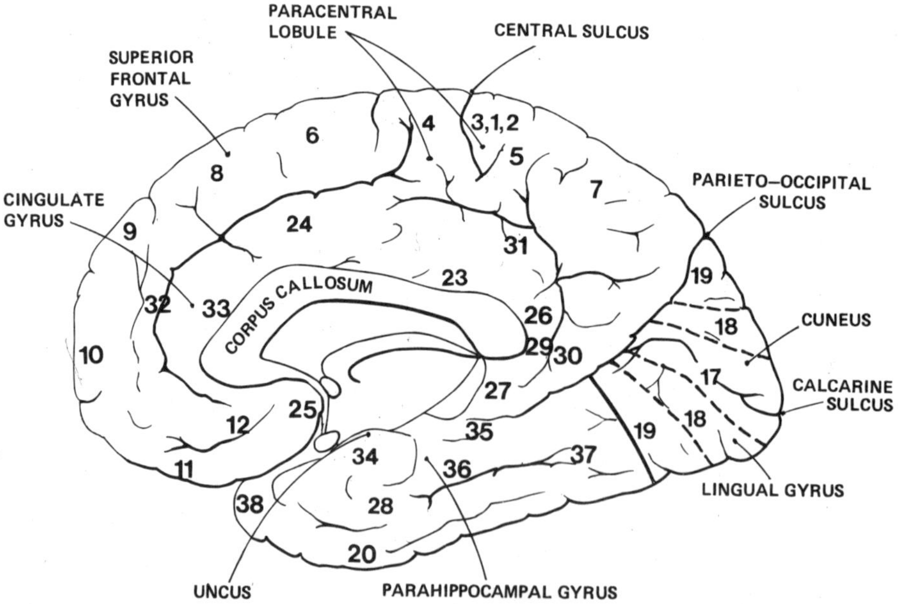

■ **FIGURE 20-2.** A medial view of the surface of the cerebral hemisphere showing the numbered Brodmann's areas of the cerebral cortex.

parietal lobe, and the posterior parts of the temporal lobe. The heteromodal association areas of the temporal lobe consist of extensions from the parietal lobe on both the medial and lateral surfaces of the hemisphere. Lesions of the heteromodal areas result in complex defects involving both cognitive and affective (emotional) components.

Mesocortex, Allocortex, and Corticoid Areas

The **mesocortex** consists of the **paralimbic areas,** which surround the medial and basal parts of the cerebral hemispheres. The five paralimbic areas are as follows:

1. Cingulate complex (cingulate gyrus, retrosplenial area, and subcallosal area, which includes the paraterminal gyrus).
2. Parahippocampal gyrus.
3. Temporal pole.
4. Insula.
5. Caudal orbitofrontal cortex.

The mesocortex contains three to six layers of neurons: six in zones that lie adjacent to isocortex and three in zones next to the allocortex. The **allocortex** consists of the **hippocampal formation** and the **piriform** or **primary olfactory cortex.** Allocortical areas contain three cell layers.

The **corticoid areas** include the **septal region** (deep to the paraterminal gyrus), the **substantia innominata,** and parts of the **amygdaloid complex.** These regions lie at the base of the forebrain and contain simple, poorly differentiated cortex, which nonetheless shares the neurotransmitter and connectional characteristics of other cortical areas. Allocortical and corticoid areas together make up the limbic telencephalon. (See Chapter 21.)

Cortical Networks and Information Processing

Our current understanding of information processing in the cerebral cortex stems from the concept of networks. This view has effectively replaced the concept of serial, unidirectional processing from primary sensory to association to motor areas, in the manner of an elaborate reflex arc. With increasing knowledge of anatomic connections in the primate cortex, and the activity patterns of various cortical areas from human imaging studies, the concept of **parallel processing in large-scale functional networks** has emerged. This model of cortical function takes into account that heteromodal association areas interconnect reciprocally not only with the unimodal sensory association areas and with each other, but also with the paralimbic and limbic areas necessary for learning, memory, and motivation (Fig. 20–3). The resulting concept focuses on essentially simultaneous activation of the various nodes in a cortical network and in the related subcortical structures during cognitive tasks.

Separate but overlapping **networks for language, attention, learning and memory, face-object recognition,** and **comportment** have been proposed. Functional imaging studies have assisted in clarifying not only the normal function of these networks, but also the basis for neurologic and psychiatric disorders in their function. These studies reveal the integral relationship of particular cortical areas with specific parts of the thalamus (described here), the basal ganglia (see Chapter 17), and the cerebellum (see Chapter 16).

Thalamus

The **diencephalon** is an egg-shaped mass of gray matter deep in the brain rostral to the midbrain. Its components include the **thalamus,** the largest subdivision, the **subthalamus** (the subthalamic nucleus is described with the basal ganglia in Chapter 17), and the **hypothalamus** and **epithalamus,** both of which are described with the limbic system in Chapter 21.

The **third ventricle** separates the right half of the thalamus from the left half, and the tela choroidea, which forms the roof of this ventricle, bears a choroid plexus. In most, but not all, human brains, a small area called the **massa intermedia** or **interthalamic adhesion** joins the two halves of the thalamus.

The **internal medullary lamina** subdivides the thalamus of each hemisphere into three unequal parts (Fig. 20–4). This band of myelinated fibers separates the **medial** and **lateral nuclear groups** from the **ventral nuclear group** and bifurcates at its rostral extent to encompass an **anterior nuclear group.** The internal medullary

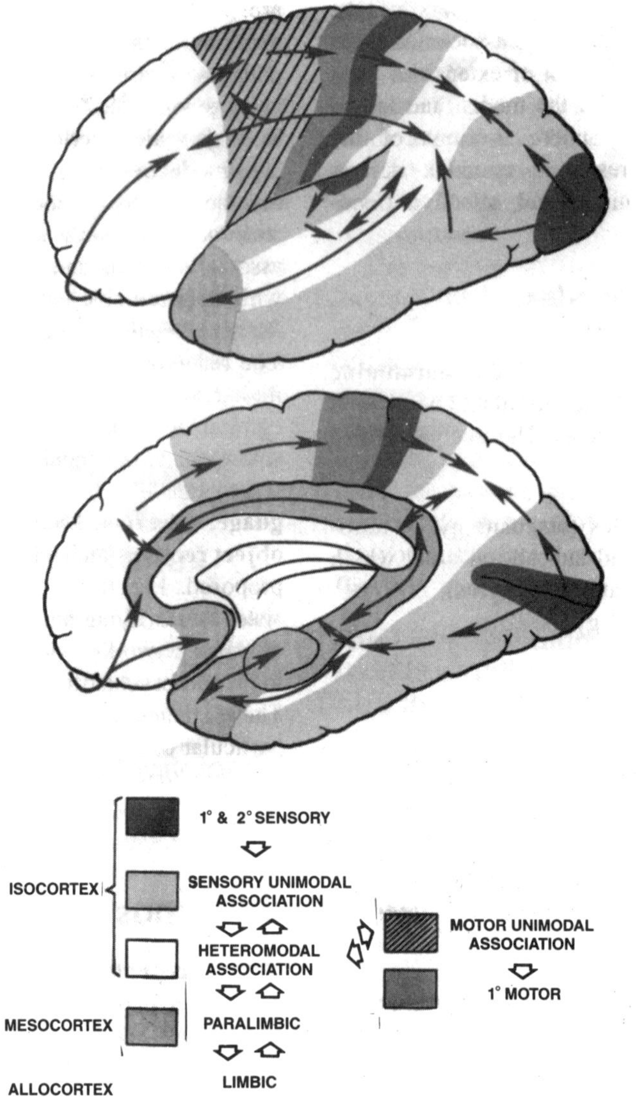

■ **FIGURE 20-3.** A simplified view of information processing across the cerebral cortex. This diagram contrasts the primarily unidirectional flow of sensory information through primary and unimodal association areas with the heavily integrated processing within and between heteromodal association, paralimbic, and limbic areas. In the processing of long-term memory, the flow of activation is bidirectional at every level. (Adapted from Mesulam, MM: Principles of Behavioral and Cognitive Neurology, ed 2. Oxford University Press, New York, 2000.)

lamina encloses the centromedian and other **intralaminar nuclei.** A thin sheet of cells called the **thalamic reticular nucleus** forms the lateral wall of the thalamus. This cell group separates the lateral group of nuclei from the posterior limb of the internal capsule. Another narrow band of cells making up the **midline nuclei** resides on the medial wall of the thalamus, adjacent to the third ventricle.

The thalamus serves as the station for processing and relaying neuronal activity from all types of peripheral sensory receptors, from the basal ganglia, and from the cerebellum to the cerebral cortex. With the exception of the reticular nucleus, all thalamic nuclei project to the cerebral cortex (thalamocortical fibers) and receive afferents (corticothalamic fibers) from the same cortical regions to which they project.

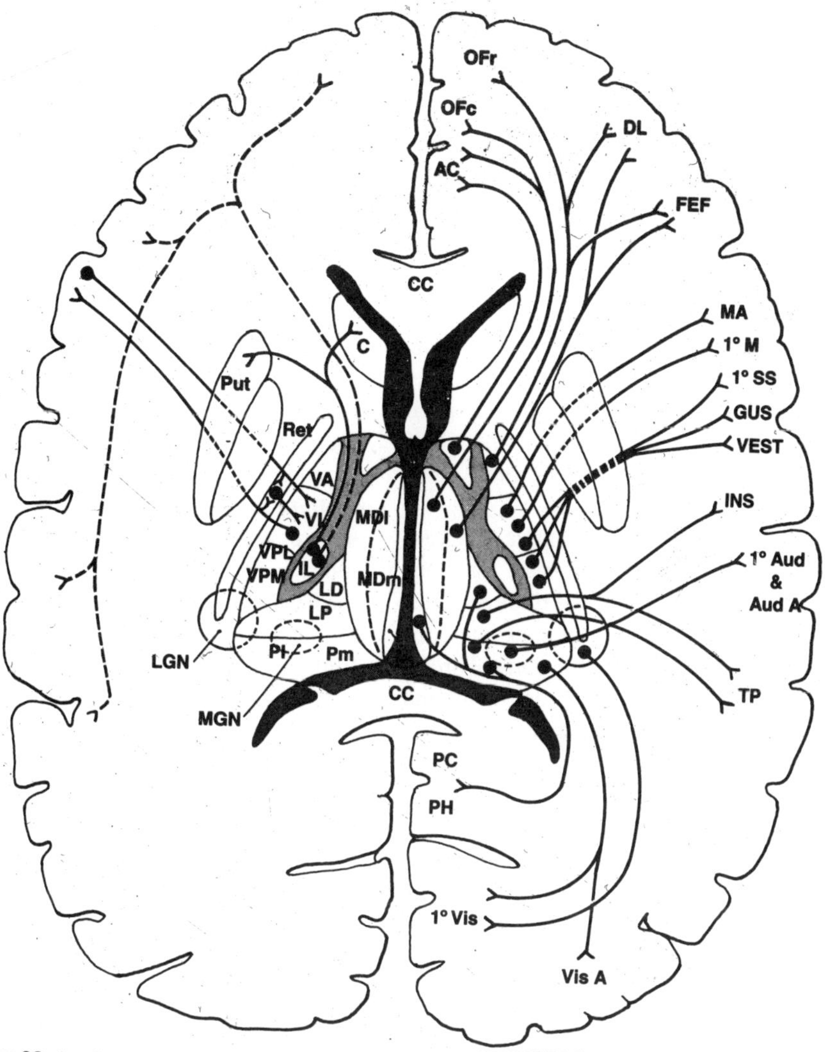

■ **FIGURE 20–4.** Schematic diagram of the relationships of the nuclear groups of the thalamus. *(Right)* The topographic thalamocortical projections of the anterior, medial, ventral, and lateral nuclear groups. Reciprocal corticothalamic connections are not shown. *(Left)* The relationship of reticular nucleus to the thalamocortical and corticothalamic connections of one nucleus (VL) is shown as an example. The intralaminar nuclei project to the striatum (including the ventral striatum) and diffusely to the frontal, parietal, and temporal lobes. The light-shaded area is the internal medullary lamina. A = anterior nuclear group; AC = anterior cingulated area; Aud = auditory cortex; AudA = auditory association cortex; C = caudate; cc = corpus callosum; DL = dorsolateral prefrontal cortex; FEF = frontal eye field; GUS = gustatory cortex; IL = intralaminar nuclei; INS = insula; LD = lateral dorsal nucleus; LGN = lateral geniculate nucleus; LP = lateral posterior nucleus; M = motor cortex; MA = motor association cortex; MDl = lateral part of mediodorsal nucleus; MDm = medial part of mediodorsal nucleus; MGN = medial geniculate nucleus; Mi = midline nuclei; OFc = caudal orbitofrontal cortex; OFr = rostral orbitofrontal cortex; PC = posterior cingulate; PH = parahippocampal cortex; Pl = lateral pulvinar; Pm = medial pulvinar; Put = putamen; Ret = reticular thalamic nucleus; SS = somatosensory cortex; TP = temporoparietal association cortex; VA = ventral anterior nucleus; VEST = vestibular cortex; Vis = visual cortex; Vis A = visual association cortex; VL = ventral lateral nucleus; VPL = ventral posterolateral nucleus; VPM = ventral posteromedial nucleus. (Adapted from Nieuwenhuys, R, Voogd, J, and van Huijzen, C: The Human Central Nervous System, ed 3. Springer-Verlag, New York, 1988.)

Thalamocortical Connections

Topographic Pattern of Thalamocortical Connections

The pattern of the extensive reciprocal connections between thalamus and cortex follows essentially a topographic distribution, with rostromedial and caudolateral parts of the thalamus interconnected with corresponding regions of the cortical mantle. Within this topographic organization, however, individual thalamic nuclei (or more accurately, subdivisions of individual thalamic nuclei) subserve individual modality-specific, heteromodal, or paralimbic-limbic cortical regions.

Figure 20–4 provides a schematic diagram illustrating the topographic pattern of thalamocortical relations. Collectively, the midline, anterior, and medial nuclei of the thalamus interconnect with the limbic and paralimbic cortical areas, as well as with the heteromodal regions of the prefrontal cortex. The ventral thalamic nuclei project in rostrocaudal order to the modality-specific areas of the frontal lobe (motor cortex), parietal lobe (somatosensory, taste, and vestibular cortices), temporal lobe (auditory cortex), and occipital lobes (visual cortex). The nuclei of the lateral nuclear group reciprocate connections with the heteromodal cortex of the posterior parietal and temporal lobes and the unimodal association cortex for vision.

Internal Capsule

The thalamocortical fiber system comprises one part of the total of afferent and efferent fibers of the cerebral cortex. Beneath the cortex, these ascending and descending fibers form the **corona radiata** in the medullary substance of the hemisphere. As they course ventrally from the frontal lobe, the most rostral fibers pass down between the head of the caudate nucleus and the rostral end of the lentiform nucleus, to form the **anterior limb of the internal capsule.** Caudally, fibers passing between the thalamus and the lentiform nucleus form the **posterior limb of the internal**

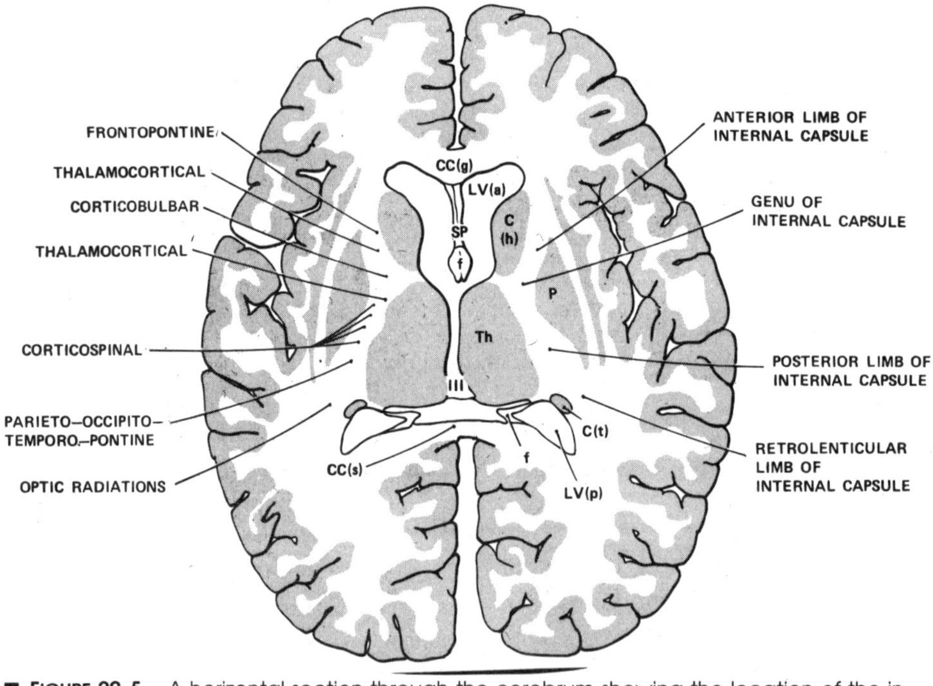

■ **FIGURE 20-5.** A horizontal section through the cerebrum showing the location of the internal capsule fibers (*right*) and the various bundles that make up the capsule (*left*). CC(g) = corpus callosum, genu; CC(s) = corpus callosum, splenium; C(h) = caudate head; C(t) = caudate tail; f = fornix; LV(a) = lateral ventricle, anterior horn; LV(p) = lateral ventricle, posterior horn; P = putamen; SP = septum pellucidum; Th = thalamus; III = third ventricle.

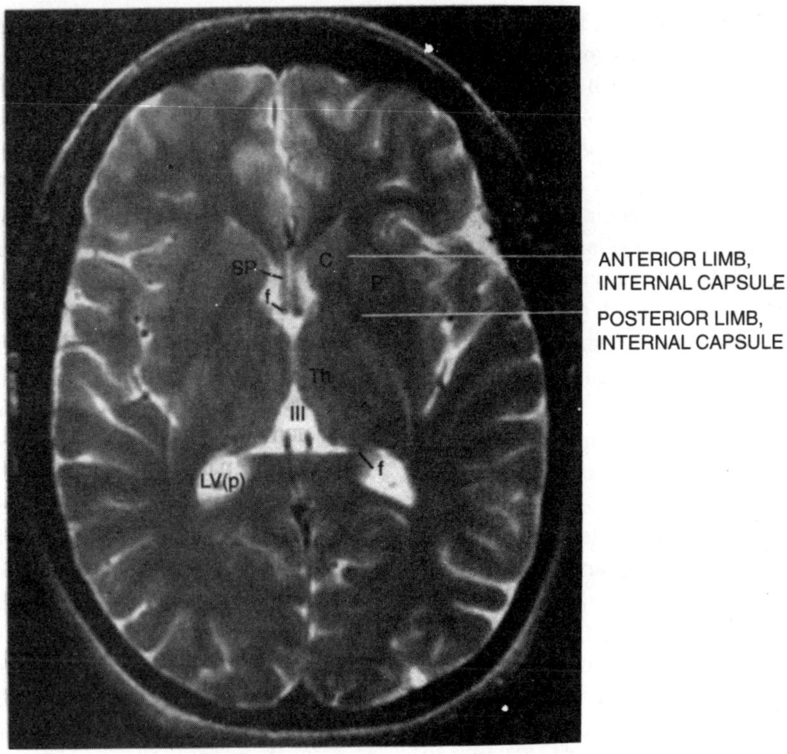

■ **FIGURE 20–6.** A T2-weighted magnetic resonance image of a neurologically normal adult in the axial plane. Compare with Figure 20–5.

capsule. At the level of the interventricular foramen, the transition between the anterior and posterior limbs forms the **genu (knee)** of the internal capsule (Figs. 20–5 and 20–6). Descending fibers of the corticospinal tract pass through the posterior limb of the internal capsule. The corticobulbar fibers, which control the muscles of the head, run rostral to the corticospinal fibers. Motor fibers to the upper extremity pass rostral to those to the lower extremity. Fibers passing to and from the frontal lobe, other than pyramidal fibers (e.g., connections of the midline, anterior, and mediodorsal thalamic nuclei with the prefrontal cortex), make up the anterior limb of the internal capsule. Fibers connecting the ventral thalamus with the parietal lobe occupy the posterior part of the posterior limb of the internal capsule. Optic radiation fibers occupy the **retrolenticular portion of the internal capsule** (i.e., ''behind'' the lentiform nucleus) (see Fig. 20–5 and 18–3). Auditory radiation fibers project through the **sublenticular part of the internal capsule** (i.e., ''beneath'' the lentiform nucleus), which is below the plane of section in the brain slice pictured in Figure 20–5.

Thalamic Nuclei with Subcortical and Diffuse Cortical Connections

The **midline nuclei** of the thalamus consist of diffuse, small nuclei surrounding the third ventricle. They project to paralimbic and limbic cortices and to the limbic sector of the basal ganglia, the ventral striatum.

The **intralaminar nuclei** consist of numerous, small, diffuse collections of nerve cells within the internal medullary lamina. In the caudal aspect of the lamina, two circumscribed intralaminar nuclei can be delineated: the **centromedian nucleus,** which lies adjacent to the ventral posterior complex, and the **parafascicular nucleus,** located just medial to the centromedian nucleus. Like the midline nuclei, the intralaminar nuclei interconnect with basal ganglia circuits. The centromedian nucleus receives fibers from the globus pallidus and area 4 of the cerebrum and projects to the putamen. The parafascicular nucleus receives fibers from area 6 of the cerebrum. Its axons project to the caudate nucleus. In addition, both the centromedian and parafascicular cell groups form topographically organized, diffuse projections to the frontal and parietal lobes important in activating the cortex. The intralaminar nuclei represent the rostral extent of the ascending reticular activating system. They receive bilateral input from the brain stem reticular formation and the anterolateral system of the spinal cord. (See Chapter 6.)

Actually derived from the subthalamus, the **thalamic reticular nucleus** consists of a thin layer of cells sandwiched between the posterior limb of the internal capsule and the external medullary lamina. Unique among thalamic nuclei, it does not project to the cerebral cortex, but rather, it sends fibers to the thalamic nuclei, the brain stem reticular formation, and other parts of the thalamic reticular nucleus. Nearly all thalamic efferents to the cortex must pass through this lateral sheet of cells, and, in doing so, they send collaterals to its neurons. Similarly, corticothalamic projections to the thalamic nuclei pass through the reticular nucleus, where collateral branches form synapses with its cells. Thus, although not directly connected to the cortex, the reticular nucleus monitors both thalamocortical and corticothalamic activity. Although still undefined, its function appears related to the regulation of thalamic activity. Many thalamic reticular nucleus neurons contain gamma-aminobutyric acid, a finding suggesting that these neurons have largely inhibitory effects.

Functional Cortical Regions

The specific connections of individual nuclei of the anterior, medial, ventral, and lateral thalamic cell groups are described in the following sections, in connection with their cortical targets.

Primary Motor and Motor Association Areas

MI corresponds to Brodmann's area 4. Located in the precentral gyrus on the convexity of the cerebral hemisphere, it extends from the fissure of Sylvius laterally into the interhemispheric fissure medially. Neurons of MI influence the motor system directly through the corticospinal and corticobulbar tracts and indirectly through their projections to the red nucleus and the reticular formation. (See Chapter 8.) These neurons also project to and, in turn, receive influences from, recurrent loops through the cerebellum (see Chapter 16) and the basal ganglia (see Chapter 17). MI contains a somatotopic distribution of neurons; that is, the arrangement of neurons follows a sequence reflecting their order of terminations in the brain stem and spinal cord (Fig. 20–7). Nevertheless, unequal amounts of cortex innervate various parts of the body. The parts of the body capable of fine or delicate movement possess a large cortical representation; large numbers of cortical neurons control them, whereas the parts capable only of gross movements have a small cortical representation.

In addition to the somatotopic arrangement, the organization of the primary motor cortex includes radially arranged columns of neurons. Each vertical column consists of a functional entity responsible for directing a group of muscles acting on a single joint. With this organization, the columns of the cortex represent movements, not individual muscles. Individual neurons within these clusters do innervate individual muscles; hence clusters of neurons in different combinations among the columns innervate individual muscles repeatedly. Neurons of the motor cortex having axons in the corticospinal tract function chiefly in the control of the distal muscles of the limbs.

The primary motor cortex interconnects reciprocally with the **caudal (posterior) part of the ventral lateral nucleus** of the thalamus. This portion of the ventral lateral nucleus receives its major input from the deep cerebellar nuclei.

Lesions in MI result immediately in paresis of the contralateral musculature with hypotonia (i.e., decreased resistance to passive manipulation) and diminished muscle stretch reflexes. In a few weeks, muscle strength partially recovers, the affected musculature develops spasticity (i.e., increased resistance to passive manipulation), the muscle stretch reflexes become enhanced, and an extensor plantar response **(Babinski's sign)** appears. In the chronic state, the affected hand and fingers show slowness of movement and loss of dexterity. This is a kinetic apraxia, which is described later in this chapter.

A unimodal cortex devoted to motor planning, the **motor association cortex,** consists of Brodmann's area 6 and parts of areas 8 and 44. The

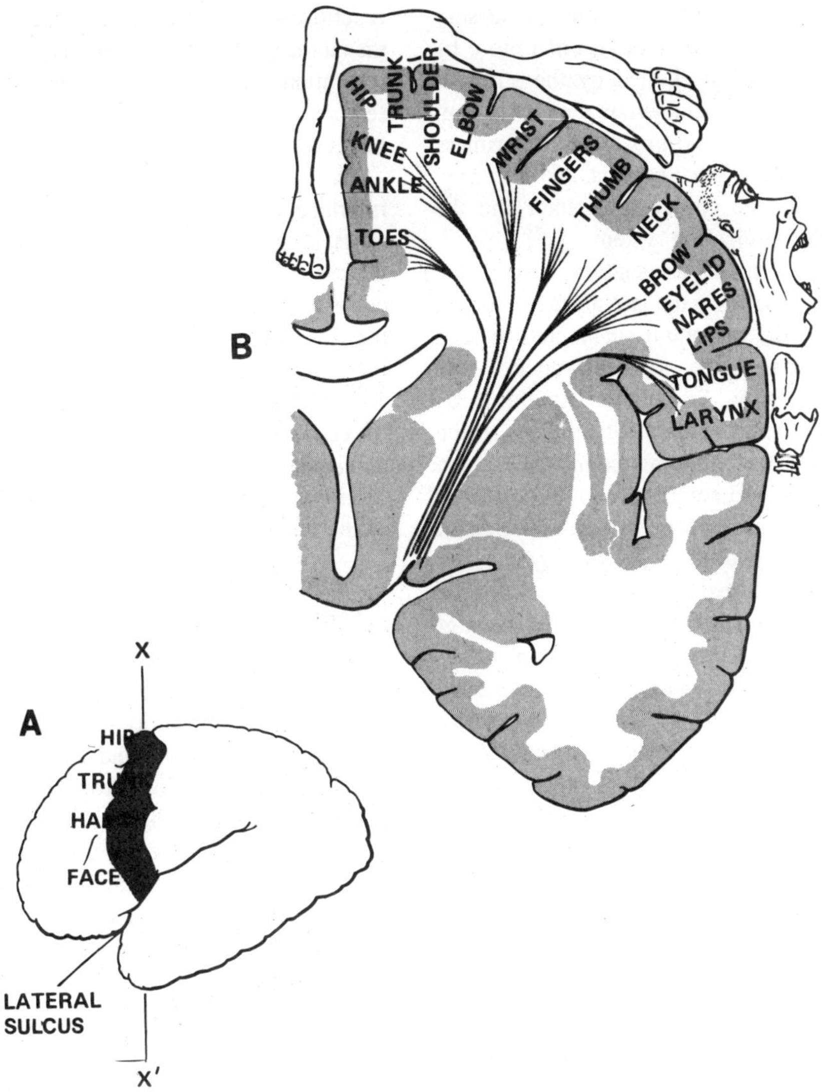

■ **FIGURE 20–7.** **(A)** Lateral surface of the left cerebral hemisphere. The precentral gyrus is *colored,* and the functional organization of upper motor neurons is indicated. **(B)** A coronal section taken through X to X′ provides a more detailed representation of the opposite side of the body in the motor area. (Adapted from Penfield, W, and Rasmussen, H: The Cerebral Cortex in Man. Macmillan, New York, 1950.)

motor association cortex includes the supplementary motor area (MII), the premotor area, the frontal eye fields, and the posterior part of Broca's area.

Located on the medial surface of the frontal lobe in area 6, just anterior to the MI, MII contains a complete somatotopic representation of the body, as shown by the results of electrical stimulation in animals and humans. MII participates in the advance planning and sequencing of movements, particularly for movements involving both sides of the body. Imaging studies demonstrate that this area becomes active when a person thinks about a movement, in the absence of any motor activation.

The **premotor area** in Brodmann's area 6, is immediately in front of area 4 on the lateral surface of the hemisphere. Neurons in both the premotor area and MII receive input from sensory unimodal and heteromodal association cortices. Accordingly, they respond to sensory stimuli, but the response is determined more by the type of movement elicited by the stimulus than by the sensory characteristics of the stimulus. Both these areas also project to the primary motor cortex and the basal ganglia, and they send their axons into the corticospinal tract and the pontocerebellar projection system.

Parts of the motor association cortex, the **frontal eye fields,** lie on the lateral surface of the hemisphere in the precentral sulcus and include the caudal parts of the adjacent superior and middle frontal gyri. Stimulation of this area results in conjugate deviation of the eyes to the opposite side. This region interconnects with the parietal eye field and contributes to all volitional and visually guided saccades, as well as to pursuit and vergence movements of the eyes. (See Chapter 19.) The primary thalamic nucleus of the motor association cortex, the **oralis portion of the ventral lateral nucleus,** contains a small-celled component and a large-celled component that receive fibers from the globus pallidus and the substantia nigra pars reticulata, respectively.

Lesions of the supplementary and premotor cortices result in complex defects of movement in the absence of weakness. Experimental animals with lesions in area 6 lose the ability to alter the type of limb and body movement in response to different types of sensory inputs. Visual guidance of motor performance also becomes impaired. Unilateral lesions that include the frontal eye field result in defective scanning and exploration of the opposite side of the visual environment.

Primary Sensory and Unimodal Sensory Association Areas

The sensory areas for somatic sensation, audition, and vision occupy large areas of the parietal, temporal, and occipital isocortex. Research on structural and functional relationships in the cerebral cortex has rapidly changed our view of its organization. For purposes of this discussion, the term **primary sensory cortex** refers to both primary and secondary areas of earlier descriptions. Each of these areas contains a topographic map of the receptor surface (the body wall, organ of Corti, and retina, respectively). The cells of the adjacent unimodal sensory areas exhibit fundamentally different response characteristics, but they also contain a topographic organization. In primates, these unimodal areas contain multiple repetitions of the somatosensory, auditory, and visual receptor surfaces, although the topographic resolution diminishes, and the extraction of features of categories and individual stimuli increases.

The vestibular and gustatory cortices lie at the interface between isocortical and mesocortical areas in the operculum, where the parietal somatosensory cortex merges with the insular cortex. The detailed structure and functions of these areas have been defined less fully than those for somatosensory, visual, and auditory areas. The olfactory cortex consists of an allocortical (three-layered) area on the ventral surface of the hemisphere. Its organization and pattern of connections necessarily differ markedly from those of the other sensory regions.

Primary Somatosensory and Unimodal Somatosensory Association Areas

The **primary somatosensory area (SI)** includes Brodmann's areas 3, 1, and 2 on the postcentral gyrus. It lies in continuity with a **secondary area (SII)** on the operculum and dorsal insula. These areas receive projections from the posterior part of the **ventral posterolateral nucleus** and from the **ventral posteromedial nucleus** of the thalamus. The ventral posterolateral nucleus transmits information from the medial lemniscus and the spinothalamic tract, and the ventral posteromedial nucleus transmits information from the trigeminothalamic tract. Many cells in these thalamic nuclei have both place- and modality-specific responses to stimuli and small receptive fields, and the functional organization of SI reflects these characteristics. The somatotopic organization of SI consists of a mirror image of the adjacent MI. Muscle spindle afferents activate neurons of area 3a (the most rostral strip of area 3, in the depths of the central sulcus), cutaneous afferents stimulate area 3b (caudal to 3a) and area 1, and joint receptors activate area 2. Active tactile exploration provides especially strong stimulation of the neurons of these areas. The cells of SII have larger receptive fields and respond to touch, pressure, and position of the limbs and pain from both sides of the body. Lesions of SI result in impairment of "cortical sensation," or tactile discrimination. This includes deficits in two-point discrimination, precise localization of tactile stimuli, position sense, and stereognosis. The ability to recognize the primary modalities of sensation (i.e., touch, pain, and temperature) remain preserved but poorly localized in human patients with lesions of SI.

The **somatosensory unimodal association area** lies in the superior parietal lobule (area 5 and the anterior part of area 7). Most of the neurons in this region respond only to somatosensory stimuli. They interconnect with the **lateral posterior nucleus of the thalamus.** This area subserves touch localization, exploration of the environment with the body surface, synthesis of personal and extrapersonal space, and memory of the somesthetic environment. Neurons of this region project to the heteromodal association area in the posterior part of area 7 and the inferior parietal lobule.

Primary Auditory and Unimodal Auditory Association Areas

The transverse temporal gyri (Heschl's gyri) lie within the lateral fissure, continuous with the superior part of the superior temporal gyrus. Brodmann's area 41, the anterior gyrus, corresponds to the **primary auditory area (AI).** Area 42, the **secondary auditory area (AII),** lies posterior to area 41, and it usually occupies the more posterior transverse gyrus and part of the adjacent planum temporale. Both these areas receive auditory information through the auditory radiations from the **medial geniculate nucleus.** AI contains a tonotopic organization; low-frequency sounds receive processing more rostrally and laterally than do high-frequency sounds. Neurons of AI respond not only to the frequency but also to the localization of sound. The ascending auditory pathway has many decussations in the brain stem; thus, the AI area of each hemisphere receives information from both ears, although the input from the contralateral ear is more heavily represented than input from the ipsilateral ear. Unilateral lesions of AI cannot be detected clinically and can be discovered only with specialized tests such as auditory evoked potentials or dichotic listening tasks. Complete cortical deafness results only from bilateral damage to the AI area and the adjacent auditory association areas of both cerebral hemispheres.

The **auditory unimodal association area** lies in area 22 of the superior temporal gyrus. As in the primary auditory cortex, the neurons in this area interconnect with the **medial geniculate nucleus** and respond only to auditory stimuli. They discriminate auditory frequencies and the sequence, or pattern, of sounds. The area also participates in the retention of auditory information. Neurons in this region project to the heteromodal association areas in the prefrontal and temporoparietal areas of cerebral cortex and also to the paralimbic and limbic structures of the temporal lobe.

In the human, bilateral lesions of the auditory association areas or a unilateral left-sided lesion that disconnects area 22 from Wernicke's area result in **pure word deafness.** Patients with this disorder cannot understand or repeat spoken language, but they respond appropriately to environmental sounds (a finding indicating that they are not deaf), and they can understand written language (a finding indicating they are not aphasic).

Primary Visual and Unimodal Visual Association Areas

The striate cortex (area 17), which lies along the banks of the calcarine fissure medially and extends onto the occipital pole, constitutes the **primary visual cortex.** This area receives visual input from the retina through the **lateral geniculate nucleus.** The striate area of each hemisphere receives information from the contralateral half of the binocular visual field. The dorsal parts of the striate cortex, in the cuneus, respond to stimuli in the contralateral lower hemifield. The ventral parts of the striate cortex, in the lingual gyrus, respond to input from the contralateral upper hemifield. Neurons of the striate cortex integrate information from the homologous areas of the two eyes and respond to the shape of objects as well as to their color, size, location, and direction of movement. The **secondary visual cortex,** Brodmann's area 18, surrounds the striate cortex. It, too, contains a representation of the contralateral half of the visual field. In humans, focal lesions of the striate cortex result in visual field defects that reflect this retinotopic organization of the cortex. (See Chapter 18.) Complete bilateral destruction of the striate cortex results in **cortical blindness.** In this condition, the pupillary light reflexes remain intact, but the patient possesses no useful vision. Some patients with cortical blindness claim that they can see when clearly they cannot. This condition bears the term **Anton's syndrome** and results from lesions that destroy area 17 and the peristriate, unimodal visual association cortex in areas 18 and 19.

The **visual unimodal association area** includes the peristriate cortex (areas 18 and 19) and areas on the middle and inferior temporal gyri (areas 20, 21, and 37). Neurons in the visual unimodal association area respond only to visual stimuli and can respond to complex aspects of visual stimuli such as form, motion, and color. The middle temporal visual area at the occipitotemporoparietal junction (areas 19, 37, and 39) analyzes the speed and direction of moving stimuli. (See Chapter 19.) These areas receive thalamic input from the **inferior and lateral parts of the pulvinar** (Figs. 20–4 and 20–8). In experimental animals, lesions of this area result in defects of depth perception, distance judgment, movement, spatial orientation, and hue discrimination thresholds. In humans, lesions in areas 20, 21, and 37 can result in discrete deficits in naming of visual stimuli that affect some categories of objects and not others. For example, a patient may easily recognize and name manufactured tools but cannot identify correctly items of food or types of animals.

Primary Vestibular Areas

Experimental evidence indicates that **areas at the boundaries of the somatosensory cortex, 3a and 2V,** respond to stimulation of the vestibular apparatus. These two areas of the somatosensory cortex also receive information about muscle spindle stimulation and joint movement, respectively. They interconnect with the **ventral posterolateral and ventral lateral thalamic nuclei.** Other areas that have been implicated in the conscious sense of gravity and acceleration include an area near SII, at the parietoinsular interface, and a part of area 7 in the posterior parietal lobe.

Primary Taste Area

The **primary taste area** or gustatory cortical area resides in the parietal operculum and adjacent anterior insular cortex (Brodmann's area 43; Fig. 20–1). This area receives taste information from the ipsilateral side of the tongue through the **parvocellular division of the ventral posteromedial nucleus of the thalamus** (Fig. 20–4).

Primary Olfactory Area

In spite of its name, the **primary olfactory cortex** differs from the sensory areas discussed earlier in the pattern of its connections. This area of allocortex receives processed olfactory signals from the olfactory bulb and relays these signals directly to other limbic areas. The primary olfactory cortex also relays olfactory signals

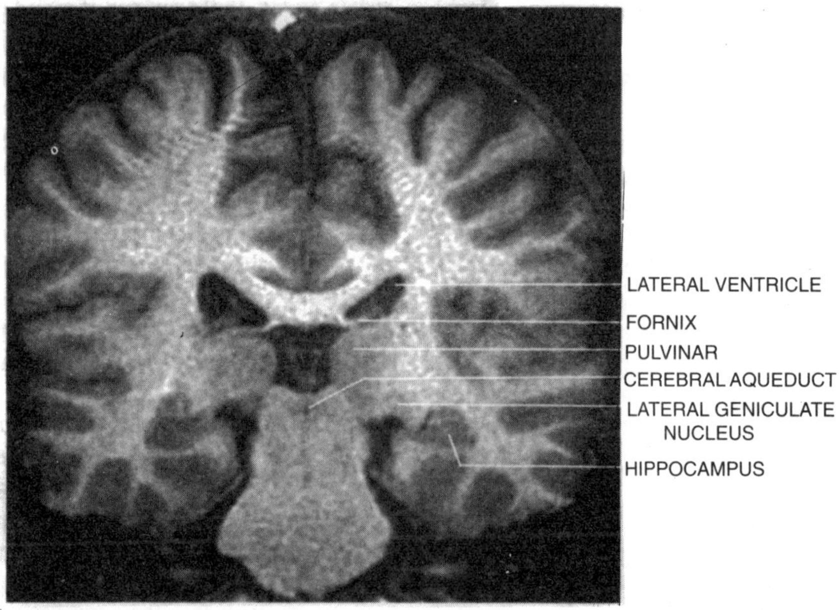

■ **FIGURE 20–8.** A T1-weighted (spoiled gradient echo) magnetic resonance image from a neurologically normal adult. This coronal sequence shows the lateral geniculate nucleus and pulvinar in the posterior thalamus.

directly to the **lateral orbitofrontal cortex** and to part of the **insula,** as well as to the magnocellular or **medial portion of the mediodorsal nucleus of the thalamus,** which reciprocally interconnects with the orbitofrontal area of the isocortex. The allocortical primary olfactory cortex therefore provides input into a set of thalamocortical-corticothalamic connections that resemble those of other sensory systems. In experimental animals, lesions in the pathway from the primary olfactory cortex through the thalamus to the orbitofrontal cortex have shown that this pathway participates in complex olfactory discrimination learning.

Heteromodal Association Areas

MI, MII, SI, and SII and the unimodal association areas participate only in single modality information processing. In the next stage of information processing, termed heteromodal, several different sensory modalities converge onto and can activate single neurons. Many neurons in heteromodal regions also change their discharge rate during specific motor acts, a finding indicating that these neurons integrate complex sensory inputs with motor output. Regions within the two major heteromodal association areas interconnect, and the networks of these connections form the basis for a variety of cognitive processes, including language. The heteromodal cortices also have extensive connections with paralimbic and limbic structures and therefore participate in learning, memory, mood, and motivation. Injury to heteromodal areas leads to complex neurologic disorders with combinations of cognitive defects and emotional disturbances. The two major heteromodal association areas include (1) the temporoparietal areas and (2) the prefrontal areas.

Temporoparietal Association Area

The **temporoparietal heteromodal association area** occupies a strip of cortex extending from the middle and caudal superior temporal gyri into the inferior parietal lobule and the posterior part of the superior parietal lobe. It includes both lateral and medial surfaces of the posterior parietal cortex, and on the medial side it continues into the posterior part of the temporal lobe. This strip thus abuts the auditory cortex of the lateral temporal lobe, the somatosensory cortex of the anterior parietal lobe, the visual cortex of the occipital lobe, and the paralimbic cortices on the medial surface of the hemisphere. The temporoparietal association cortex receives input from all these adjacent sensory areas and has both input and output relations with the paralimbic cortex. The activity of its cells reflects these connections, because many neurons within this region respond to a single sensory modality, whereas neighboring neurons respond to a single sensory modality of another type or to multiple types of sensory modalities. In addition, many of these neurons alter their responses during performance of tasks with a strong motivational component such as a reward. The thalamic nuclei most heavily connected with the temporoparietal area include the **medial part of the pulvinar nucleus** and the **lateral posterior nucleus.**

In experimental animals, unilateral lesions in these areas result in neglect of objects and stimuli in personal and extrapersonal space on the contralateral side of the body. Bilateral lesions in animals lead to impairment in exploring extrapersonal space, with defects in determining spatial relationships between objects and negotiating relatively simple mazes. Visual, auditory, and somatosensory perceptions remain intact, but these sensory modalities cannot be integrated.

Lesions of the temporoparietal heteromodal association areas in the human result in complex disturbances that depend on the side of the lesion. Damage in the left cerebral hemisphere leads to disorders of language and disturbed spatial integration. An important part of the temporal heteromodal association area in the left hemisphere, **Wernicke's area,** lies in the posterior part of the superior temporal gyrus (Brodmann's area 22). This area integrates the sensory modalities needed to understand written and spoken language. Injury results in **Wernicke's aphasia,** which is described later in this chapter. Complex disorders result from left cerebral hemisphere lesions that spare Wernicke's area but damage the angular gyrus (Brodmann's area 39) in the inferior parietal lobe. These consist of varying combinations of the following:

1. Alexia (inability to read).
2. Anomia (inability to name objects).
3. Constructional apraxia (inability to construct simple figures such as a clock or a house with pencil and paper).
4. Agraphia (inability to write).

5. Finger agnosia (inability to name individual fingers).
6. Confusion between the left and right sides of personal and extrapersonal space.

A subset of these disorders, the combination of acalculia, agraphia, finger agnosia, and right-left disorientation, has been termed the **Gerstmann syndrome;** however, it seldom appears in isolation. Lesions of the left cerebral hemisphere that spare Wernicke's area but affect the supramarginal gyrus (Brodmann's area 40) in the inferior parietal lobule result in conduction aphasia. This disorder is described later.

Unilateral damage to the temporoparietal heteromodal association area in the right cerebral hemisphere causes disturbances in the integration of personal and extrapersonal space, referred to as **sensory neglect.** Such lesions result in dressing apraxia (difficulty in dressing, particularly the left side of the body), constructional apraxia (difficulty in constructing simple figures with pencil and paper, usually with inattention to the left side of the figure), neglect of the left side of personal and extrapersonal space, and lack of insight about these difficulties.

Bilateral lesions of the temporoparietal heteromodal association areas lead to complex disorders including visual, spatial, and language defects. One such disorder, **Balint's syndrome,** usually results from bilateral lesions of the posterior parietal lobe. This consists of (1) inability to gaze toward the peripheral field (even though eye movements are intact), (2) difficulty in reaching out and touching objects accurately with visual guidance, and (3) inattention to objects in the peripheral parts of the visual field.

In addition to the cognitive, perceptive, and motor disturbances resulting from lesions of the temporoparietal heteromodal association areas, affective disorders also appear. Mood alterations ranging from anger to apathy can be seen with these disturbances. These emotional disturbances result from interruption of the connections between heteromodal association areas and parts of the limbic system.

Prefrontal Cortex

The largest part of the frontal lobe, the prefrontal region, lies rostral to the motor areas. The **prefrontal heteromodal association area** makes up most of this region. It includes Brodmann's areas 8 through 10, parts of 11 and 12, and 45 through 47. A small area on the ventral surface of the frontal lobe, the orbital cortex, interconnects principally with the limbic lobe and is discussed as part of the paralimbic cortex. The prefrontal heteromodal association area has major connections with other areas of cortex, notably the temporoparietal association cortex and the motor association areas of the frontal lobe, as well as the paralimbic cortex. The prefrontal heteromodal area interconnects reciprocally with the **lateral part of the mediodorsal nucleus of the thalamus** and with the **ventral anterior nucleus,** which receives input from the reticular formation. The prefrontal area also sends projections to the basal ganglia through the head of the caudate nucleus.

The neurons of the prefrontal cortex respond to many different types of sensory inputs and thus can be characterized as heteromodal neurons, but they also respond to the behavioral importance of the inputs. A neuron responding strongly to a sensory input that has been associated with a pleasant reward may respond differently when the same input has been associated with a noxious stimulus. Thus, the neurons of the prefrontal region appear to integrate motivational events with complex sensory stimuli. Neurons in this area also serve to inhibit motor responses when a task requires delaying the response. The ventromedial component of the prefrontal cortex participates in emotional processing and in planning and decision making.

Injury to the prefrontal cortex in experimental animals impairs the ability to perform tasks requiring the animal to alternate responses to stimuli with a delay. Unilateral ablation of the frontal eye fields in animals results in neglect of stimuli in the opposite side of extrapersonal space. In humans, lesions of the prefrontal cortex disrupt some of the most complex aspects of behavior. Unilateral lesions of either side lead to neglect of the contralateral side of extrapersonal space. Bilateral lesions cause markedly disturbed behavior. These patients become unconcerned with their illness and may appear depressed or inappropriately jocular. Their social graces and concern for others disappear. They may eat from the floor, drop food on their clothing without concern, and ignore the ordinary standards of cleanliness. Often they appear apathetic, although they may be irascible. They cannot exercise foresight or good judgment and have essentially no insight. They can be distracted easily and cannot perform complex tasks requiring appropriate sequencing of several actions or responses. These disorders have been termed the **frontal lobe syndrome** and also the **dysexecutive syndrome.**

Paralimbic Areas

The **paralimbic areas** consist primarily of mesocortical areas. With the limbic cortex, they form a continuous ring of tissue at the medial edge of the cerebral hemisphere (the limbic lobe) that extends laterally to include the insula. The areas of Brodmann that make up this ring of cortex include the following:

1. The temporal pole (area 38).
2. The insula.
3. The caudal orbitofrontal cortex (caudal parts of areas 11 and 12).
4. The parahippocampal regions (areas 27, 28, 34, and 35).
5. The retrosplenial area (areas 26, 29, and 30), cingulate gyrus (areas 23, 24, 31, and 33), and the precallosal and subcallosal regions (areas 32 and 25).

The paralimbic areas receive information from heteromodal association areas of the isocortex, limbic cortex, and **anterior, laterodorsal, midline, and medial nuclei of the thalamus.** The medial nuclei heavily interconnected with the paralimbic cortex include the **medial part of the mediodorsal nucleus** and the **medial part of the pulvinar.**

The paralimbic areas participate in memory and learning, drive and affect, and social behavior. Through their direct impact on the hypothalamus, these areas influence homeostasis. (See Chapter 21.) Damage to the parahippocampal cortex as well as to the hippocampus and amygdala leads to severe disorders of memory. Damage to the paralimbic areas of the orbitofrontal region and to the amygdala results in changes in mood and social behavior. In some patients, this damage leads to severe apathy. The paralimbic areas of the orbitofrontal and insular regions also participate in processing olfactory and gustatory information, as noted previously in this chapter.

Limbic Areas

The **limbic cortex,** which consists of **allocortex,** includes the (1) hippocampal formation and (2) primary olfactory (pyriform) cortex. The **corticoid areas,** which contain no discernible layering of cells, include the (1) amygdala, (2) septal area, and (3) substantia innominata. Many of these areas cannot be seen on the medial or ventral surface of the hemisphere because, although they are directly continuous with the paralimbic cortex, they are folded under, so they appear deep to the medial edge of the paralimbic cortex.

A specific group of neurons extending through several limbic areas provides excitatory cholinergic innervation for the entire surface of the cerebral cortex, particularly the paralimbic areas. These include the medial septal nucleus, the vertical and horizontal nuclei of the diagonal band of Broca, and the nucleus basalis of Meynert in the substantia innominata. (See Fig. 23–1.)

Limbic structures participate in both explicit memory (the hippocampus) and associative, or emotional, memory (the amygdala). The **anterior thalamic nuclei,** the **medial part of the mediodorsal nucleus,** and the **medial pulvinar** connect directly to the hippocampus, primary olfactory cortex, and amygdala. The limbic cortex provides input to basal ganglia through projections to the ventromedial part of the head of the caudate nucleus and to the ventral striatum. (For additional discussion of the limbic areas of the cortex, see Chapter 21.)

Disorders of Cortical Networks

Agnosias

The process of comprehension (''knowing'' or ''gnosis'') entails a comparison of present sensory phenomena with past experience. For example, the visual association areas must be called on when a person recognizes an old friend in a crowd. **Agnosia** consists of a failure to recognize stimuli when the appropriate sensory systems function adequately. Agnosia commonly occurs in visual, tactile, and auditory forms.

Visual agnosia can be defined as the failure to recognize objects visually in the absence of a defect of visual acuity or intellectual impairment.

The patient often can see the object clearly but cannot recognize or identify it visually. In a pure visual agnosia, the same object can be identified by other sensibilities such as touch. The most striking example of this, **prosopagnosia,** consists of an agnosia for familiar faces. Bilateral lesions of the temporal aspect of visual unimodal association areas usually underlie visual agnosia.

Tactile agnosia consists of the inability to recognize objects by touch when tactile and proprioceptive sensibilities remain intact in the part of the body being tested. Patients with tactile agnosia often have disturbances of body image. Lesions of the supramarginal gyrus (area 40) usually underlie tactile agnosia.

Auditory agnosia involves the failure of a patient with intact hearing to recognize specific sounds, including speech, music, or familiar noises. Bilateral lesions of the posterior part of the superior temporal convolution (area 22) are responsible for this condition.

Apraxias

Apraxia can be defined as loss of the ability to carry out correctly certain movements in response to stimuli that normally elicit these movements. This deficit occurs in the absence of weakness, sensory loss, or disturbance of language comprehension. Accomplishing a complex act requires the integrity of a large part of the cerebral cortex. There must first be an idea or a mental formulation of the plan to carry out the movement. This formulation must then be transferred by association fibers to the motor system, where it can be executed. Apraxias usually result from lesions interrupting connections between the site of formulation of a motor act and the motor areas responsible for its execution.

Ideomotor apraxia consists of the inability to perform a complex motor task despite awareness of the task the patient intends to perform. Patients with this disorder can perform many complex acts automatically but cannot carry out the same acts on command. A lesion of the supramarginal gyrus of the dominant parietal lobe underlies this disorder.

Ideational apraxia refers to failures in carrying out sequences of acts, although individual movements can be made correctly. This form of apraxia results from lesions in the dominant parietal lobe or the corpus callosum.

Kinetic (motor) apraxia involves the inability to execute fine acquired movements and results from disease of the contralateral frontal lobe. **Gait apraxia** consists of difficulty in initiating and continuing smoothly the movements needed for walking. It results from bilateral disease of the frontal lobes. Typically, the patient appears to have the feet "glued to the floor," because the patient makes a series of incomplete walking movements of the legs, then may stride for one or two steps, only to develop another series of incomplete ambulatory movements.

Aphasias

Facile use of language and speech is a remarkable attribute of the human brain—one that no other animal shares. **Language** refers to the vocabulary and syntactic rules needed for communication. **Speech** refers to the production of spoken language. **Dysarthria** can be defined as a disturbance in the execution of speech and often occurs without a disorder of language. **Aphonia** involves the inability to produce sounds. **Aphasia** consists of a disorder of language caused by a defect in either the production or the comprehension of vocabulary or syntax.

Beginning early in life, nearly everyone selectively develops one hemisphere of the brain more intensively than the other in the processes required for language. Usually, the left side of the brain assumes the leading role, and the person becomes right-handed. Right-handedness indicates the preferential use of the right hand in most or all unimanual activities, and it is usually associated with preferential use of the right eye for monocular visual functions and the right foot for motor acts such as kicking. Approximately 90% of people in the United States use the right hand preferentially, and essentially all of them have left-hemisphere dominance for language. About 10% of people use the left hand preferentially, but about half of them nevertheless have left-hemisphere dominance. The remaining left-handed people have right-hemisphere dominance or mixed left and right dominance. Aphasia appears only if a lesion involves the language areas of the dominant hemisphere. Children display a preference for the use of the right or left hand from an early age, so it is unclear when cerebral dominance for language actually occurs. In any case, cerebral dominance for language is a plastic phenomenon; that is, it can be changed, up to the age of about 7 years. For example, a right-handed child 5 years of age who suffers an injury in the language areas of the left cerebral hemisphere will lose speech initially, but will learn to speak again in 1 or 2 years. An adult cannot recover speech to this extent after damage to the language areas of the left hemisphere.

Three regions of the dominant cerebral hemisphere serve important roles in aphasia: **Broca's area, Wernicke's area,** and the intervening area of parietal lobe (the parietal operculum). Broca's area, the anterior speech region, lies in the inferior frontal gyrus just rostral to the site of the motor representation of the face (Fig. 20–9). The region includes Brodmann's areas 44, 45, and 47. As mentioned previously, Wernicke's area lies in the posterior part of the superior temporal gyrus on the convexity of the brain and extends onto the upper surface of the temporal lobe. The posterior part of Brodmann's area 22 lies central to Wernicke's area. Wernicke's area connects with Broca's area through a series of neuronal relays in the cerebral cortex from the temporal lobe around the posterior end of the fissure of Sylvius into the lower parietal lobe and running forward into the frontal lobe. Functionally, Wernicke's area provides the capacity to recognize speech patterns relayed from the left primary auditory cortex. Information about incoming speech patterns moves to Broca's area, which generates the proper pattern of signals to the speech musculature for the production of meaningful speech. Three general forms of aphasia have been recognized that relate to Broca's area, Wernicke's area, and the intervening cerebral cortex.

Lesions of Broca's area lead to **nonfluent** (also termed **motor, anterior,** or **Broca's) aphasia** (Fig. 20–9). The patient produces spoken language slowly and effortfully, with poorly produced sounds and ungrammatical, telegraphic speech that deletes many prepositions, nouns, and verbs. The patient has extreme difficulty in expressing certain grammatical words and phrases. The phrase, "no ifs, ands, or buts" proves to be particularly difficult for affected persons to speak. Phrases or sentences can be repeated only poorly. The patient usually comprehends spoken and written language, but becomes frustrated and discouraged by the difficulty with speech. Vascular lesions of Broca's area often involve the underlying white matter and

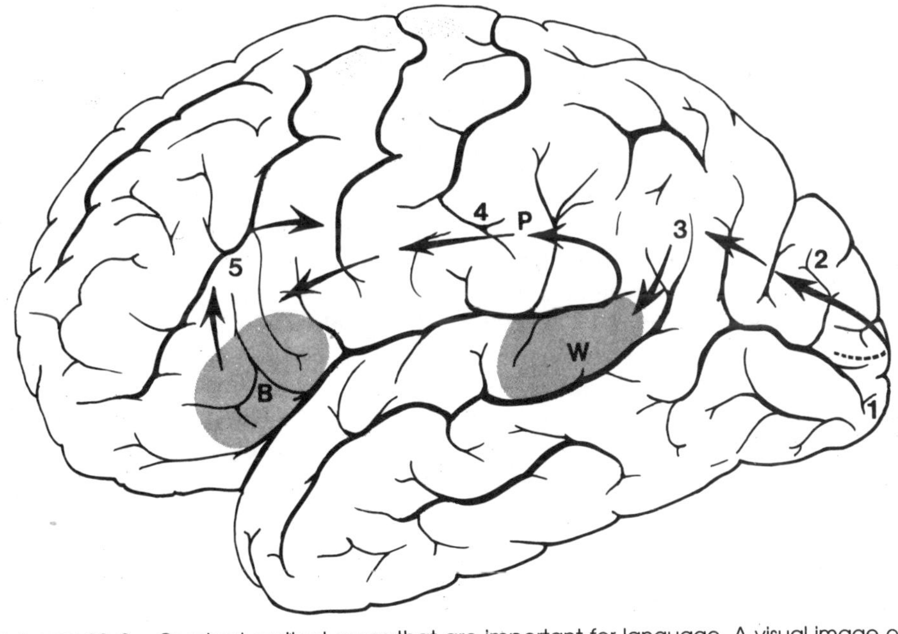

■ **FIGURE 20–9.** Cerebral cortical areas that are important for language. A visual image of a word is projected from the calcarine cortex **(1)** into the visual association areas 18 and 19 **(2)** to the region of the angular gyrus **(3).** Information is then transferred to Wernicke's area (W) to arouse the learned auditory form of the word. This information is then transferred by corticocortical connections **(4)** across the parietal operculum (P) to Broca's area (B), which contains programs that control **(5)** the cortical motor region in the precentral gyrus involved in speech.

thereby damage the internal capsule. Consequently, right hemiplegia usually accompanies Broca's aphasia.

Lesions of Wernicke's area lead to **fluent** (also termed **sensory, posterior,** or **Wernicke's) aphasia** (Fig. 20–9). The patient produces spoken language more rapidly than normal, with preserved grammatical construction. The patient cannot find the correct words to express thoughts, however, and may omit words or use circumlocutions, may use words without precise meanings, or may substitute words. Substitutions of one word for another are called **verbal paraphasias. Literal paraphasia** involves the substitution of a well-articulated but inappropriate phoneme in a word (e.g., saying pork for cork). Words may be produced that consist of random collections of sounds; these are termed **neologisms.** The patient has poor comprehension of speech and poor repetition of phrases or sentences. The patient often does not recognize the speech difficulty and may show no concern about it. Because lesions of Wernicke's area are far removed from MI and the internal capsule, patients with Wernicke's aphasia usually do not have hemiplegia.

Lesions of the conduction pathway from Wernicke's area to Broca's area cause **conduction aphasia** by disconnecting the speech recognition area from the speech execution area. This condition usually causes fluent aphasia with poor repetition of spoken language. Despite phonetic errors, comprehension of spoken language usually remains preserved.

Posteriorly placed vascular lesions affecting speech may damage the angular gyrus (area 39) in association with injury to Wernicke's area. Infarction of the angular gyrus of the dominant hemisphere results in loss of the ability to read **(alexia)** and write **(agraphia)** in the absence of primary visual or motor impairment.

The preceding paragraphs describe localization of the regions that control various aspects of language. Individual patients vary greatly, however, in the precise location of small subregions of cortex that control various language skills within these large areas. Individual brains also appear to vary in the number of cortical loci within these regions that control language. As a consequence of this individual variability, partial lesions of these general cortical regions in the dominant hemisphere may not produce predictable language deficits. The effects of any given lesion depend on the number and distribution of language processing sites within Broca's area and Wernicke's areas in the afflicted individual patient.

Case Follow-up

The man with the right-sided weakness and nonfluent aphasia was thought to have ischemia (diminished blood flow) of the anterior portion of the left cerebral hemisphere affecting Broca's area and the underlying white matter, with extension to the internal capsule. An imaging study of the head with computed tomography revealed no evidence of hemorrhage in the brain, and because the patient had been seen within 3 hours of the onset of his difficulty, he was given intravenous tissue plasminogen activator. This medication has the capacity of breaking down already formed clots of blood in the vasculature. The result was a gradual return of strength in the right limbs and full recovery of language functions over the next 24 hours. Further evaluation of the patient revealed that he had two untreated risk factors for stroke: high blood pressure and hypercholesterolemia. These disorders were treated with antihypertensive medication and a cholesterol-lowering agent. He was also given one aspirin per day as prophylaxis against further strokes. He continues to do well 5 years after this event.

21

Limbic System

Overview

The **limbic system** integrates our experience of the external world with the fundamental physiologic processes that keep us alive. At this most basic level of function, limbic circuits coordinate reflexes and behaviors through which we maintain our internal environment "within normal limits," a process called **homeostasis.** The limbic system achieves this through feedback signals from sensory receptors (primarily in the viscera) to neurons that regulate (1) the endocrine system, (2) the autonomic nervous system, and (3) homeostatic behaviors. Often ignored in descriptions of homeostasis, **behavior** serves as the primary mechanism by which the body achieves homeostasis. We achieve nutrient assimilation, water balance, and thermoregulation by procuring and eating food, finding and drinking fluids, and seeking a more comfortable environment (going into the shade or turning on an air conditioner to cool off). Sleeping behavior is also essential for our survival.

In parallel with the regulation of homeostatic mechanisms for individual survival, the limbic system integrates endocrine function and autonomic activity with **social behaviors** that are essential for survival of the species. These include reproduction, parenting behavior, and territorial aggression. The circuits linking the limbic telencephalon with the hypothalamus and the brain stem most directly control these social functions. Finally, paralimbic and limbic cortices, particularly the hippocampal formation and the amygdala, play essential roles in **learning and memory.**

Telencephalic Limbic System

The limbic system can be defined best by its functions. The anatomic circuits required to carry out these functions extend from the cortex to the brain stem, and no single anatomic definition of this extensive system has been accepted universally. In the telencephalon, the limbic structures include the mesocortex or **paralimbic cortex** (the parahippocampal, cingulate and paraterminal gyri, and the caudal orbitofrontal, insular, and temporal pole cortices), the allocortex or **limbic cortex** (hippocampal formation and primary olfactory cortex), and the **corticoid areas** (amygdala, septal area, and substantia innominata). These limbic regions participate in two fundamentally different sets of connections: (1) intracortical networks for emotion, comportment, attention, and memory and (2) subcortical pathways through the hypothalamus and brain stem that regulate homeostasis and social behaviors.

Hippocampal Formation

Structure

The **hippocampal formation** consists of a three-layered allocortical structure folded into the most medial edge of the parahippocampal gyrus, where the hippocampal formation and the parahippocampal gyrus are directly continuous with each other (Fig. 21–1B and C). In the part of the temporal lobe illustrated in Figure 21–1C, the medial edge of the parahippocampal gyrus forms Brodmann's area 28, or the **entorhinal cortex.**

The **hippocampal formation** includes three parallel zones or strips, and each of these zones

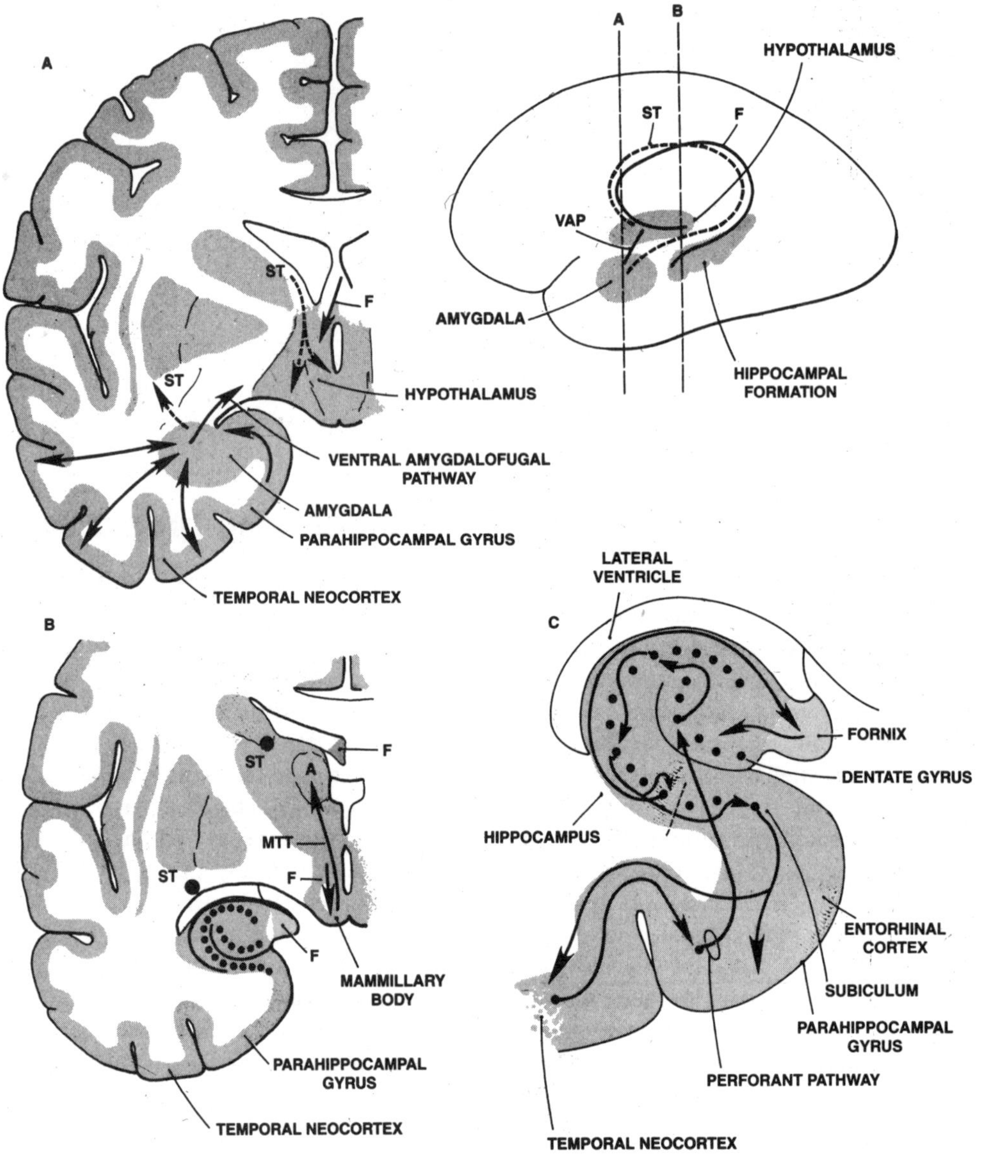

■ **FIGURE 21-1.** The amygdala and hippocampal formation. The lateral view of the hemisphere in the upper right shows the position of these limbic structures and their major efferent pathways. **(A)** and **(B)** on this small diagram indicate the levels of the corresponding coronal sections illustrated in **A** and **B** on the *left*. The drawing on the *lower right* **(C)** provides an enlarged view of the hippocampal formation. A = anterior nucleus of the thalamus; F = fornix; MTT = mammillothalamic tract; ST = stria terminalis; VAP = ventral amygdaloid pathway. (Adapted from Heimer, L: The Human Brain and Spinal Cord. Springer-Verlag, New York, 1983.)

contains three-layered cortex. The zones appear to have been folded in on one another at the medial edge of the hemisphere. They include the following: (1) the **subiculum,** which resides in direct continuity with the entorhinal cortex of the parahippocampal gyrus; (2) the **hippocampus** proper **(Ammon's horn);** and (3) the **dentate gyrus.** This folded cortical structure forms the floor of the inferior horn of the lateral ventricle from the amygdala to the splenium of the corpus callosum.

Connections

The hippocampal formation articulates with other brain areas through two main fiber pathways: the **perforant pathway** and the **fornix** (Fig. 21–1).

Both these pathways carry the afferent as well as the efferent projections of the hippocampal formation. The organization of this brain area into three subunits (subiculum, hippocampus, and dentate gyrus) relates not only to its cytoarchitecture but also to its circuitry. Inputs from other brain areas move serially through each of these components of the hippocampal formation. Afferent information from the fornix and the perforant pathway initially enters the dentate gyrus and then moves into the hippocampus. The hippocampus projects information to the subiculum, which provides the major source of efferent fibers from this region, although some output also originates in the hippocampus proper.

Through the fornix, the hippocampal formation connects reciprocally with the septal area, the thalamus (particularly the anterior nuclear group), and the hypothalamus, where many of its fibers terminate in the mammillary bodies. Through the perforant pathway, the hippocampal formation articulates reciprocally with the entorhinal cortex (see Fig. 21–1C). The entorhinal area receives direct olfactory input from the olfactory bulb and primary olfactory cortex, but in the human its major inputs come from association areas of the temporal lobe, consisting of indirect visual, auditory, and multimodal sensory inputs. These inputs provide highly processed information about objects, individuals, settings, and events, rather than elemental sensory stimuli.

The Hippocampal Formation Is Important for Learning and Memory

Although we know a great deal about the connections, neurotransmitters, and electrophysiologic properties of the hippocampal formation, we are just beginning to comprehend its functions. Experimental and clinical observations clearly indicate the importance of this formation in **learning and memory,** particularly in explicit or declarative memory. Through its connections with networks of the isocortex, and its integration with the amygdala and other limbic areas, the hippocampus builds cognitive maps through which humans recognize their location in space and time and their relation to external objects and events, both present and past.

Some people with long-standing, severe temporal lobe epilepsy have sustained bilateral damage to the hippocampal formation, either as a result of the disease, or in a few cases, in conjunction with surgical resections to relieve the seizures. These people have severe deficits in declarative memory. In patients who have had surgical lesions, the deficits usually include profound anterograde amnesia, or the inability to learn new information, in spite of normal, or only mildly impaired, memory for information and events that occurred preoperatively. Combined with clinical observations of this type, studies on experimental animals suggest that the hippocampus participates in the consolidation of new information. Memory formation requires the hippocampus, but memories do not appear to be stored in the structure. The storage of information probably occurs in the relevant cortical circuits or networks (i.e., the cortical circuits that were activated by the incoming sensory stimuli).

Amygdala

A spherical mass of neurons within the temporal lobe, the **amygdala** (Figs. 21–1 and 21–2), forms an external bulge on the parahippocampal gyrus called the **uncus** (see Figs. 1–6 and 20–2). The amygdala consists of a matrix of nuclei that can be subdivided into three functional units: basolateral, central, and corticomedial divisions. Each of the three divisions, in turn, consists of one or more individual amygdaloid nuclei.

Basolateral Division

The **basolateral amygdala** includes the lateral nucleus and several nuclei in the basal group. Collectively, the lateral and basolateral nuclei receive highly processed sensory information from the heteromodal sensory association area of the temporal lobes and connect reciprocally with paralimbic cortex, especially the orbitofrontal cortex (the ventral and ventromedial parts of the frontal lobe) and temporal pole. (See Chapter 20.) In the primate brain, major inputs from the temporal lobe and minor inputs from the insula provide the amygdala with integrated gustatory, viscerosensory, and somatosensory information. In nonprimate mammals, afferents from the insula are the predominant inputs. The temporal lobe connections also give the basolateral amygdala complex sensory information for use in visual and auditory recognition of objects and individuals.

In the basolateral amygdala, the neuronal morphology, connections, and neurotransmitters show striking similarities to those of the cerebral cortex. As in other types of cortex, the basolateral amygdala projection cells employ glutamate as a neurotransmitter; there are numerous gamma-

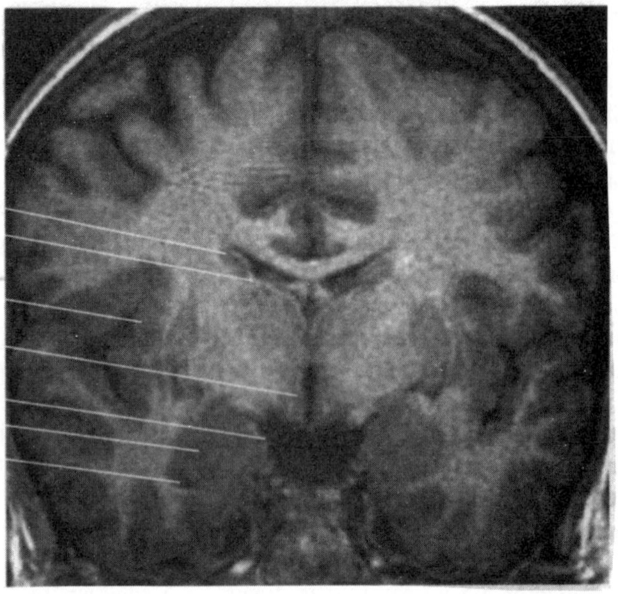

■ **FIGURE 21-2.** A T1-weighted magnetic resonance image from a neurologically normal adult. This image shows a coronal plane through the amygdala. Compare with Figure 21-1A.

aminobutyric acid–ergic interneurons; and the area receives important cholinergic activation from the basal forebrain. (See Chapter 23.) The connections of this amygdaloid area also show cortical characteristics. These connections include principally other areas of cortex, but also the thalamus (especially the mediodorsal and midline nuclei) and the striatum (primarily the nucleus accumbens). The basolateral nuclei also send important intra-amygdalar projections to the corticomedial and central amygdaloid nuclei. Thus, through the basolateral amygdala, the corticomedial and central nuclei gain access to highly processed sensory input, especially auditory and visual information.

Central Nucleus

The **central nucleus** of the amygdala articulates most intimately with the brain stem and hypothalamus, through which it receives sensory information from the body wall and the viscera and, in turn, modulates visceral and cardiovascular functions. Through these connections, the central amygdala plays an important role in coordination of emotional and autonomic responses. This nucleus also serves a key function in the complex limbic circuitry that responds to and regulates fear and stress.

Corticomedial Amygdala

The **corticomedial amygdala,** which includes the medial nucleus and several cortical nuclei, receives its primary input from the olfactory bulb and primary olfactory cortex and reciprocates these connections. The efferent connections of the corticomedial amygdala, however, are focused on the hypothalamus. Through these connections, the corticomedial amygdala modulates and integrates pituitary function and social behaviors (see later). In nonprimate mammals, the olfactory connections of this area of the amygdala provide essential contributions to the regulation of endocrine function and social behaviors. In primates, other sensory inputs, especially visual, relayed through the basolateral amygdala, play equally important roles in these functions.

Extended Amygdala

Two pathways, the **stria terminalis** and the **ventral amygdaloid pathway,** connect the central and corticomedial nuclei with the hypothalamus and brain stem (Fig. 21–1A). These pathways form a ring of fibers linking the corticomedial and central cell groups of the amygdala with cell groups in the substantia innominata and the bed nucleus of the stria terminalis, at the rostral end of the hypothalamus. This ring of cells and fibers is termed the **extended amygdala.**

The Amygdala Modulates Emotion and Associates Memory with Emotion

Experimental lesions of the amygdala in nonhuman primates evoke a series of behaviors known as the Kluver-Bucy syndrome. Monkeys with large amygdala lesions often display (1) inappropriately directed and increased amounts of sexual behavior, (2) loss of aggressiveness, and (3) compulsive oral exploration of objects in their environment.

Lesion and imaging studies in humans demonstrate that the amygdala performs important functions in **linking emotional and motivational responses to external stimuli;** that is, it functions in both the perception and the production of emotion. Most of the available data associate the amygdala with negative affect, but some evidence suggests that it participates in positive emotional reactions, although fewer studies have evaluated this aspect of its function. Specifically, the amygdala appears to contribute to learning and memory and serves a function in **associative memory.** It may also participate in declarative memory for complex emotional stimuli, because patients with amygdala damage show deficits in this aspect of behavior.

The roles of the amygdala in motivation and affect undoubtedly stem from its connections with cortical networks involving the prefrontal and paralimbic cortices and the ventral striatum. Through its connections with the hypothalamus, the amygdala also performs important functions in homeostatic regulation of autonomic, endocrine, and immune processes.

Hypothalamus

In the ventral diencephalon, the **hypothalamus** forms the floor and the ventral part of the walls of the third ventricle. The shallow **hypothalamic sulcus** on the wall of the third ventricle demarcates the hypothalamus from the thalamus.

The hypothalamus forms the ventral surface of the brain from the level of the **optic chiasm** to the rostral midbrain. The **tuber cinereum** occupies the portion of the hypothalamic floor between the optic chiasm and the mammillary bodies. The **infundibulum,** or stalk of the pituitary, extends ventrally from the tuber cinereum to the pars nervosa of the hypophysis. The lumen of the third ventricle may evaginate into the infundibulum for a variable distance, to form the infundibular recess (see Figs. 1–3 and 1–4). A part of the tuber cinereum, the **median eminence,** extends between the optic chiasm and the infundibulum. The paired, spherical **mammillary bodies** reside caudal to the tuber cinereum and rostral to the interpeduncular fossa of the midbrain.

Subdivisions: Regions and Zones

The hypothalamus consists primarily of gray matter formed into a matrix of nuclei. The matrix can be divided rostrocaudally into four regions: the **preoptic region,** which is most rostral; the **anterior hypothalamus;** the **tuberal region;** and the **mammillary region,** which is most caudal (Fig. 21–3).

The hypothalamic matrix can also be divided into three parasagittal zones. From medial to lateral, they are the periventricular, medial, and lateral. The **periventricular zone** consists of a narrow lamina of evenly distributed cells adjacent to the third ventricle. The suprachiasmatic, paraventricular, and arcuate nuclei are the most conspicuous cell groups within this narrow zone. The **medial zone,** in contrast, contains numerous, well-differentiated cell groups, which are described in the following sections of this chapter. The **lateral zone** contains sparsely distributed neurons and, like the periventricular zone, includes only a few discrete nuclei, notably the lateral tuberal nuclei. A parasagittal plane through the fornix forms the boundary between the medial and lateral zones. A bundle of fibers, the fornix, connects the hypothalamus with the hippocampus. It enters the hypothalamus at the anterior commissure and passes ventrally and caudally to the mammillary bodies.

Hypothalamic Nuclei

Although discrete nuclei can be identified in the human hypothalamus, particularly in the medial zone, little definitive information has been obtained about their connections and functions. At present, we must make assumptions about functions of these cell groups in the human based on studies in other mammals. Many of these assumptions are noted later in this chapter, and some are described in specific sections on hypothalamic functions. Most remain to be verified in the human.

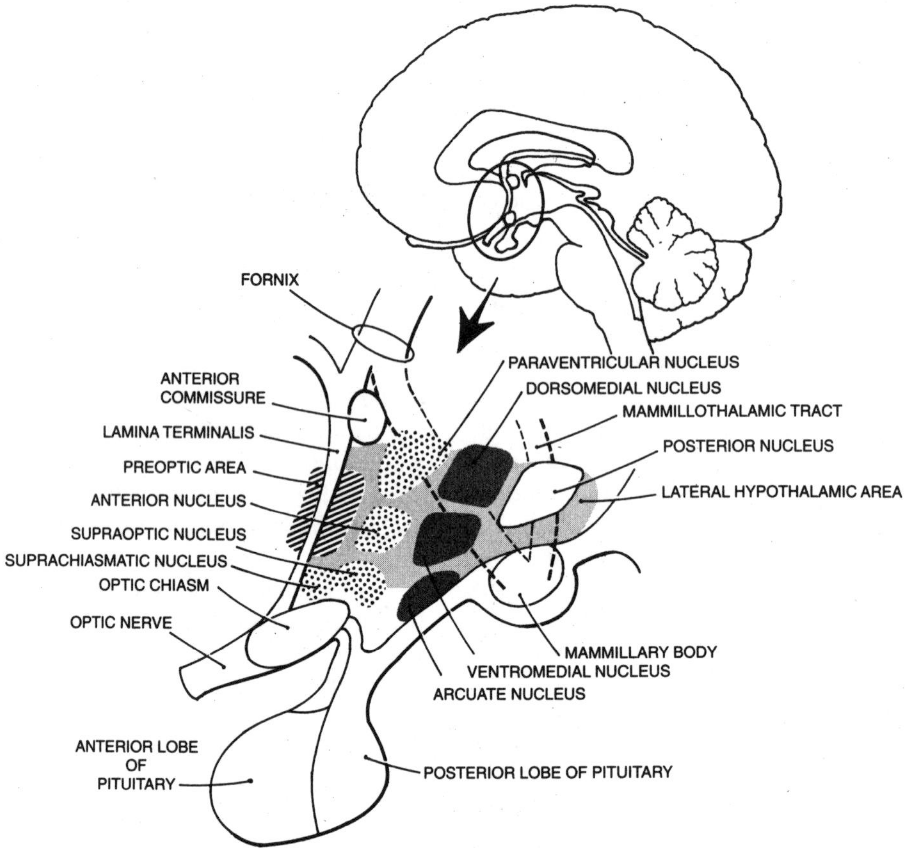

■ **FIGURE 21–3.** The major nuclei of the human hypothalamus. The nuclei of the medial zone are depicted in groups corresponding to the four regions: *cross-hatching* = preoptic region; *stippled area* = anterior hypothalamus; *dark gray* = tuberal region; *white* = mammillary region. The adjacent lateral hypothalamus is shown in light gray. Between the lateral and the medial hypothalamic nuclei run the fibers of the fornix and the mammillothalamic tract. These tracts are shown in *dashed lines.*

Preoptic Area

The **preoptic area** begins developmentally as a part of the telencephalon. With the lamina terminalis, it forms the rostral wall of the brain from which the two telencephalic hemispheres extend laterally. Nevertheless, the preoptic area cannot be distinguished histologically from the hypothalamus and functions in such close association with it that many authorities describe it as part of the hypothalamus. The preoptic area consists of a periventricular zone, a **medial preoptic area** in the medial zone, and a **lateral preoptic area** in the lateral zone. It extends caudally to an imaginary line running from the interventricular foramen to the midportion of the optic chiasm. Neurons in the medial and lateral preoptic areas contribute to circuits that control sexual behavior, parental behavior, thermoregulation, and sleep-waking cycles.

Anterior Hypothalamic Area

The **anterior hypothalamus** lies caudal to the preoptic area, and some descriptions combine the two. The anterior hypothalamus contains several distinctive nuclear groups, including the suprachiasmatic, supraoptic, and paraventricular nuclei, as well as the more diffuse anterior hypothalamic nucleus and lateral hypothalamic area (Fig. 21–3).

The **suprachiasmatic nucleus** resides immediately dorsal to the center of the optic chiasm, where it receives retinal input directly from the chiasm. This nucleus serves as the primary circadian clock of the brain. Its retinal input entrains the natural oscillatory rhythm of its cells, which, in turn, provide outputs that influence circadian cycles for sleep, locomotion, and hormone secretion. In most mammals, pathways through hypothalamic and brain stem nuclei mediate these functions. These pathways provide input to the sympathetic nervous system, which directly regulates melatonin secretion from the pineal gland.

The **supraoptic and paraventricular nuclei** of this area develop from the same anlage. Both these nuclei include **magnocellular neurosecretory cells,** which have axons that terminate in the posterior pituitary, where they secrete oxytocin and vasopressin into the systemic circulation. The paraventricular nucleus actually includes a composite of cell groups that individually belong to several different, important functional circuits. Two of these circuits regulate water balance and responses to stress. The paraventricular nucleus also contains parvocellular cell groups with axons that project to other limbic centers, where they use oxytocin and vasopressin, as well as other substances, as neurotransmitters. Some of these parvocellular neurons connect directly with the preganglionic sympathetic neurons in the spinal cord. The **anterior hypothalamic nucleus,** a defined nucleus within the anterior hypothalamus, has been implicated in circuits that control body temperature and aggressive behavior.

Tuberal Region

In the **tuberal region** of the human hypothalamus, a cell-sparse capsule surrounds the best differentiated of the medial cell groups, the **ventromedial nucleus.** Like its counterpart in other mammals, the ventromedial nucleus consists of two somewhat separate subnuclei. The **arcuate nucleus** lies in the floor and ventral walls of the third ventricle, adjacent to the ventromedial nucleus and in the periventricular zone. Like other nuclei of the zone, this nucleus plays an important role in regulating the anterior pituitary. Neurons in the ventromedial nucleus and the adjacent arcuate nucleus belong to circuits that control sexual behavior and food intake and nutrient metabolism. Located above the ventromedial nucleus, the **dorsomedial nucleus** cannot be distinguished easily from the adjacent lateral hypothalamic area. The **lateral tuberal nuclei** can be defined easily within the lateral area. Histaminergic neurons of the tuberal nuclei (along with other aminergic neurons) become active during arousal. Neurons in the lateral preoptic area that are uniquely active during sleep inhibit the histaminergic neurons. Both these cell groups belong to a system that extends from the hypothalamus into the brain stem and that integrates sleep-waking cycles.

Mammillary Region

The medial mammillary nucleus is the most prominent structure in the **mammillary region.** The **tuberomammillary nuclei** and the **posterior hypothalamus** surround the **mammillary bodies.** A distinctive group of large cells in the lateral zone of the mammillary region blends rostrally with the lateral tuberal nuclei and caudally with the fields of Forel in the subthalamus. These cells constitute a caudal extension of the basal nucleus of Meynert and provide cholinergic projections to the isocortex (see Chapter 23) and noncholinergic projections to the remaining allocortex. Other cells in this lateral hypothalamic group give rise to descending projections to the brain stem and spinal cord.

Fiber Connections of the Hypothalamus

The hypothalamus maintains direct connections with the telencephalic limbic system, with cranial nerve nuclei and the reticular formation in the brain stem, and with the spinal cord. Pathways connecting the hypothalamus with telencephalic limbic system structures include the stria terminalis, the ventral amygdaloid pathway, and the fornix (see the earlier section on the telencephalic limbic system).

Numerous different fiber systems connect the hypothalamus with the brain stem and spinal cord. The largest of these, the **medial forebrain bundle (MFB),** consists of a diffuse tract extending from the septal area through the lateral hypothalamic zone to the brain stem, with heavy connections to the reticular formation. A particularly important set of fibers arises from cells in the paraventricular nucleus and lateral hypothalamus and descends through the MFB to visceral sensory neurons in the nucleus solitarius. These fibers also project to preganglionic parasympathetic nuclei in the dorsal motor nucleus of the vagus and nucleus ambiguus, and to both sympathetic and parasympathetic cell groups in the spinal cord. Many fibers join the MFB, and others leave it in all areas through which the traet travels. Hence this system provides both afferent and efferent connections for the hypothalamus.

Several smaller fiber bundles also connect the hypothalamus with the brain stem. The **mammillary peduncle** carries input from the tegmentum of the midbrain to the mammillary bodies, and the **dorsal longitudinal fasciculus** parallels the MFB but passes through the medial zone of the hypothalamus.

A fiber bundle that arises from neurons of the mammillary body, the **fasciculus mammillary princeps,** passes dorsally for a very short distance and then bifurcates into two collateral systems. The **mammillothalamic tract,** the much larger of the two in humans, projects to the anterior nuclear group of the thalamus. The second, the **mammillotegmental tract,** turns caudally and terminates in the tegmentum of the midbrain.

Hypothalamic Functions

The hypothalamus integrates descending influences from the cerebral cortex (e.g., through the hippocampal formation and amygdala) with ascending influences from the spinal cord and brain stem (from somatic and visceral sensory systems and the reticular formation). With this integrated information, the hypothalamus coordinates visceral function with a constellation of behaviors that both the individual and the species need for survival.

For example, coordination of sexual behavior with neuroendocrine regulation of the gonads and reproductive organs ensures survival of the species. Coordination of feeding and drinking behavior with gastrointestinal and renal function ensures the survival of the individual. Similarly, thermoregulatory behavior must be coordinated with endocrine regulation of metabolism, peripheral vascular tone, and sweating for control of body temperature within the narrow range compatible with human life. The hypothalamus and limbic system also influence many aspects of emotional expression, such as anger, placidity, fear, social attraction, and affiliation, some of which are associated with survival behaviors, but all of which can occur independently.

Controlling all these complex behaviors requires integration of the endocrine system and the autonomic nervous system with the somatic motor system. The **hypothalamus regulates endocrine activity** through the vascular system of the pituitary (see later). In return, vital information reaches the hypothalamus, not only through neural connections, but also through the bloodstream. Specialized receptors in the hypothalamus monitor the temperature and osmolarity as well as the concentrations of circulating hormones and glucose levels of the blood.

The hypothalamus **controls the autonomic nervous system** by neural pathways that project to the reticular formation and by direct projections from the hypothalamus through the MFB to the parasympathetic and sympathetic neurons in the cranial nerve nuclei and the spinal cord. Ascending viscerosensory pathways from the spinal cord and brain stem provide reciprocal connections to the hypothalamus.

Finally, the hypothalamus **organizes homeostatic and social behavioral patterns** such as eating, drinking, sexual activity, parental behavior, aggression, and sleeping and waking. The fundamental neural circuits for these complex behavioral sequences exist within the limbic system and its connections with the basal ganglia and midbrain locomotor control centers. To the degree that humans use their ability to plan long-term goal-directed activities, preparation of the context for these limbic-driven behaviors obviously requires the isocortex as well, particularly the prefrontal cortex.

Endocrine Activity: Hypothalamic-Pituitary Relationships

Cells in the **supraoptic and paraventricular nuclei** of the hypothalamus produce the peptide hormones **oxytocin** and **vasopressin** (antidiuretic hormone). The **hypothalamohypophyseal tract** transports these hormones into the posterior pituitary (neurohypophysis). Neurons of the hypothalamic nuclei produce both hormones initially as prohormones. During transport along the axons of the neurons, cleavage of the hormones occurs, yielding a **neurophysin** with oxytocin and another neurophysin with vasopressin. Axon terminals in the posterior pituitary release the hormones and neurophysins directly into the systemic circulation. Vasopressin stimulates water reabsorption by the kidney, and oxytocin stimulates uterine contraction and milk ejection.

Cells in the hypothalamus also control the anterior pituitary, but by a fundamentally different mechanism. Cells primarily localized in the **arcuate nucleus** (in primates) and other parts of the **periventricular zone of the hypothalamus** produce peptide-releasing hormones (or, in some cases, release-inhibiting hormones), transport the hormones to their terminals, and secrete them into capillaries in the median eminence and pituitary stalk. These capillaries collect into very short portal veins that deliver the releasing hormones to cells of the anterior pituitary **(adenohypophysis).** In response to the appropriate releasing hormones, subpopulations of cells of the anterior pituitary synthesize and secrete thyroid-stimulating hormone, follicle-stimulating hormone, luteinizing hormone, growth hormone, adrenocorticotropic hormone, and prolactin. Collectively termed **trophic hormones,** these substances stimulate their target tissues. In response, many of the target tissues (e.g., thyroid, adrenal glands) produce hormones that serve as negative feedback regulators of the hypothalamus and pituitary. This is not true, however, of the regulation of growth hormone and prolactin, which a balance of stimulating and inhibiting substances from the hypothalamus controls. Prolactin-releasing hormone, for example, produces and releases prolactin, and the release of dopamine from hypothalamic neurons into the hypophyseal portal system inhibits the secretion of prolactin. Similarly, the inhibitory action of somatostatin cells in part regulates the release of growth hormone.

Reproductive Physiology and Behavior

Neurons in the **preoptic region, anterior hypothalamus, ventromedial nucleus,** and **arcuate nucleus** of the hypothalamus participate in **gonadal regulation and sexual behavior** in the male and female. Anatomic and physiologic differentiation of these brain areas occurs in response to gonadal hormones circulating before birth and leads to a postpubertal pattern of cyclical (female) or noncyclical (male) secretion of gonadotropin-releasing hormone. In the human, neurons in the arcuate nucleus and throughout the extent of the periventricular zone synthesize gonadotropin-releasing hormone, transport it down their axons, and secrete it into the portal capillaries in the infundibulum. Through this pathway, the hypothalamus regulates the pituitary-gonadal axis.

Neurons in the **medial preoptic area, anterior hypothalamus,** and **ventromedial nucleus** profoundly influence sexual behavior. The pathways coordinating sexual behavior emerge from the hypothalamus and project to locomotor sites in the midbrain, to the reticular formation, and to the parasympathetic and sympathetic preganglionic neurons that control genital reflexes. (See Chapter 5.)

The neuronal inputs to the preoptic area and hypothalamus that regulate sexual behavior come from the amygdala and the brain stem. In addition, the blood-borne gonadal hormones, estrogen and progesterone or testosterone, provide feedback to the brain. Androgen and estrogen receptors occur abundantly in neurons of all limbic areas that control reproduction, including the amygdala, the periventricular and medial zones of the hypothalamus, and the brain stem.

Body Temperature

The **preoptic region** and the **anterior hypothalamic area** participate in **temperature** regulation. Receptors for core body temperature (the temperature of the blood supplied to the hypothalamus) in the anterior hypothalamus integrate core temperature data with information about body surface temperature delivered over spinoreticular-reticulohypothalamic pathways. Damage to the preoptic area/anterior hypothalamus, or pyrogenic molecules reaching this area, interfere with heat dissipation (move to a cooler environment, peripheral vasodilation, sweating) and produce chronic hyperthermia. Integration between the preoptic area/anterior hypothalamus and the posterior hypothalamus achieves heat conservation. Lesions in the posterior hypothalamus prevent mammals from generating heat (seeking of cover or a source of external heat, peripheral vasoconstriction, shivering) and result in hypothermia in cold environments.

Food Intake

Like body temperature, body weight appears to be regulated around a set point, but unlike body temperature, the normal range of body weight varies greatly across individuals and within individuals as a result of age, dietary changes, exercise level, and psychological factors such as stress. Correspondingly, the **food intake** system is much more complicated than the thermoregulatory system, both in terms of the number of signals that control the central mechanisms and the number of brain areas that contribute to these mechanisms.

Glucose receptors in the ventromedial and arcuate nuclei of the hypothalamus stimulate an immediate increase in food intake in response to drastic reductions in blood glucose concentration. Adipose tissue provides a more indirect measure of the body's nutritional status by producing the peptide hormone leptin in proportion to the amount of available stored fat. Acting directly, and through a variety of intermediate hormones and neuropeptide systems, leptin inhibits food intake mechanisms. Its direct action on neuropeptide Y neurons in the arcuate nucleus plays a major role in food intake. Along with other neuronal groups in the hypothalamus, these neuropeptide Y neurons and their projections to the paraventricular and dorsomedial nuclei stimulate food intake and inhibit thermogenesis. These groups include galanin neurons, as well as melanin-concentrating hormone-producing cells in the lateral hypothalamus. Hypothalamic neuronal systems that inhibit food intake and stimulate thermogenesis include the corticotrophin-releasing hormone cells of the paraventricular nucleus and neuropeptides produced both in the brain and in the gastrointestinal system (the gut-brain peptides) such as cholecystokinin.

In addition to the interactions of these regulatory cell groups within the hypothalamus and their responses to nutrient signals from the body, neural signals through viscerosensory pathways from the taste buds and gastrointestinal tract directly modulate eating behavior. The close connection between food intake and anabolic mechanisms ties these behaviors not only to temperature regulation, but also to growth, to responses to stress, and to reproduction (particularly in females) and to the hormones and neural systems that regulate these activities.

Emotion

The hypothalamus clearly regulates the autonomic discharge of nerve impulses that evoke the physical expressions of **emotion:** acceleration of the heart rate, elevation of blood pressure, flushing or pallor of the skin, sweating, "goose-pimpling" of the skin, dryness of the mouth, and disturbances of the gastrointestinal tract. Emotional experience, however, includes the subjective phenomenon of feelings, which relate to functions of the cerebral cortex. Pathways that connect the cerebral cortex and hypothalamus, particularly pathways through the amygdala, participate in both the experience and the physiologic reactions of emotions.

Our understanding of the brain circuitry responsible for emotion and affective behaviors remains limited, but functional imaging studies have provided strong support for earlier observations in patients with lesions. These studies highlight the importance of the prefrontal cortex. They further suggest that separate sectors of the prefrontal area mediate positive and negative emotional states and that these functions are lateralized within the brain. The working hypothesis states that activity in the dorsolateral prefrontal cortex in the left hemisphere generates a state of happiness or positive affect, and activation of the right prefrontal cortex, especially in the ventromedial orbital area, leads to sadness or disgust.

The emphasis on negative affect relating to the medial orbitofrontal cortex is consistent with the known connections of this area to the amygdala and with data linking activation of the amygdala specifically to negative emotions such as fear. This, however, may be too restrictive a view of the function of orbitofrontal-amygdala connections. Less evidence has been collected concerning the role of the amygdala in positive emotions.

Epithalamus

The most dorsal division of the diencephalon, the **epithalamus,** contains the pineal body (epiphysis), the habenular nuclei and habenular commissure, the posterior commissure, the striae medullaris, and the roof of the third ventricle.

Pineal Body

The dorsal diverticulum of the diencephalon, the **pineal body,** consists of a cone-shaped structure that overlies the tectum of the midbrain. Microscopically, the pineal body contains glial cells (i.e., astrocytes) and parenchymal cells (i.e., pinealocytes). The pineal body contains no neurons, but has abundant nerve fiber terminals of postganglionic sympathetic neurons in the superior cervical ganglion. We understand the function of the pineal body better in other vertebrates than in the human. In many vertebrates, the secretions of the pinealocytes, including **melatonin,** participate in regulating circadian rhythms and in the cyclical maintenance and regression of the gonads associated with seasonal breeding.

Calcareous accumulations (i.e., corpora arenacea) appear conspicuously in the pineal body after middle age. Because the pineal body normally lies in the midline and its calcifications can be seen in skull radiographs, its position can be a useful diagnostic aid.

Habenula

The **habenular nuclei** reside in the dorsal margin of the base of the pineal body. Afferent fibers to the habenula originate in the septal area, the ventral pallidum (see Chapter 17), the lateral hypothalamus, and the brain stem, including the interpeduncular nucleus, the raphe nuclei, and the ventral tegmental area. The brain stem afferents reach the habenula through the **habenulopeduncular tract,** whereas the **stria medullaris** carries the more rostral afferents. The stria medullaris forms a small ridge on the dorsomedial margin of the thalamus. The efferent fibers of the habenula in the **habenulopeduncular tract,** or **fasciculus retroflexus,** form a conspicuous, dense bundle that terminates in the interpeduncular nucleus in the ventral midline area of the midbrain. Fibers from the interpeduncular nucleus include ascending projections to the thalamus, hypothalamus, and septal area and descending fibers that terminate in the central gray matter and serotonergic raphe nuclei of the brain stem. The **habenular commissure** consists of stria medullaris fibers crossing over to the contralateral habenular nuclei. Located ventral to the base of the pineal body, the **posterior commissure** carries decussating fibers of the superior colliculi and pretectum (visual reflex fibers), and possibly fibers from other sources.

22

Olfaction

The **olfactory system** consists of the **olfactory nerves, bulbs,** and **tracts,** a portion of the anterior perforated substance called the **olfactory tubercle,** the **piriform region of the cortex or primary olfactory cortex,** and portions of the **entorhinal cortex of the parahippocampal gyrus** and the **corticomedial division of the amygdala.** Macrosmatic vertebrates such as carnivores and rodents use this system prominently for locating food and communicating with other members of the species. Microsmatic vertebrates such as primates use visual and auditory senses more extensively than the olfactory system for these purposes.

Olfactory Receptors

The peripheral olfactory receptors reside in a specialized area of the nasal mucosa designated the **olfactory epithelium.** In humans, this tissue consists of pseudostratified columnar olfactory epithelium located on the superior concha, the roof of the nasal chamber, and the upper portion of the nasal septum. The receptor cells consist of bipolar neurons, bearing cilia from their dendritic endings at the surface of the olfactory epithelium. The chemical moieties that serve as olfactory stimuli alter the membrane potential of the receptor neurons primarily through ligand-receptor–mediated second-messenger mechanisms that lead to opening of cyclic nucleotide-gated ion channels in the ciliary membrane. The receptor molecules on the olfactory cilia belong to a superfamily of more than 1000 different receptor proteins.

Coding of discrete stimuli for discrimination of different odorants appears to be a product of the differential expression of these receptor proteins in receptor cells across the surface of the mucosa, combined with selective convergence of axons from functionally related receptor cells to target cells in the olfactory bulb. Grouped into fascicles, the receptor cell axons pass through the fenestrae of the **cribriform plate** as the **olfactory nerve.** The olfactory nerve terminates in an extension of the telencephalon, the **olfactory bulb.**

Olfactory Bulbs and Their Projections

The paired olfactory bulbs rest on the cribriform plate. Layers of different neuronal cell types make the laminar architecture of the bulb prominent in histologic preparations of most vertebrate brains, although this organization appears less distinct in humans. The bulb contains several types of neurons, including interneurons and **mitral cells.** The mitral cells receive direct synaptic input from **olfactory nerve fibers** and project their axons into the **lateral olfactory tract.**

The **anterior olfactory nucleus,** in the **olfactory stalk,** consists of groups of neurons (Fig. 22–1). One of these groups constitutes the origin of the **olfactory portion of the anterior commissure** (Fig. 22–2). These cells receive input from the ipsilateral olfactory bulb and send their axons across the anterior commissure to the contralateral olfactory bulb.

The olfactory stalk lies in the **olfactory sulcus** of the frontal lobe, lateral to the gyrus rectus of the orbitofrontal cortex. The olfactory tract in the stalk bifurcates into medial and lateral striae. Some of the fibers of the **medial olfactory stria** consist of the axons of anterior olfactory nucleus neurons, which enter the rostral portion of the anterior commissure to be returned to the opposite

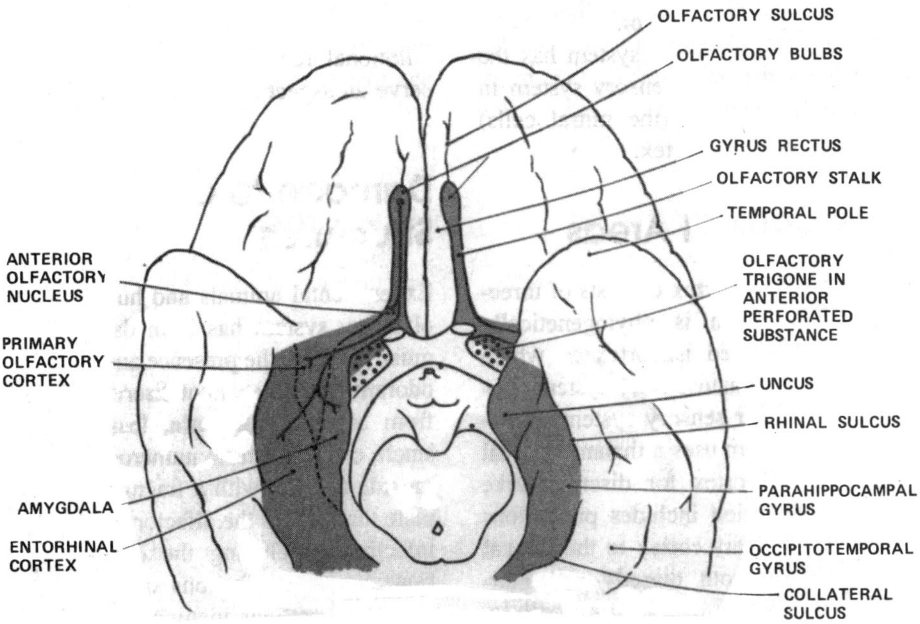

■ **FIGURE 22–1.** The structures of the olfactory system. On the *left*, the temporal lobe has been pulled to the left to expose more of the ventral surface of the brain. The projections of the mitral cells of the olfactory bulb are indicated in *color*.

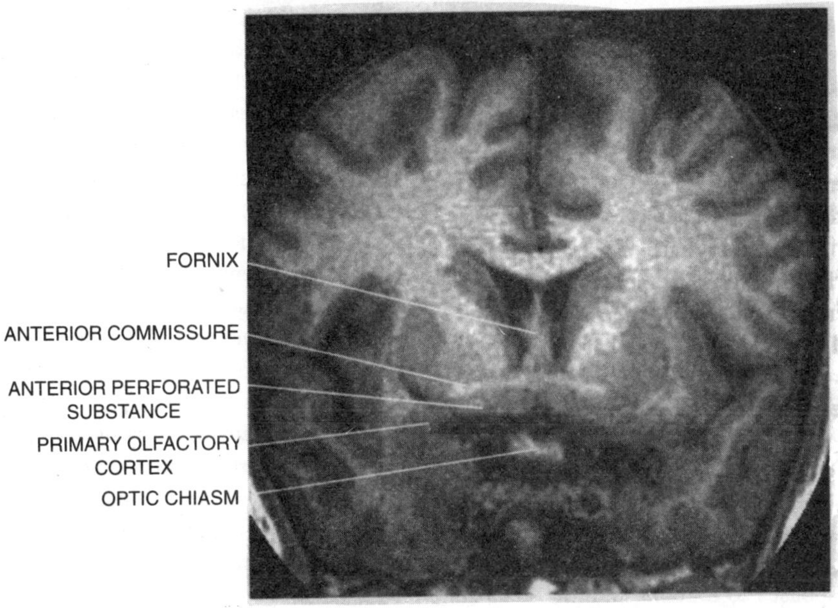

■ **FIGURE 22–2.** A T1-weighted (spoiled gradient echo) magnetic resonance image of a neurologically normal adult. This coronal sequence shows the anterior commissure beneath the fornix and the anterior perforated substance, part of which is the olfactory tubercle.

olfactory bulb. The remaining fibers, which terminate in the ipsilateral **olfactory tubercle** within the anterior perforated substance, consist of mitral cell axons from the olfactory bulb. Mitral cells project only ipsilaterally (See Fig. 22–1).

Composed primarily of mitral cell axons, the **lateral stria,** or **lateral olfactory tract,** delivers terminals to the lateral margin of the anterior perforated substance, the **piriform cortex (primary olfactory cortex),** a small rostral portion of the

entorhinal cortex, and the **corticomedial amygdala** (Fig. 22–1). The olfactory system has the distinction of being the only sensory system in which second-order neurons (the mitral cells) project directly to cerebral cortex.

Olfactory Cortical Areas

The **primary olfactory cortex** consists of three-layered allocortex, which is phylogenetically older than the six-layered isocortex in which visual, auditory, and somatosensory systems terminate. Like these other sensory systems, however, the olfactory system uses a thalamocortical connection to the isocortex for discriminative functions. This connection includes projections from the primary olfactory cortex to the **lateral orbitofrontal cortex,** both directly and indirectly, through projections to the magnocellular portion of the **dorsomedial nucleus of the thalamus.** Corticocortical connections between the temporal pole and the orbitofrontal cortex may also be important in olfactory discrimination.

In macrosmatic vertebrates, olfactory impulses that reach the **corticomedial amygdala** participate in the control of social behaviors. These behaviors include sexual, aggressive, and parental responses to other members of the same species. In microsmatic vertebrates such as primates, however, the behavioral significance of olfactory projections to the amygdala in primates has not been clarified. Similarly, the function of the olfactory input to the hippocampus through the **entorhinal cortex** remains unclear. In both these pathways, olfactory information probably becomes integrated with visual, auditory, and somatosensory impulses arriving from the respective association cortices. In addition, through connections with the amygdala, the hippocampus likely participates in the integration of multisensory inputs into appropriate emotional and physiologic responses to external stimuli. This may provide the groundwork for developing learned emotional responses to specific stimuli, which serve an aspect of motivation.

Damage to Olfactory Structures

Experimental animals and humans in which the olfactory system has been damaged can distinguish between the presence and the absence of an odorant, but they cannot discriminate one odorant from another. **Anosmia,** loss of the sense of smell, can result from numerous disorders. These include trauma, with a fracture of the cribriform plate that injures the olfactory bulbs or tracts, and infections, including the common cold, other systemic viral infections such as viral hepatitis, syphilis, bacterial meningitis, abscesses of the frontal lobe, and osteomyelitis of the frontal or ethmoid regions. Other causes include the following: neoplasms, such as olfactory groove meningiomas and frontal lobe gliomas; metabolic diseases, such as pernicious anemia and disorders of zinc metabolism; and drug ingestion, especially amphetamines or cocaine. People with complete anosmia lose the ability to recognize flavors because the olfactory and taste systems function together in the perception of flavors. **Hyperosmia,** an increase in olfactory sensitivity, occurs commonly in early pregnancy and also occurs frequently in conversion disorders and in some psychoses.

The subarachnoid space on the cranial side of the cribriform plate lies closely approximated to the olfactory mucosa. A fracture through the cribriform plate that tears the mucosa can result in a leak of cerebrospinal fluid through the nose **(cerebrospinal fluid rhinorrhea).** This condition can result in meningitis caused by the spread of microorganisms from the nose to the cerebrospinal fluid.

23

Chemical Neuroanatomy

Neurons in the human nervous system communicate primarily by releasing neuroactive substances or **neurotransmitters** at chemical synapses. Neurons also release neurotransmitters into the extracellular space of the neuropil in sites that do not contain specialized postsynaptic receptors directly adjacent to the release site. In both cases, synaptic and nonsynaptic (volume) chemical transmission, the distribution and number of specific **receptors** for these chemicals determine their actions. This chapter necessarily deals with a limited set of the full range of chemical signals and signal transduction mechanisms found in the nervous system. Information on the interactions of neurotransmitters within specific neuronal systems (e.g., cerebellum, basal ganglia) can be found in preceding chapters.

Characteristics of Neurotransmitter Molecules

The chemicals that have been tentatively or definitively identified as neurotransmitters include several different classes of compounds and dozens of individual molecules. Most neurotransmitters fall into one of four different groups of compounds: **acetylcholine** (ACh), a derivative of the lipid cholesterol; **biogenic amines** or **monoamines,** derived from aromatic amino acids; **neuropeptides,** which consist of short chains of amino acids; and **amino acids** themselves. To qualify as a neurotransmitter, a compound must fulfill specific criteria. The compound must be synthesized in the presynaptic neuron, stored in presynaptic vesicles, and released by calcium-dependent mechanisms from the presynaptic neuron. Moreover, the compound must be active at selective receptors on a postsynaptic element, where it alters the membrane potential, and it must be removed from the extracellular space by reuptake into the presynaptic cell or by biochemical degradation. The neurotransmitters discussed in this chapter satisfy these criteria.

Most neurons release not only neurotransmitters, but also other types of neuromediators. For example, neurons often produce an amino acid neurotransmitter in combination with a neuropeptide. In some cases, these substances appear to be acting cooperatively, to provide for both rapid action by the amino acid and subsequent long-duration effects by the peptide. In other cases, the two substances may have different actions and may be released under quite different circumstances (e.g., in relation to different patterns of neuronal firing).

Functional Characterization of Neurotransmitter Receptors

Although the factors that control the synthesis and release of a neurotransmitter at a chemical synapse influence the action of the neurotransmitter, the **receptors** on the postsynaptic cell determine the nature of that action, specifically by the types of membrane channels coupled to the receptors. Both the amount of neurotransmitter released and the number of receptors present influence the intensity of the action of a neuroactive substance. Chemical synapses, and chemical systems in the brain, therefore can be characterized not only by the transmitter released but also by the subtype or subtypes of receptors available for that transmitter. Experimentally, the selective binding of specific pharmacologic agents acting as agonists or antagonists of the transmitter defines these subtypes.

In general, two different mechanisms account for the actions of neurotransmitters at their receptors, and individual receptor subtypes have been characterized accordingly. At **ionotropic receptors,** neurotransmitters produce rapid, phasic responses by altering the state of ion channels in the postsynaptic membrane. Activation of ionic receptors rapidly excites or inhibits the postsynaptic membrane, depending on the types of ions admitted by the channel that has opened. In contrast, neurotransmitters at **G-protein–coupled (metabotropic) receptors** evoke slowly responding, longer-lasting effects. Some of these act directly on ion channels; others contain linkages to a variety of second messengers, through which a cascade of enzymatic reactions alters the metabolism of the postsynaptic cell. The receptor subtypes identified for ACh and the amino acid neurotransmitters glutamate and gamma-aminobutyric acid (GABA) use both these receptor mechanisms. However, the receptors identified to date for monoamines and neuropeptides are all G-protein–coupled receptors, with the exception of the ionotropic 5-HT_3 serotonin receptor.

Acetylcholine

Acetylcholine Production and Acetylcholine Receptors

The synthesis of **ACh** results from the combination of acetylcoenzyme A and choline in a reaction catalyzed by the enzyme **choline acetyltransferase.** The enzyme **acetylcholinesterase** destroys ACh on its release from a presynaptic terminal. Cholinergic receptors include muscarinic and nicotinic groups. Although metabotropic, the **muscarinic receptors** (M_1 to M_5) can have the ultimate action of opening or closing potassium, calcium, or chloride channels, depending on their location in the central nervous system (CNS). At least seven different types of **nicotinic receptors** have been found in muscle, neurons of the autonomic ganglia, and CNS neurons, and all are ionotropic.

Acetylcholine Neurons Are Found in the Peripheral and Central Nervous Systems

ACh serves as the primary neurotransmitter of motor neurons of the peripheral nervous system. **All alpha, beta, and gamma motoneurons** of the brain stem and spinal cord release ACh at the neuromuscular junction. Within the spinal cord, axon collaterals of the alpha motoneurons activate Renshaw cells at cholinergic synapses. **All preganglionic sympathetic and parasympathetic neurons** release ACh in the autonomic ganglia. In these locations, the primary cholinergic receptor is **nicotinic.** Additionally, **all postganglionic parasympathetic neurons** and one population of postganglionic sympathetic fibers, those to the sweat glands of the skin, are cholinergic. At these postsynaptic autonomic sites, **muscarinic receptors** predominate.

Except for somatic and autonomic motoneurons in the cranial nerve nuclei, ACh neurons within the brain consist of a cluster of nuclear groups in the ventral forebrain and hypothalamus, a smaller group of nuclei in the tegmentum of the brain stem, and interneurons of the striatum (Fig. 23–1). In the brain areas that receive input from these cells, **muscarinic receptors** predominate. The projection neurons of the ventral forebrain include those in the **medial septum,** the **nucleus of the diagonal band of Broca,** the **basal nucleus of Meynert,** and a limited number of neurons in the **lateral hypothalamus.** These neurons give rise to an extensive system of axons to the entire cerebral cortex, to the hippocampal formation and olfactory bulb from the more rostral neurons in the septal area and diagonal band, and to the isocortex from the basal nucleus. The basal nucleus of Meynert also provides cholinergic fibers to the basolateral amygdala. These widespread projections to the cerebral cortex activate the cortex and enhance its responsiveness to incoming sensory information. They form an important part of cortical arousal during **attention, learning, and memory.** A decrease in density in this system occurs as a normal part of aging, and a marked decrease in the number of terminals in the cerebral cortex has been found in the dementia of Alzheimer's disease, although this is only part of the complex pathologic spectrum of this disease.

Cholinergic neurons in the **pedunculopontine and laterodorsal tegmental nuclei** project rostrally to the thalamus and to the ACh neurons in the lateral hypothalamus and basal forebrain and caudally to the cerebellum and the pontine and medullary reticular formation. The connections with the more rostral ACh neurons and the thalamic projections constitute important links in the **reticular activating system,** which partici-

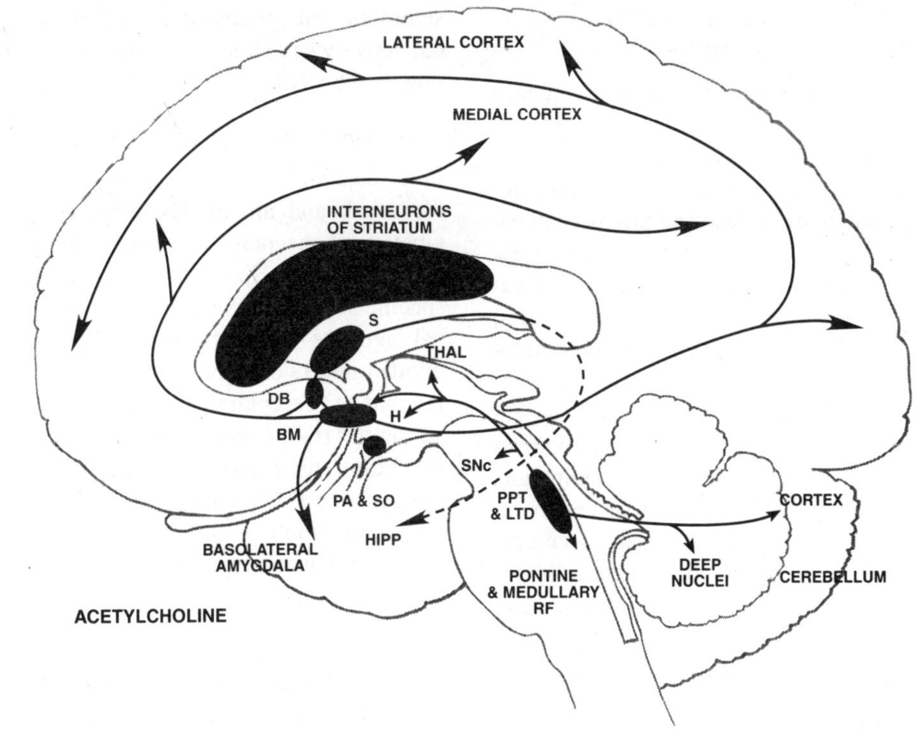

■ **FIGURE 23–1.** The location of the acetylcholine neurons in the central nervous system and their projections. Areas containing cell bodies are shown and are labeled in *color.* The projection pathways of these neurons are indicated with *colored arrows.* The regions that receive the cholinergic input are labeled in *black.* BM = basal nucleus of Meynert; DB = diagonal band of Broca; H = hypothalamus; HIPP = hippocampal formation; PA & SO = paraventricular and supraoptic nuclei of the hypo-thalamus; PPT & LTD = pedunculopontine tegmental nucleus and laterodorsal tegmental nucleus; RF = reticular formation; S = septum; SNc = substantia nigra pars compacta; THAL = thalamus.

pates in **arousal** and **wakefulness.** The caudal projections to the reticular formation initiate the eye movements of rapid-eye-movement, or **REM sleep.** Dreaming occurs during REM sleep, along with rapid lateral conjugate movements of the eyes and virtual paralysis of the somatic musculature.

The pedunculopontine and laterodorsal nuclei also project into the basal ganglia circuits of the frontal lobe, including both the dorsal and ventral striatopallidal systems and the substantia nigra pars compacta. The cholinergic **interneurons of the striatum** excite the striatal projection neurons and serve an important function in motor control. (See Chapter 17.) Excessive activation of cholinergic neurons relative to dopaminergic terminals in the striatum contributes to parkinsonism, and blockade of cholinergic transmission in this structure can ameliorate the symptoms of Parkinson's disease.

Another group of cholinergic neurons in the CNS arises in the medial **habenula** nucleus of the epithalamus. These neurons project to the interpeduncular nucleus. The functions of these neurons are not known.

Finally, choline acetyltransferase immunoreactive neurons have been localized in the magnocellular neuronal populations of the **paraventricular and supraoptic nuclei of the hypothalamus** and in the **posterior lateral hypothalamus.**

Monoamines

The monoamines, or biogenic amines, that have been identified as neurotransmitters include the following: the catecholamines **dopamine, norepinephrine,** and **epinephrine;** the indoleamine **serotonin;** and **histamine.**

Synthesis of Catecholamines, Serotonin, and Histamine

In the brain and sympathetic ganglia, a sequence of enzymatic steps converts the amino acid precursor **tyrosine** into several **catecholamines.** The first and rate-limiting step in this synthesis requires **tyrosine hydroxylase** and produces dopamine. In the presence of the appropriate enzymes, including **dopamine beta-hydroxylase,** dopamine can be converted to norepinephrine, and it, in turn, in the presence of **phenylethanolamine-*N*-methyl-transferase** (PNMT), can be converted to epinephrine. The functions of the enzymes in this metabolic sequence provide a method by which presumptive dopaminergic, noradrenergic, and adrenergic neurons and axons can be identified in the human brain. Neuronal elements that stain immunohistochemically for tyrosine hydroxylase but not for dopamine beta-hydroxylase are considered dopaminergic. Elements that stain for tyrosine hydroxylase and dopamine beta-hydroxylase but not for PNMT are presumed to be noradrenergic. Elements that are labeled with PNMT are identified as adrenergic. In the human brain, the dopaminergic and adrenergic neurons contain melanin pigment and often can be visualized microscopically without special stains. The brain and other tissues of the body (the neural plexus of the gastrointestinal tract) produce **serotonin** from the amino acid **tryptophan.** The brain and other body tissues synthesize **histamine** from **histidine.**

Reuptake and Degradation

Reuptake into the presynaptic ending and enzymatic **degradation** limit the activity of the monoamine neurotransmitters. Reuptake into the presynaptic ending leads to recycling into vesicles for future use. Both monoamine oxidase and catechol-*O*-methyl transferase deactivate monoamines, the former primarily inside the presynaptic terminal and on the postsynaptic membrane and the latter in the synaptic cleft.

Dopamine

Found only in the CNS, dopamine neurons characteristically form small cell groups that send their axons through relatively short projection routes to discrete targets. In these respects, they differ from the centralized norepinephrine and serotonin cell groups of the brain stem, which collectively have long axons and diffuse distribution in the CNS.

Dopamine Receptors

Five dopamine receptor subtypes have been identified, and all are G-protein–coupled (metabotropic) receptors that affect the activity of adenyl cyclase. However, on the basis of their specific actions on this enzyme and their individual agonists and antagonists, they have been divided into two major subgroups, for which the D1 and D2 receptors serve as prototypes. Activation of D1-like postsynaptic receptors (D1 and D5) results in excitation, whereas activation of postsynaptic D2-like receptors (D2, D3 and D4) causes inhibition. A special group of D2 receptors found on dopaminergic cells and terminals functions as autoreceptors that can reduce firing rate, dopamine synthesis, and dopamine release.

Dopaminergic Cell Groups throughout the Brain and Their Projections

In some of its sites, interneurons use dopamine as a neurotransmitter. These sites include the **retina** and the **olfactory bulb,** where the dopamine neurons selectively inhibit transmission of sensory information to enhance the signal-to-noise ratio. Known as **lateral inhibition,** this physiologic process constitutes an important part of information processing in all sensory systems.

Projection neurons found in the diencephalon and the brain stem use dopamine as a neurotransmitter. In the arcuate and periventricular nuclei of the hypothalamus, dopamine cell bodies give rise to the **tuberoinfundibular and tuberohypophysial dopamine projections,** which inhibit the release of prolactin and melanocyte-stimulating hormone from the anterior and intermediate lobes of the pituitary, respectively. The **incertohypothalamic projections,** which connect the zona incerta in the posterior diencephalon with the anterior hypothalamus, medial preoptic area, and septal area, contribute to pathways that regulate sexual and other social behaviors. A third diencephalic dopamine projection system exerts a major influence on visceral function. This system arises from neurons in the caudal diencephalon that send descending axons to the locus ceruleus, parabrachial nucleus, dorsal motor nucleus of the vagus, nucleus solitarius, and the preganglionic autonomic neurons of the spinal cord.

Longer dopamine projection systems arise from the **substantia nigra compacta** and the **ventral tegmental area (VTA)** of the midbrain (Fig. 23–2). The former, the **nigrostriatal dopamine system,** serves a particularly important function in motor control. **Parkinson's disease** results from the progressive degeneration of these neurons and the consequent loss of their input to neurons of the caudate nucleus and putamen. (See Chapter 17.) The VTA projections include two anatomically, biochemically, and electrophysiologically heterogeneous systems. The **mesotelencephalic** system projects to the prefrontal, cingulate, and entorhinal cortices. In contrast to the nigrostriatal system and the **mesolimbic system** (from the VTA to nucleus accumbens, olfactory tubercle and cortex, amygdala, and septum), the mesotelencephalic system lacks dopamine autoreceptors. The mesotelencephalic system shows less response to dopamine agonists and antagonists, and it has higher levels of physiologic activity and dopamine turnover. In addition, this system responds very differently to long-term treatment with antipsychotic drugs than the other two systems. These differences appear to be important in the role of the mesotelencephalic system in schizophrenia, but the etiology and pathophysiology of this complex set of diseases remain to be elucidated.

Norepinephrine

Norepinephrine Cells Are Localized in Sympathetic Ganglia and in the Brain Stem

Found in **sympathetic ganglia,** peripheral nervous system **norepinephrine,** or noradrenaline, cell bodies give rise to all of the postganglionic fibers except those to sweat glands. CNS norepinephrine cell bodies are confined to the pons and medulla. They send their highly branched axons to all parts of the brain (Fig. 23–3). The norepi-

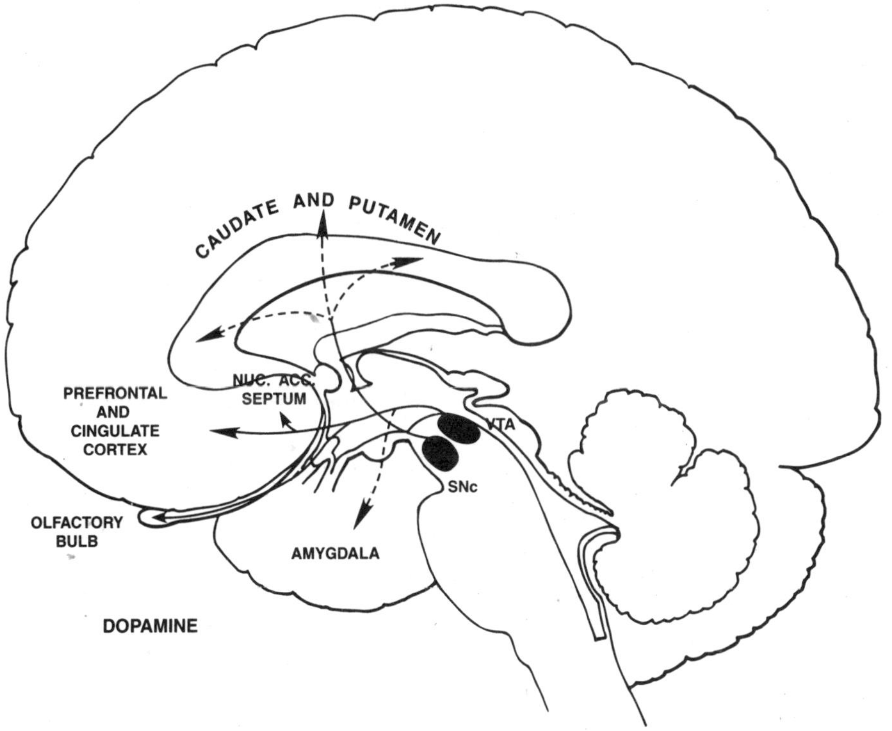

■ **FIGURE 23–2.** The locations and projections of two of the major dopaminergic systems in the brain are illustrated in *color.* Areas containing cell bodies are shown and labeled in *color.* The projection pathways of these neurons are indicated with *colored arrows.* The regions that receive the input are labeled in *black.* Other dopaminergic systems are described in the text. NUC. ACC. = nucleus accumbens; SN = substantia nigra; VTA = ventral tegmental area.

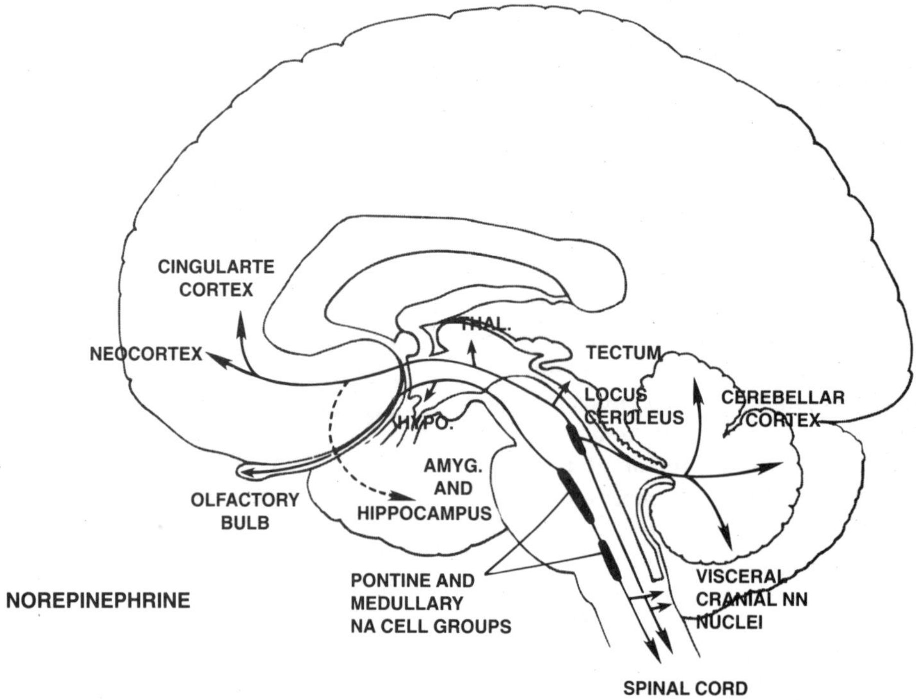

■ **FIGURE 23–3.** Norepinephrine (noradrenaline) neurons in the brain stem and their projections are illustrated in *color.* Areas containing cell bodies are shown and labeled in *color.* The projection pathways of these neurons are indicated with *colored arrows.* The regions that receive the input are labeled in *black.* AMYG. = amygdala; HYPO. = hypothalamus; NA = norepinephrine; NN = nerves; THAL. = thalamus.

nephrine cell bodies of the medulla reside in the **medullary reticular formation,** closely associated with the dorsal motor nucleus of X and the nucleus solitarius. In the pons, norepinephrine neurons lie in the central gray area surrounding the fourth ventricle and in the locus ceruleus.

Although the **locus ceruleus** contains only several hundred neurons, it sends axons to all parts of the CNS, including rostrally to the forebrain, dorsally to the cerebellum, and caudally to the medulla and spinal cord. The rostral projections of the locus ceruleus follow three different routes: the **central tegmental tract,** the **dorsal longitudinal fasciculus,** and the **medial forebrain bundle.** (These three tracts are not shown separately in Figure 23–3.) These pathways terminate extensively in the tectum, thalamus, and outermost (molecular) layer of the cerebral cortex, including the hippocampus. A projection through the superior cerebellar peduncle leads to a similar terminal field in the molecular layer of the cerebellar cortex. The **lateral tegmental norepinephrine cell groups** project to the hypothalamus, where they influence cardiovascular and endocrine systems, and to the spinal cord, where they regulate pain transmission and autonomic reflexes.

Alpha- and Beta-Adrenergic Receptors

Numerous tissues of the body contain abundant receptors for norepinephrine as mediators of adrenal hormone actions. These metabotropic receptors have been divided into two groups, **alpha and beta receptors,** and both have several subtypes that are coupled to different G-proteins. Of these, the beta receptors predominate in the brain, where beta-1 receptors occur in highest density in the cerebral cortex and beta-2 receptors in the cerebellum. However, both in the brain and other tissues, especially the heart, beta-1 and beta-2 receptors coexist in the same location.

The physiologic effects of norepinephrine release have been studied primarily in relation to locus ceruleus activation, which produces widespread inhibition of spontaneous discharge in the postsynaptic neurons. Thus, like the action of dopamine in the retina and olfactory bulb, norepinephrine may enhance the signal-to-noise ratio in its terminal field. This influence spreads widely, not only because of the extensive branching of locus ceruleus axons, but also because varicosities along the axons and axonal terminals secrete norepinephrine into the neuropil. In the cerebral cortex, beta-adrenergic receptors mediate this action. Through this system, the locus ceruleus enhances responsiveness to unfamiliar or surprising stimuli and participates in arousal and vigilance.

Epinephrine

In the periphery, both the adrenal medulla and postganglionic sympathetic nerve endings release norepinephrine and epinephrine. In the CNS, epinephrine neurons (identified by their PNMT immunoreactivity in the human brain) reside only in the lower brain stem, specifically within the **dorsal tegmentum** near the floor of the fourth ventricle and in the **lateral reticular nucleus** in the ventrolateral tegmentum (Fig. 23-5A). The ascending projections from these cells comprise part of the central tegmental tract and, in the human, appear to project primarily to the locus ceruleus, parabrachial nucleus, and the midbrain periaqueductal gray area. In most mammals, caudal projections of the adrenergic cells into the spinal cord terminate in the intermediolateral cell column of sympathetic neurons. Epinephrine, like norepinephrine, acts at both alpha- and beta-adrenergic receptors.

Serotonin

The indolamine serotonin (5-hydroxytryptamine, or 5-HT) can be found in many cells of the body (e.g., mast cells, platelets, and enterochromaffin cells of the gut) and in neurons of the CNS. Synthesized from tryptophan, it is released from synaptic vesicles in neuronal endings. Active reuptake into the same terminal principally limits the action of serotonin in the synaptic cleft, with enzymatic digestion playing only a secondary role.

Many serotonin receptor subtypes have been identified and grouped into five families: 5-HT_1 to 5-HT_5. Of these, all but the 5-HT_3 receptors are G-protein–coupled receptors.

Serotonin Cells Are Localized in the Raphe Nuclei of the Brain Stem Tegmentum

Cell bodies of origin for the serotonin pathways reside only in the brain stem. Most of these neurons lie within the eight **raphe nuclei,** which extend along the midline throughout the length of the brain stem, bounded laterally by nuclei of the medial zone of the reticular formation (Fig. 23–4). The efferent projections of the raphe nuclei have a topographic organization. The rostral nuclear groups project rostrally to the forebrain. The caudal raphe nuclei send their axons into the spinal cord, where they terminate in laminae I and II in the intermediolateral cell column and in the ventral horn. The centrally located cell groups, overlapping with the rostrally and caudally projecting groups, innervate brain stem nuclei and the cerebellum. Serotonin endings also can be found in the ependyma lining the ventricles.

Axons of the rostral raphe nuclei ascend in the **medial forebrain bundle** and distribute to the diencephalon and to both the striatum and the cortex of the telencephalon. In the cerebral cortex, the 5-HT terminals ramify less extensively than the norepinephrine terminals, but both 5-HT and norepinephrine terminal systems project rather diffusely, in contrast to the discrete and topographically organized endings of the dopamine system. Serotonin terminals cluster particularly densely in limbic cortical areas and in the sensory cortical areas such as the primary visual cortex.

Multiple factors influence the firing of the raphe nuclei, including pain stimuli and changes in blood pressure and body temperature. Through its diffuse projections, the serotonin system, in turn, influences multiple systems. In the spinal cord, for example, descending raphe-spinal axons inhibit afferent input from pain fibers and facilitate motoneurons. The ascending serotonin pathways participate in hypothalamic (temperature regulation, sleep, eating), limbic (emotion), and isocortical (sensory processing) functions. Presumably because of their action in the limbic system, serotonin reuptake inhibitors have therapeutic effects on both depression and obsessive-compulsive disorders.

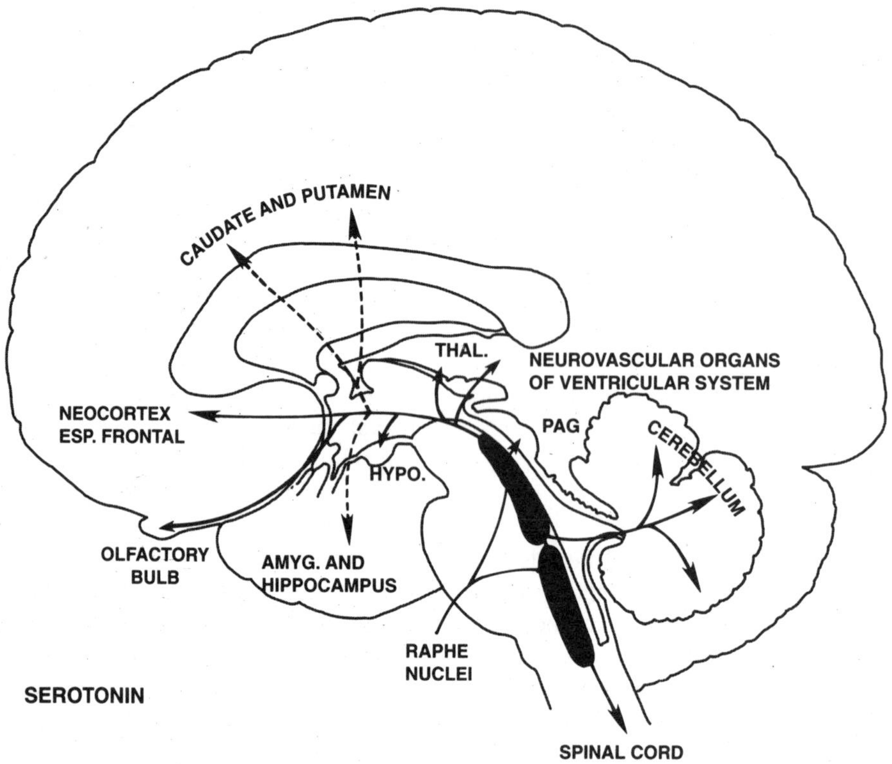

■ **FIGURE 23–4.** Serotonin fibers arising from the raphe nuclei of the brain stem are illustrated in *color.* Areas containing cell bodies are shown and labeled in *color.* The projection pathways of these neurons are indicated with *colored arrows.* The regions that receive the input are labeled in *black.* AMYG. = amygdala; HYPO. = hypothalamus; PAG = periaqueductal gray area; THAL. = thalamus.

Neuropeptides

Neurons that produce **neuropeptides** for release at their terminals employ a fundamentally different system for neurotransmitter synthesis, storage, and release than do neurons that produce ACh and monoamines. Enzymatic alterations of molecules delivered to the cell produce ACh and monoamines in axon terminals. In contrast, RNA-directed preparation of a protein precursor produces neuropeptides de novo in the cell body, and peptidases later cleave the precursors to generate the active peptides. In many cases, this cleavage process produces more than one neurally active peptide. The cell synthesizes the precursor and packages it in vesicles within the cell body and subsequently transports it to the terminals. Hence this process occurs relatively slowly compared with the mechanisms through which monoamines and choline can be recaptured from the synaptic cleft, then synthesized and packaged in recycled vesicles in the terminals. Diffusion and destruction by extracellular peptidases remove neuropeptides from the synaptic cleft.

Often, a single precursor molecule produces more than one neuroactive peptide, and multiple closely related precursor molecules, coded by different genes, form "families" of neuropeptides, such as opioid peptides. Correspondingly, multiple receptor subtypes have been identified for single neuropeptides, and in many cases different genes also code these receptors. Most neuropeptide receptors are G-protein–coupled receptors, but they exhibit differential sensitivity to their endogenous peptide ligands. In addition, they vary in the intracellular systems to which they are coupled and in their physiologic properties.

Neuropeptides also differ from other groups of transmitters in the variability of their distribution in different species. Given this variability, it is particularly important to have information derived from human brains. However, definitive localization of the cell bodies containing neuropeptides is difficult to obtain from human postmortem material. Even under experimental conditions, neuropeptide-producing cell bodies often can be visualized only when blocking axonal transport has artificially caused the peptide to accumulate. Thus, the descriptions of neuropeptide systems in this chapter summarize the current state of knowledge, with the caveat that definitive information from the human brain remains limited.

Opioid Peptides

The **opioid peptides** constitute an entire class of transmitters. They consist of three "classical" genetically distinct peptide families and a fourth, less-studied group. The classical opioid peptide neurotransmitters come from three precursors: **pro-opiomelanocortin,** the beta-endorphin/adrenocorticotropic hormone precursor; **proenkephalin,** which is actually one of the gut-brain peptides; and **prodynorphin.** Each of these precursors can be cleaved into several active peptides that are differentially produced and regulated in different brain areas. In addition, a single peptide contains several biologically active sites, and multiple opioid receptors have been identified. The newest member of the opioid family is orphanin FQ, or nociceptin.

The opioid transmitters appear to be important in neural systems that respond to stress, including pain pathways and cardiovascular control circuits. Opioid cells and terminals have been localized in multiple sites along the neural systems that process somatic and visceral pain information, particularly in the dorsal horn of the spinal cord and in the periaqueductal gray. The opiatergic system also participates in regulating hypothalamopituitary neuroendocrine function, and abundant opioid cells and terminals can be found in the limbic system.

All three of the opioid peptide precursors can produce **enkephalin.** Met-enkephalin originates from both pro-opiomelanocortin and proenkephalin, whereas leu-enkephalin comes from both proenkephalin and prodynorphin. Viewed together, met-enkephalin and leu-enkephalin neurons appear widely distributed in the CNS. Figure 23–5B shows the location of some of the major groups of enkephalin cell bodies in the striatum, limbic system, and raphe nuclei of the brain stem. One of these groups, the striatal neurons, projects to the external segment of the globus pallidus and to the substantia nigra. In these cells, the enkephalin coexists with GABA. In many other areas, the enkephalin-containing neurons are interneurons. This includes the cerebral cortex (not illustrated in Fig. 23–5B).

Limbic system structures and the hypothalamus contain heavy concentrations of **dynorphin** cells as well as enkephalin cells. Dynorphin cells appear in fewer structures in the CNS than enkephalin cells, but in more structures than beta-endorphin neurons.

Beta-endorphin cell bodies can be found almost exclusively in the hypothalamus (Fig. 23–5C). One group of beta-endorphin neurons has been found in some species in the nucleus solitarius of the medulla.

Opioid Receptors

Opioid receptors are metabotropic. The best-studied receptor subtypes—mu, delta, and kappa receptors—preferentially bind beta-endorphin, enkephalins, and dynorphins, respectively. Although preferential, the binding appears not to be exclusive, because each of the three receptor subtypes has been found in areas containing few, if any, projections from cells that produce the preferred ligand. Mu receptors appear to be the most abundant and widely distributed opioid receptors in the human brain. All three opioid receptor subtypes can be found in the neocortex, limbic cortex, basal ganglia, and cerebellum, but they show differential distributions within these areas.

Cloning of the opioid-receptor-like (ORL-1) protein actually preceded identification of its ligand, orphanin FQ, and determination of the human sequence for orphanin FQ. Both ligand and receptor show anatomic distributions in the rat brain similar to those of the dynorphins, which are closely related.

Gut-Brain Peptides

Certain **peptides** initially identified in the gastrointestinal tract have been localized in specific cell groups within the brain. These include substance P, cholecystokinin, vasoactive intestinal peptide, somatostatin, and neurotensin. **Substance P** belongs to the family of neuropeptides called neurokinins, which are the tachykinins of the mammalian nervous system. An undecapeptide for which the amino acid sequence has been known for some time, substance P induces a long

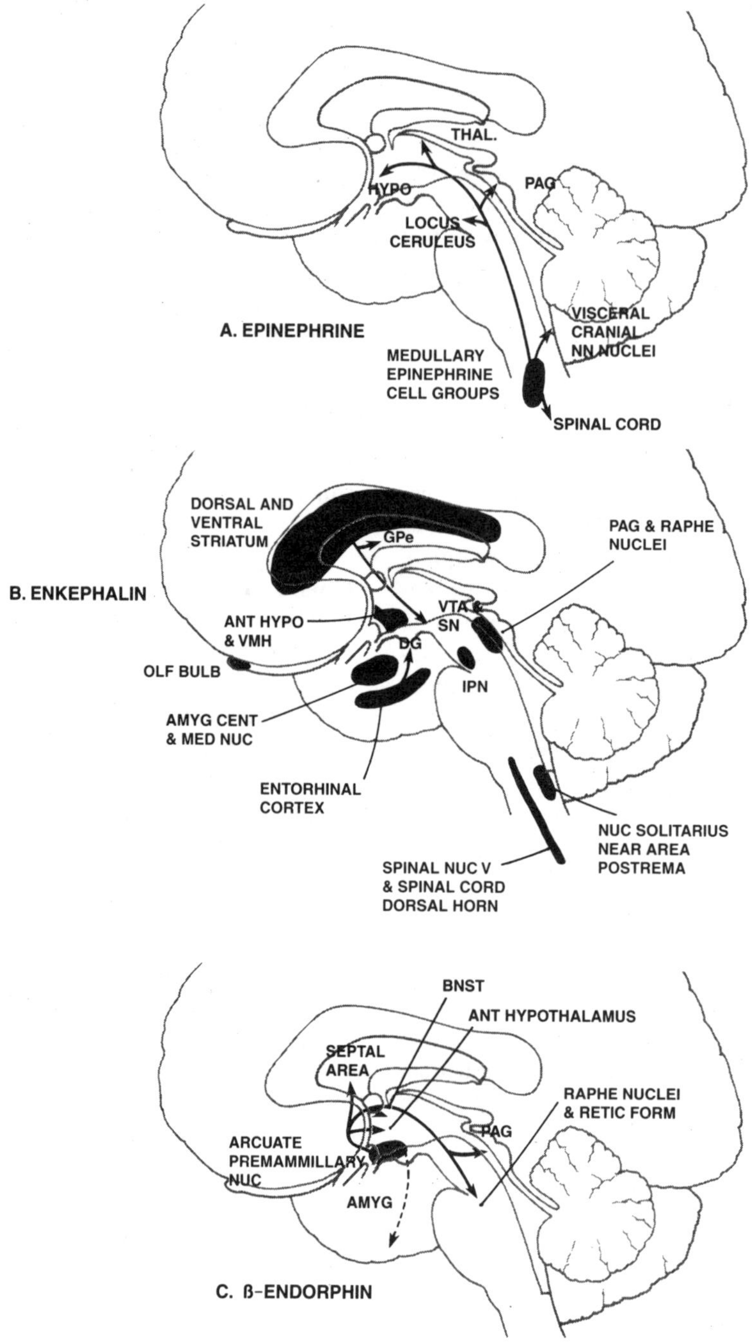

■ **FIGURE 23–5.** **(A)** to **(F)** Composite of a variety of central nervous systems producing epinephrine, peptides, and amino acids as neurotransmitters. *Colored areas* indicate the locations of cell bodies; *colored arrows* show projections away from the area of origin. Areas of termination of these projections are labeled in *black.* AMYG = amygdala; AMYG CENT & MED NUC = central and medial nuclei of the amygdala; ANT HYPO = anterior hypothalamus; BNST = bed nucleus of the stria terminalis; DG = dentate gyrus; ENTO CORTEX = entorhinal cortex; GPe = globus pallidus pars externa; GPi = globus pallidus pars interna; H or HIPP = hippocampal formation; HYPO = hypothalamus; IPN = interpeduncular nucleus; NUC SOL = nucleus solitarius; PAG = periaqueductal gray area; RN = red nucleus; RETIC FORM = reticular formation; SN = substantia nigra; SpV = spinal nucleus of V; SUBS GEL = substantia gelatinosa; THAL = thalamus; VMH = ventromedial nucleus of the hypothalamus; VTA = ventral tegmental area.

(Continued)

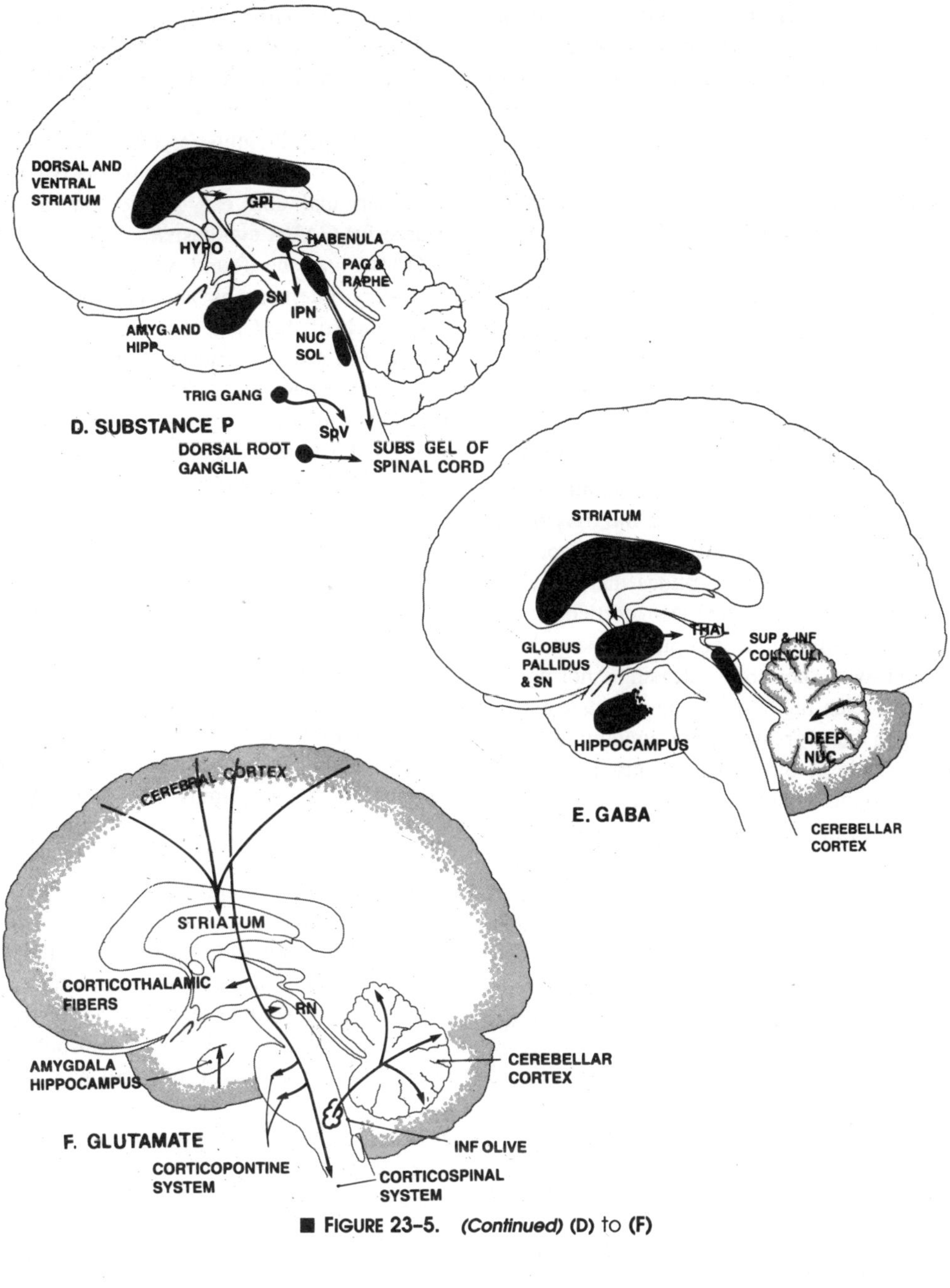

■ **FIGURE 23–5.** *(Continued)* **(D)** to **(F)**

duration of excitation in the CNS areas where it is active. In one of these areas, the substantia gelatinosa of the spinal cord, dorsal root ganglion cells conveying information from Aδ and C fibers secrete substance P as well as glutamate. Enkephalins from interneurons in the superficial dorsal horn inhibit the secretion of substance P and block pain transmission at this site. In addition, a specific population of neurons in the striatum that projects to the internal segment of the globus pallidus and the substantia nigra pars reticulata contains substance P. These cells, like enkephalinergic striatal cells, contain GABA as well as the neuropeptide.

Figure 23–5D shows other areas where radioimmunoassay and immunohistochemical studies have demonstrated high concentrations of this peptide. Figure 23–5D does not show areas where substance P fibers and terminals have been found, but the origin of these neuronal elements remains undetermined. These areas include the anterior nucleus, centromedian nucleus, and ventral posteromedial nucleus of the thalamus, as well as the deep layers of the superior colliculus and the parabrachial nucleus of the brain stem. Substance P binds, with differences in potency, to three neurokinin receptor subtypes, all of which consist of G-protein–coupled receptors.

Hypophysiotrophic Peptides

A third group of neuropeptides that act as neuromodulators in the brain consists of the peptides first identified as neuroendocrine secretory products. Neurons that control pituitary function produce these peptides. They include the following: peptides released into systemic circulation from the pituitary—vasopressin, oxytocin, adrenocorticotropic hormone, and melanocyte-stimulating hormone; and peptides that serve as hypothalamic releasing hormones—corticotropin-releasing hormone, gonadotropin-releasing hormone, growth hormone–releasing hormone, thyrotropin-releasing hormone, and somatostatin.

Although many of the neurons containing these peptides reside in the hypothalamus, they have also been found in numerous other areas of the brain. Moreover, their axons project not only to the neurohypophysis and median eminence, but also to distant areas of the CNS, including the spinal cord. Only some of the specific projection systems of these peptidergic cells have been determined.

Like other peptidergic systems, hypophysiotrophic peptides have multiple receptor subtypes. For example, three vasopressin receptors and five somatostatin receptors have been identified.

Amino Acids

Abundantly present in the CNS, amino acid neurotransmitters act at more synapses than any of the other transmitters identified to date. The major molecules in this group include the inhibitory transmitters GABA, glycine, and taurine and the excitatory amino acids glutamate and aspartate.

Gamma-Aminobutyric Acid and Glycine

In mammals, GABA can be found almost exclusively in the CNS. The presynaptic terminal produces it from glucose through the GABA shunt of the Krebs cycle. Glutamic acid decarboxylase converts the immediate precursor, L-glutamic acid, to GABA. The inactivation of GABA includes its uptake into glial cells, where conversion to glutamine creates a molecule that can be transported back into the GABA presynaptic terminal and can provide an additional source for GABA synthesis.

GABA can be found widely distributed in inhibitory interneurons and projection neurons over much of the CNS. Two of the best-known sites of GABAergic neurons include the cerebellar cortex, where Purkinje cells produce GABA for inhibition of the deep nuclei, and the striatum, where GABAergic cells project to the substantia nigra and globus pallidus (Fig. 23–5E). In **Huntington's disease,** loss of GABAergic neurons in the caudate nucleus and putamen reduces the GABA-mediated inhibition of other basal ganglia nuclei. The globus pallidus projections to the thalamus and subthalamic nucleus use GABA as the major transmitter. (See Chapter 17.)

GABAergic inhibitory interneurons also play important roles in the circuitry of the cerebral cortex, cerebellar cortex, olfactory bulb, hippocampus, and hypothalamus, most of which are not shown in Figure 23–5E. In many of these cell populations, GABA coexists with a variety of neuropeptides. Although cells containing GABA and a neuropeptide account for less than 20% of the total population of GABA neurons, more than 90% of the substance P, cholecystokinin, neuropeptide Y, and somatostatin cells in the monkey brain also produce GABA as a transmitter. The GABAergic neurons of the thalamic reticular nucleus constitute a major component of the circuitry that generates slow-wave sleep. (See Chapter 20.)

Two major types of GABA receptors have been identified: ionotropic $GABA_A$ receptors, which mediate chloride conductance through the membrane, and G-protein–coupled $GABA_B$ receptors, which inhibit cyclic adenosine monophosphate production. Distributed throughout the brain, $GABA_A$ receptors mediate the sedative effects of benzodiazepines and the actions of barbiturates. They also appear to be a major site of anesthetic action.

Like GABA, glycine functions as an inhibitory neurotransmitter in the CNS through its effect on chloride ion channels, but unlike GABA, which has a wide distribution in the brain, glycine appears to be used primarily by inhibitory neurons in the spinal cord and brain stem. The brain stem auditory pathways contain abundant amounts of glycine.

Glutamate and Aspartate

The most plentiful amino acid transmitter in the adult CNS, glutamic acid (glutamate) does not cross the blood-brain barrier and must be synthesized from glucose in a metabolic pathway that includes glutaminase. Glutamate functions as an excitatory neurotransmitter in many areas of the CNS. Initially, its status as a neurotransmitter was difficult to establish because of its widespread distribution and its role in other metabolic pathways (e.g., synthesis of GABA). Even now, the available evidence does not allow aspartate to be ruled out as the active amino acid in many cases. Consequently, the use of the term **glutamate** in the following paragraphs should be understood to mean **glutamate/aspartate.** In the particular case of climbing fibers projecting from the inferior olive to the cerebellum, data from nonhuman primates convincingly identify aspartate as the neurotransmitter.

The highest concentrations of glutamate synapses in the mammalian brain appear in the cerebral cortex, particularly in the hippocampal formation, and in the striatum. The hippocampal formation not only receives glutamatergic input from the entorhinal cortex, but also contains pyramidal cells in the hippocampus proper that use glutamate as a transmitter. In the isocortex, glutaminase-immunoreactive neurons have been localized in layers V and VI, the layers of origin of the corticostriate, corticopontine, corticobulbar, corticospinal, and corticothalamic pathways. The striatum receives excitatory glutamatergic inputs from all areas of the cortex (Fig. 23–5F). Changes in this corticostriatal system may, in fact, be the first step in the development of Huntington's disease and may be a clue to the involvement of glutamatergic pathways in other neurodegenerative disorders.

Although normal brain function requires the excitation provided by these fibers, hyperactivation of the excitatory amino acid systems, or failure of the normal rapid uptake mechanisms for glutamate, can be more deleterious than inactivation of the pathways. Both experimental and clinical data demonstrate that, in excess, these amino acids can function as excitotoxins, causing neuronal cell death. Reduced reuptake by a glial glutamate transporter appears to be an important mechanism underlying excitotoxicity in **amyotrophic lateral sclerosis** (also known as Lou Gehrig's disease).

Like other neurotransmitter systems, glutamate acts at a variety of different receptors that can be defined by their specific agonists. These include both ionotropic and G-protein–coupled receptors. The three types of ionotropic receptors include AMPA (α-amino-3-hydroxy-5-methylisoxazole-4-propionic acid), kainate, and *N*-methyl-D-aspartate. More than a dozen genes encode subunits for these ionotropic receptors. Eight glutamate receptors are coupled to G proteins and are known as metabotropic glutamate receptors ($mGluR_{1\text{-}8}$). Glutamate appears to participate in many normal physiologic processes, including long-term potentiation, which has been implicated in memory. Glutamate has also been implicated in many pathologic conditions such as stroke, epilepsy, and head injury, in addition to amyotrophic lateral sclerosis and Huntington's disease, as mentioned earlier. Hence intense research currently focuses on the functions of the various glutamate pathways and receptors.

SECTION 6

Circulation of Blood and Cerebrospinal Fluid

24

Cerebral Arteries Supplying the Forebrain

Anterior Circulation

Four arteries, one common carotid on each side and one vertebral on each side, provide the entire arterial supply to the brain. The carotid arteries supply the **anterior circulation,** and the vertebral arteries supply the **posterior circulation.** The posterior circulation supplies the brain stem, cerebellum, and the posterior and ventral surfaces of the cerebral hemispheres and is described in Chapter 10. This chapter deals principally with the anterior circulation, which arises from the internal carotid artery, the terminal branches of the basilar artery, and the communicating arteries that join them into the circle of Willis.

Blockage **(occlusion)** of intracerebral arteries can result from local formation of a clot in a vessel narrowed by atherosclerosis **(thrombosis)** or from propagation of a clot from another site such as the heart or a large proximal vessel **(embolus).** Occlusion of an artery results clinically in a stroke (a **neurologic deficit** of sudden onset that has a vascular cause).

Internal Carotid Artery and Its Branches

Each **common carotid artery** divides into an **external carotid artery,** which supplies the face, scalp, and meninges, and an **internal carotid artery.** The internal carotid artery supplies the orbit and a large portion of the brain. It gives off the **ophthalmic artery** and then ascends into the cranial cavity and divides into the **middle cerebral artery** and the **anterior cerebral artery.**

The Ophthalmic Artery Supplies the Eye

The first branch of the internal carotid artery, the **ophthalmic artery,** supplies arterial blood to the eye. Occlusion of this artery can lead to complete monocular blindness. **Amaurosis fugax** consists of temporary monocular blindness. It often results from emboli (small particles of cholesterol and platelets from vascular disease in the heart or carotid artery) that pass through the ophthalmic artery to the eye. This disorder often can be treated, and treatment can prevent future loss of vision.

The Middle Cerebral Artery Supplies the Lateral Surface of the Hemisphere

The **middle cerebral artery** (Fig. 24–1), a terminal branch of the internal carotid artery, enters the depth of the lateral fissure and divides into cortical branches that radiate out to supply the insula and the lateral surface of the frontal, parietal, occipital, and temporal lobes.

Occlusion of the main trunk of the middle cerebral artery causes **infarction** of a large region of the lateral surface of the brain. This leads to paralysis of the opposite side of the body, with a preponderant effect in the face and upper extremity and sensory loss in the same regions. Although the distribution of the anterior cerebral artery may be unaffected, thereby sparing the cerebral cortical representation of the lower extremity, this limb usually becomes paralyzed as well. This is because of decreased flow through the lenticulostriate artery, a branch of the middle cerebral artery, which supplies the internal capsule (see later). Concomitant symptoms include aphasia (language disturbances) or sensory neglect (failure to recognize the contralateral half of the environment), depending on which hemisphere (dominant or nondominant, respectively) has been affected. Initially, the patient develops hypotonic hemiplegia with decreased muscle stretch reflexes; with time, spastic hemiplegia evolves, with increased muscle stretch reflexes and an extensor plantar response. When individual branches of the middle cerebral artery become occluded, the symptoms remain limited to the loss of function reflecting the particular region affected. For example, occlusion of the branch of the middle cerebral artery supplying the inferior frontal gyrus on the left causes weakness in the lower part of the right face and tongue and Broca's aphasia.

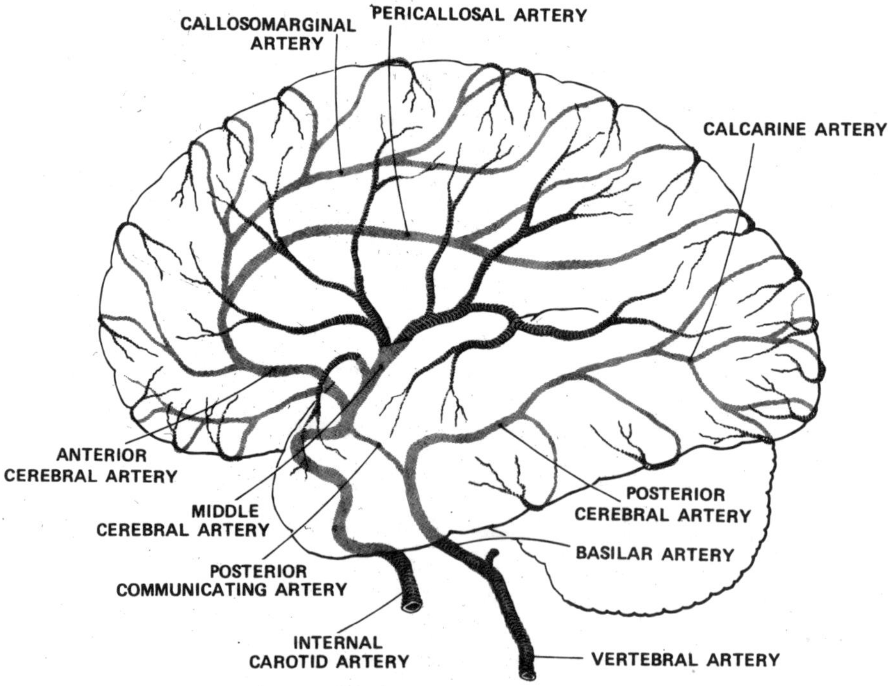

■ **FIGURE 24-1.** A left lateral view of the cerebral hemisphere showing the principal arteries. The anterior cerebral and posterior cerebral arteries reside on the medial surface and are shown as though projected through the substance of the brain.

The Anterior Cerebral Artery Supplies the Anterior Medial Surface of the Hemisphere

The **anterior cerebral artery,** one of the two terminal branches of the internal carotid artery, turns medially to enter the medial longitudinal cerebral fissure. On reaching the genu of the corpus callosum, it curves dorsally and turns backward close to the body of the corpus callosum, supplies a callosomarginal branch, and continues as the pericallosal artery. These arteries supply the medial surface of the frontal and parietal lobes and an adjoining strip of cortex along the medial edge of the lateral surface of these lobes (Figs. 24–1 and 24–2). A small recurrent branch (medial striate artery, or recurrent artery of Huebner), arising near the base of the artery, supplies the anterior limb of the internal capsule (Figs. 24–2 and 24–3). **Thrombosis** along the course of the anterior cerebral artery produces paresis and hypesthesia of the opposite lower extremity because of infarction of the paracentral lobule.

Occlusion of the Internal Carotid Artery or of a Lateral Striate Artery

Occlusion of the internal carotid artery causes infarction in the major distributions of both the middle and anterior cerebral arteries. This results in contralateral hemiplegia and sensory loss involving the face, arm, and leg, and, if the damage is in the dominant hemisphere, language disturbances (aphasia). With infarction affecting the nondominant hemisphere, language remains preserved, but the patient shows neglect of the contralateral half of the environment. Differentiating an internal carotid artery occlusion from a middle cerebral artery occlusion can be difficult, because frequently equally severe hemiplegia and hemisensory loss result from either occlusion. This is because occlusion of the middle cerebral artery frequently involves the striate arteries, thereby causing infarction in the internal capsule.

The lateral striate arteries, also termed the lenticulostriate arteries, are small branches of the middle cerebral artery. The medial striate artery, also known as the recurrent artery of Huebner, is a branch of the anterior cerebral artery. The lateral and medial striate arteries vary in position and arrangement, but together supply the internal capsule and portions of the basal ganglia (Figs. 24–2 and 24–3). Occlusion of a lateral striate artery causes infarction of the internal capsule, caudate nucleus, and putamen. Occlusion of the medial striate artery causes infarction of the internal capsule, globus pallidus, and amygdala. Because all corticospinal fibers pass through one small area of the internal capsule, a relatively small infarct (less than 1.0 cm in diameter) **(lacunar stroke)** in this structure can paralyze the lower portion of the face and the arm and leg of the opposite side of the body. Thus, a small vascular lesion in the internal capsule can have effects on the corticospinal system that mimic those seen after occlusion of the internal carotid artery. In hypertensive patients, a striate artery can rupture, resulting in **hemorrhage** in the putamen and internal capsule. A small hemorrhage produces contralateral hemiplegia, whereas a major hemorrhage can be fatal because of a marked increase of intracranial pressure (see Fig. 9–2).

Posterior Cerebral Artery and Its Branches

The basilar artery terminates in the paired posterior cerebral arteries (see Figs. 24–3 and 10–14). The **posterior cerebral arteries** curve dorsally around the cerebral peduncles and send branches to the upper brain stem and the medial and inferior aspects of the temporal lobe and the occipital lobe (Fig. 24–1). Occlusion of a posterior cerebral artery can cause multiple neurologic disorders, depending on the site of occlusion and the amount of collateral supply provided through the circle of Willis, as described later.

The most common manifestation of posterior cerebral artery **occlusion** consists of **homonymous hemianopia** because of infarction of the calcarine cortex. This results from ischemia in the territory of a distal branch of the posterior cerebral artery, the **calcarine artery.** Macular vision usually remains preserved because the occipital pole receives collateral blood supply from the middle cerebral artery. If both calcarine arteries become occluded, the patient develops **cortical blindness,** a disorder resulting from infarction of both calcarine regions. These patients have preserved pupillary reflexes to light and normal-appearing optic discs. Some patients with cortical blindness cannot recognize or admit their loss of vision, and some experience hallucinations in

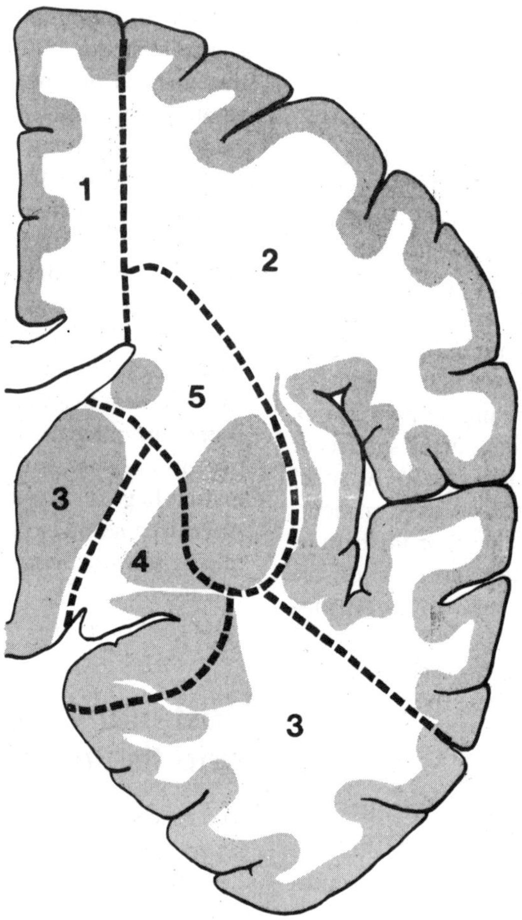

■ **FIGURE 24–2.** A cross section through the brain at about the level of the central sulcus that shows the areas of distribution of the following: **(1)** the anterior cerebral artery, including the callosomarginal and pericallosal arteries; **(2)** the middle cerebral artery; **(3)** the posterior cerebral artery to the diencephalon and inferior temporal lobe; **(4)** the medial striate artery to the internal capsule, globus pallidus, and amygdala; and **(5)** the lateral striate arteries to the caudate nucleus, putamen, and internal capsule.

their blind fields. In some patients with this disorder, macular vision remains preserved (because of collateral supply from the middle cerebral arteries), and the patient experiences tunnel vision. Differentiating these patients from those with conversion disorders can be difficult.

Posterior cerebral artery occlusion more proximally affects several **perforating branches** (posterior medial and posterior lateral groups shown in Fig. 24–3) that supply the posterior and lateral parts of the thalamus and the subthalamus (Fig. 24–2). **Occlusion** of the posterolateral thalamic branches produces partial to complete loss of sensation in the opposite half of the body, often with an accompanying paresis of the affected side of the body. In time, the **thalamic syndrome** may appear, consisting of severe, constant pain in the parts of the body that have limited sensation. Agonizingly severe, the pain often has a burning quality. The affected limbs show decreased sensations of touch, pain, and temperature. With involvement of the subthalamic nucleus, **hemichorea** or **hemiballismus** may occur. Hemiballismus usually results from occlusion limited to a small artery supplying the subthalamic nucleus alone.

Posterior cerebral artery occlusion affecting the interpeduncular branches causes infarctions of the midbrain. Common disorders include unilateral oculomotor palsy with contralateral hemiplegia from ventral mesencephalic infarction and hemiataxia or cerebellar tremor from infarction of the superior cerebellar peduncle.

Formation of the Circle of Willis and Its Central Branches

The junction of the terminal branches of the basilar artery and the two internal carotid arteries forms the **circle of Willis.** This is achieved through a pair of **posterior communicating arteries** and an **anterior communicating artery** (Fig. 24–3). All the major cerebral vessels receive blood through this arterial circle, although there are marked individual variations in the anatomy of the circle. For example, the anterior communicating and posterior communicating arteries may be atretic or hypoplastic on one side or both. Thus, patients may have markedly different symptoms, depending on the collateral circulation through the circle. As an extreme example, an occlusion of the internal carotid artery on one side may not affect the flow through the anterior and middle cerebral arteries if the communicating arteries are well developed.

The **central arteries** supply structures within the interior of the brain: diencephalon, corpus striatum, and internal capsule. These vessels arise as direct branches of the circle of Willis. They are illustrated in Figure 24–3 and may be conveniently considered in four groups:

1. The **anterior medial group** of central arteries originates from the anterior cerebral and anterior communicating arteries. Distribution through the anterior perforated substance supplies the anterior hypothalamic region (i.e., the preoptic and supraoptic regions).
2. The **posterior medial group** originates from the posterior cerebral and posterior communicating arteries. Distribution occurs through the posterior perforated substance. The rostral group supplies the tuber ci-

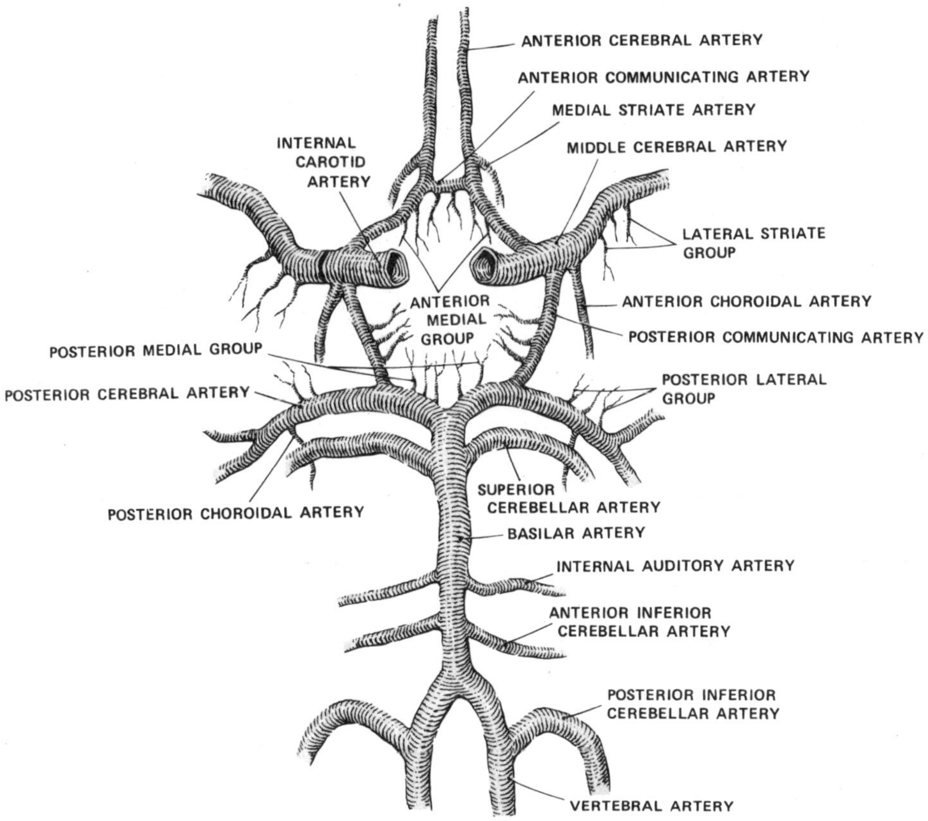

■ **FIGURE 24–3.** The origin of the branches from the circle of Willis.

nereum, infundibular stalk, and hypophysis. Deeper branches penetrate the thalamus. The caudal group supplies the mammillary bodies, subthalamus, and medial portion of the thalamus and midbrain.

3. The **anterior lateral group** consists of the **lateral striate arteries,** which originate primarily from the middle cerebral arteries, and the **medial striate artery** or **recurrent artery of Huebner,** which originates from the anterior cerebral arteries. The lateral striate arteries supply the caudate nucleus, putamen, and posterior limb of the internal capsule. The medial striate artery supplies the anterior limb of the internal capsule and adjacent components of the basal ganglia and amygdala.
4. The **posterior lateral group** originates from the posterior cerebral artery. Distribution is to the caudal portion of the thalamus (i.e., the geniculate bodies, pulvinar, and lateral nuclei).

The **anterior and posterior choroidal arteries** are also considered to be central branches. The anterior choroidal artery arises from the internal carotid or the middle cerebral artery and supplies the choroid plexus of the lateral ventricles, the hippocampus, some of the globus pallidus, and part of the posterior limb of the internal capsule. The posterior choroidal artery arises from the posterior cerebral artery and supplies the choroid plexus of the third ventricle and the dorsal surface of the thalamus.

25

Cerebrospinal Fluid

The brain and spinal cord lie suspended in **cerebrospinal fluid,** a clear, watery liquid filling the subarachnoid space surrounding them. Cerebrospinal fluid also fills the four ventricles of the brain. The total quantity of fluid in adults averages 100 to 150 mL. Production and reabsorption constantly renew the cerebrospinal fluid and replace the total volume several times daily. The fluid contains small amounts of protein, sugar, electrolytes, and a few lymphocytes (no more than 5/mm^3). It differs from plasma in that it contains very little protein, and it differs from an ultrafiltrate of plasma in that various ions (e.g., sodium and chloride) are maintained at concentrations different from those in plasma.

Formation and Circulation

The cerebrospinal fluid forms mainly by processes in the **choroid plexuses,** which are capillary networks surrounded by cuboidal or columnar epithelium projecting into the ventricles. Small plexuses in the roofs of the third and fourth ventricles supplement the two large plexuses in the floor of each lateral ventricle (Fig. 25–1). On average, cerebrospinal fluid forms at a rate of 0.37 mL/min. The production of cerebrospinal fluid is not pressure regulated; consequently, impaired reabsorption by any mechanism does not alter production.

Cerebrospinal fluid moves slowly from the ventricles into the subarachnoid spaces, from which it passes into the dural venous sinuses to be removed by the bloodstream. The fluid leaves the lateral ventricles through the **interventricular foramina (foramina of Monro),** traverses the third ventricle, and reaches the fourth ventricle by way of the **cerebral aqueduct,** which is the narrowest passageway of its entire route (Fig. 25–1). Three openings in the fourth ventricle allow cerebrospinal fluid to pass from the ventricle into the subarachnoid space outside the brain. There are two **lateral ventricular foramina (foramina of Luschka)** in the roof of the lateral recesses of the fourth ventricle and one **median ventricular foramen (foramen of Magendie)** in the midline of the roof of the fourth ventricle. The subarachnoid space, which lies between the arachnoid membrane externally and the pia mater internally, provides a route by which the fluid can flow from its site of production in the ventricles to the points of absorption. Cerebrospinal fluid flows from the outlet foramina of the fourth ventricle over the whole surface of the brain and spinal cord. In places where the brain surface is separated from the skull, cerebrospinal fluid collects within the subarachnoid space, particularly around the base of the brain. The largest of these collections, the **cisterna magna,** is located between the inferior surface of the cerebellum and the medulla. Other cisterns—pontine, interpeduncular, and chiasmatic—lie between the base of the brain and the floor of the cranial cavity. The ambient cistern lies dorsal and lateral to the midbrain.

Cerebrospinal fluid fills the tubular extension of the subarachnoid space that forms a sleeve around the spinal cord. The lower limit of this space is variable, but on average, it lies at the body of the second sacral vertebra, considerably below the end of the spinal cord. Only a small amount of cerebrospinal fluid reabsorption occurs in **spinal arachnoid villi.** Thus, the spinal subarachnoid space is in effect a blind pocket, and exchange of spinal fluid requires changes in posture to move the fluid upward over the cerebral hemispheres where reabsorption occurs.

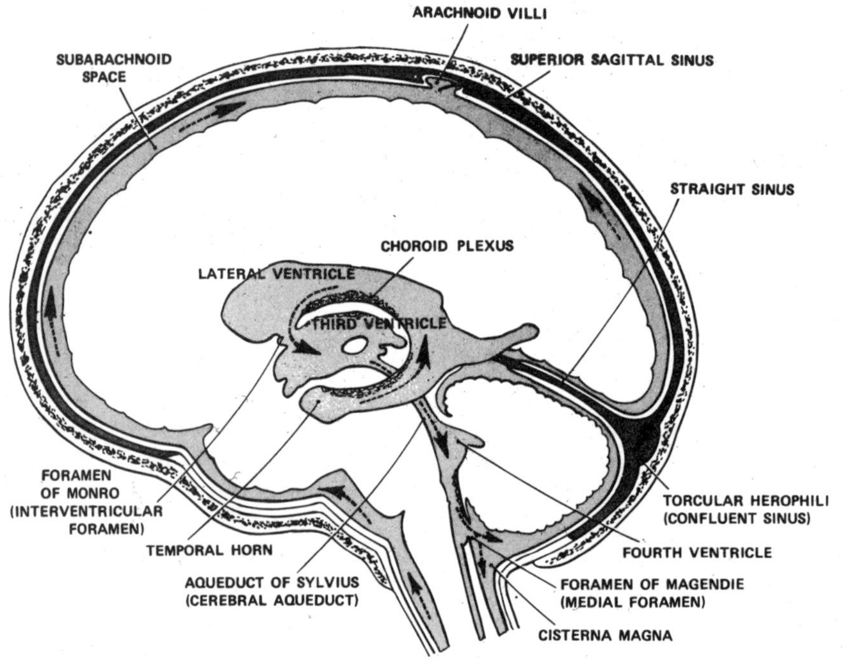

■ **FIGURE 25-1.** The circulation of the cerebrospinal fluid. The foramina of Luschka, in the lateral recesses of the fourth ventricle, are not shown.

Cerebrospinal fluid flows slowly upward from the spinal cord and basal areas of the brain over the convexities of the hemispheres until it reaches the **arachnoid villi (pacchionian granulations)** in the walls of the superior sagittal sinus. It passes through these villi into the venous bloodstream in the sinus. The arachnoid villi function as valves, allowing one-way flow of cerebrospinal fluid from the subarachnoid spaces into the venous blood. All constituents of the fluid leave with the fluid, a process termed **bulk flow.** Vessels in the sheaths of emerging cranial and spinal nerves also absorb cerebrospinal fluid from the subarachnoid space surrounding the brain stem and spinal cord. The veins and capillaries of pia mater also may remove some cerebrospinal fluid by diffusion across their walls.

The subarachnoid space extends into the substance of the nervous system through extensions around blood vessels known as perivascular spaces, or **Virchow-Robin** spaces. Every blood vessel entering the nervous system passes across the subarachnoid space and carries with it a sleeve of arachnoid immediately surrounding the vessel. As the blood vessel enters the brain, it carries both this arachnoid covering and, more externally, a sleeve of pia mater, for a short distance into the tissue. The cerebrospinal fluid of the subarachnoid space probably receives a contribution from the perivascular spaces. Small solutes diffuse freely between the extracellular fluid and the cerebrospinal fluid in these perivascular spaces and also across the ependymal surface of the ventricles, so metabolites can move from brain tissue to the subarachnoid space. Within the depths of the central nervous system (CNS), the layers of pia and arachnoid fuse; therefore, the perivascular space does not continue to the level of the capillary beds.

Composition and Function

A combination of capillary filtration and active epithelial secretion leads to the formation of cerebrospinal fluid. The fluid is similar to an ultrafiltrate of blood plasma but contains lower concentrations of potassium, bicarbonate, calcium, and glucose and higher concentrations of magnesium and chloride. The pH of cerebrospinal fluid is lower than that of blood.

Cerebrospinal fluid has several functions. First, it preserves homeostasis in the nervous system. The constituents of cerebrospinal fluid are in equilibrium with brain extracellular fluid and thus maintain a constant external environment for cells of the nervous system. Second, the fluid provides buoyancy for the brain, decreases the weight of the brain on the skull, and serves as a mechanical cushion, protecting the brain from impact with the bones of the skull. Finally, the fluid drains unwanted substances away from the brain. This is important because the brain has few, if any, lymphatic vessels.

Blood-Brain Barrier

The brain readily absorbs some substances from the blood, such as glucose and oxygen, but it cannot absorb other substances. The barrier to passage of molecules from the blood into the brain is known as the **blood-brain barrier.** This is a physical barrier resulting from a combination of membrane properties and cellular transport systems. A similar barrier exists between blood and cerebrospinal fluid and is called the **blood–cerebrospinal fluid barrier.** The blood-brain barrier provides selective mechanisms for exclusion or transport of any given solute depending on the functional characteristics of brain capillaries and the biochemical characteristics of the solute. The primary locus of the blood-brain barrier is the capillary endothelium. Brain capillaries are unique in having (1) **tight junctions** between capillary endothelial cells, (2) few pinocytotic vesicles, (3) foot processes of astrocytes encasing capillaries, and (4) an exceptionally high number of mitochondria (and thus the capability for high levels of oxidative metabolism) in the endothelial cells. These features make brain capillary endothelium unique, functioning more like a secretory membrane than the capillary endothelium in other organs.

Several characteristics of solutes affect their ability to penetrate the blood-brain barrier. These characteristics determine how well drugs enter the CNS.

1. Small molecules enter the CNS more rapidly than large molecules.
2. Larger proteins do not enter the CNS at all.
3. Ordinarily, substances bound to serum protein cannot penetrate the CNS.
4. Substances that are highly soluble in lipid enter the CNS more readily than those that are poorly soluble in lipid.
5. Carrier-mediated mechanisms transport some substances, such as glucose and some amino acids, into the brain. These transport systems can affect both entry and exit of substances.

The permeability barriers provide mechanisms to preserve the homeostasis of the nervous system by promoting entry of needed substances and by excluding or removing unwanted substances. The blood-brain barrier breaks down under certain conditions, including infections, stroke, brain tumors, generalized seizures, and trauma.

Brain edema refers to an enlargement of brain volume resulting from an increase of water and sodium content. Brain edema can be divided into three types: vasogenic, cellular (cytotoxic), and interstitial. **Vasogenic edema** results from increased permeability of brain capillary endothelial cells to large molecules such as plasma proteins and occurs with brain tumors, abscesses, infarctions, trauma, and hemorrhage. **Cellular (cytotoxic) edema** consists of swelling of the cellular elements of brain, including glia, neurons, and capillary endothelial cells, with an accompanying reduction in volume of the extracellular space in the brain. Cellular edema results from hypoxia, diabetic ketoacidosis, and uremia. **Interstitial (hydrocephalic) edema** refers to increased water and sodium content of the periventricular white matter because of movement of cerebrospinal fluid across ventricular walls (see later).

Pressure

Any obstruction to the normal passage of cerebrospinal fluid causes the fluid to accumulate in the ventricles and leads to a general increase of intracranial pressure. After the pressure has been elevated for days or weeks, swelling of the optic nerve head occurs and can be detected by inspecting the optic fundus with an ophthalmoscope. The high cerebrospinal fluid pressure in the subarachnoid space inside the sleeve of dura mater that surrounds the optic nerve exerts pressure on the retinal veins and optic nerve. As a result, the retinal veins become dilated, and the optic nerve head (optic disc) extends forward above the level of the retina. This condition is known as **papilledema.** Papilledema persisting for weeks or months damages the fibers of the optic nerve and leads to visual impairment. Ultimately, the disc turns chalk white, instead of its normal pale pink.

The most common cause of papilledema is **brain tumor.** Tumors far removed from the ventricles in the supratentorial cranial cavity often do not cause increased intracranial pressure or papilledema until they become large. Tumors of the brain stem and cerebellum, however, often cause increased intracranial pressure while they are still relatively small. The semirigid tentorium cerebelli forms the roof of the posterior fossa and provides little room for expansion in this compartment. Thus, tumors in this region often cause early obstruction to the flow of cerebrospinal fluid through the aqueduct or fourth ventricle and result in increased intracranial pressure. In addition to papilledema, other cardinal signs of brain tumor include persistent headache and vomiting, which often become worse in the early morning when intracranial pressure is particularly high. The headache probably results from the stretching of nerve endings in the dura mater and intracranial blood vessels. The cause of the nausea and vomiting is not clear, but stimulation of the area postrema and vagal nuclei in the floor of the fourth ventricle may be involved. The symptoms are worse on awakening in the morning and are improved by sitting or standing up because of the increased hydrostatic pressure from lying prone, with improvement on assuming the upright posture.

There are many causes of increased intracranial pressure, including **meningitis** (bacterial or viral infection of the meninges), **hypertensive encephalopathy** (severe uncontrolled high blood pressure), **venous sinus thrombosis** (a blood clot affecting one or more of the large venous sinuses in the brain), and certain **drug intoxications. Idiopathic intracranial hypertension (benign intracranial hypertension or pseudotumor cerebri)** is a disorder of unknown cause usually affecting otherwise healthy adolescent girls and young women who often are overweight and have menstrual irregularities. The disease causes headaches and papilledema resulting from a marked increase of intracranial pressure. The condition can be treated effectively and usually resolves after a few weeks or months. If untreated, the disease can impair vision and may ultimately lead to blindness.

Hydrocephalus refers to an increase in the volume of cerebrospinal fluid within the ventricular system and can be divided into noncommunicating (obstructive) hydrocephalus and communicating hydrocephalus. In **noncommunicating hydrocephalus,** an obstruction interferes with the normal flow of cerebrospinal fluid through the ventricles and subarachnoid space. Obstruction occurs most commonly at the foramina of Monro, the aqueduct of Sylvius, or the outlet of the fourth ventricle. Many pathologic processes can cause obstructive hydrocephalus, including developmental abnormalities, brain tumors, hemorrhages, and inflammatory processes. In **communicating hydrocephalus,** cerebrospinal fluid moves freely between the ventricles and subarachnoid space. Communicating hydrocephalus results from a disturbance in the circulation of cerebrospinal fluid through the subarachnoid space or in the reabsorption of cerebrospinal fluid at the arachnoid villi. Impaired reabsorption at the arachnoid villi has been described after subarachnoid hemorrhage and in conditions that markedly increase the protein content of the cerebrospinal fluid such as Guillain-Barré disease (an inflammatory polyneuritis) and certain tumors such as ependymomas. In young children with unfused cranial sutures, hydrocephalus from essentially any cause usually leads to cranial enlargement. Children with hydrocephalus often fail to achieve normal mental and motor milestones. In older children and adults, the fused sutures do not readily permit cranial enlargement. As a result, the head may be normal in size, but the intracranial pressure is elevated. In these instances, hydrocephalus may cause lethargy, headaches, vomiting, and unsteadiness of gait.

Normal-pressure hydrocephalus refers to a disorder of adults characterized by the triad of dementia, unsteady gait, and urinary incontinence. It is a type of communicating hydrocephalus most likely resulting from impaired absorption of cerebrospinal fluid through the arachnoid villi. In some cases, it occurs after an inflammatory disorder, subarachnoid hemorrhage, or head trauma, but in most cases the cause is unclear. Most likely, the cerebrospinal fluid pressure becomes increased early in the disorder, but it stabilizes within the normal range by the time the clinical disorder becomes apparent. The cerebrospinal fluid is normal in composition. Imaging studies such as computed tomography or magnetic resonance imaging show enlarged ventricles without corresponding cerebral atrophy. Imaging also may show abnormal transependymal diffusion of fluid, chiefly in the periventricular regions, which results from increased water content (edema) adjacent to the ventricles. The edema results from passage of cerebrospinal fluid from the ventricles into adjacent brain, where it is reabsorbed. A shunt to divert cerebrospinal fluid from the ventricles to the peritoneal cavity in the abdomen can relieve the symptoms of this condition. The diagnosis of normal-pressure hydrocephalus requires the identification of the clinical features and characteristic imaging study results, as well as the demonstration that the patient's gait improves substantially after removal of 30 to 50 mL of cerebrospinal fluid. Even in typical cases, however, shunting does not always improve the patient's condition.

SECTION 7

Approaches to Patients with Neurologic Symptoms

26

Clinical Evaluation of Neurologic Disorders

Physicians evaluating patients with neurologic disorders use approaches similar to those used for patients with other disorders. The evaluation includes a history followed by a physical examination, a formulation of the likely categories of disease that may be responsible with a differential diagnosis, and then a laboratory evaluation as indicated by the differential diagnosis. One major difference distinguishes the neurologic evaluation from other types of medical assessments, however, and this is the necessity of determining the **localization** of the disorder in neurologic diseases as part of the formulation. Localizing the pathologic process responsible for the symptoms and clinical signs usually permits the physician to focus the differential diagnosis sharply and thereby to restrict the number and often the costs of the diagnostic tests needed. The entire **neurologic evaluation** requires a full and complete history of the illness, physical examination and neurologic examination, and then a **formulation** that includes the probable **site of the pathologic process** and **type of pathologic process,** the **differential diagnosis,** and recommendations concerning laboratory tests for further evaluation. After completing these tasks, the physician can make a definitive diagnosis and then can plan the **management** and **treatment** and give a **prognosis.**

The **neurologic history** consists of a detailed chronologic account of the symptoms and usually provides clues to the **type of pathologic process** underlying the patient's symptoms. For example, the sudden onset of neurologic impairment (e.g., paralysis of the limbs on one side of the body) followed by gradual improvement over weeks or months suggests the possibility of a vascular disorder such as an ischemic or hemorrhagic stroke. Progressively increasing symptoms (e.g., limb weakness or cognitive dysfunction) that do not improve over time suggest a neoplastic disease such as brain tumor or a neurodegenerative disease such as Alzheimer's disease. Symptoms that appear, then improve, only to reappear (relapsing and remitting symptoms such as visual loss, ataxia, or paraparesis) suggest a demyelinating disease such as multiple sclerosis.

The **neurologic examination** provides information that assists in localizing the site of the disorder. For example, in a right-handed patient with expressive aphasia and right hemiplegia, localization will be to the left frontal lobe, including Broca's area and the white matter underlying the precentral region. Other types of aphasia, apraxia, and agnosia also commonly result from relatively focal disease of the cerebral cortex. A unilateral cranial nerve disorder associated with contralateral hemiplegia localizes to one side of the brain stem, and the cranial nerve involved assists in determining whether the disorder is in the medulla, pons, or mesencephalon. The combination of spastic paraparesis and loss of sensation below a specific level on the trunk localizes to the spinal cord, and the specific level of the cord can be determined by the level of the motor and sensory loss.

After completing the history, general physical examination, neurologic examination, and localization of the lesion, the physician adds to the formulation the category of pathologic process most likely responsible for the lesion; that is, whether it is the result of vascular disease, trauma, genetic disorder, toxins, neoplasm, degenerative changes, metabolic disorder, or demyelination. The next step is to determine the differential diagnosis, which is a short list of the specific disease processes that could account for the other elements in the formulation. Often, a correct formulation yields a short list. The physician then uses selective laboratory investigations to complete the diagnostic process. In most cases, completion of these steps results in a clear diagnosis, so appropriate management and treatment can be administered.

Since the advent of anatomic imaging techniques such as computed tomography and magnetic resonance, some physicians request imaging procedures for their patients before the history and examination are fully explored. This often results in misleading or inconclusive findings and in wasted time, effort, and funds. It is essential to obtain a full history and examination initially and then to formulate the problem before ordering any laboratory tests. Considerable time, effort, and expense can be saved in this way. Moreover, disease processes that progress rapidly, such as meningitis or encephalitis, can be evaluated and treated much more quickly if the physician focuses on the history and physical examination and does not waste time obtaining tests that may not be helpful.

Patient History

Neurologic History

Chief complaint. Obtain the patient's name, age, gender, occupation, and handedness. Record the chief complaint in the patient's own words, preferably as a direct quotation, if possible, and give the duration of the complaint. If the patient cannot provide the chief complaint, attempt to obtain it from a family member, guardian, or friend.

Present illness. Give a chronologic sequence of the present illness beginning with the first symptom, and then describe how the symptoms have changed over time. Often, patients want to discuss only other physicians' opinions about the illness and to describe the many tests that were done. Usually, this information is not helpful, and you may need to interrupt the patient repeatedly, if necessary, and to ask focused questions about the symptoms and the evolution of these symptoms over time. Make special inquiry about the following complaints:

- Changes in memory or personality
- Disturbances of consciousness
- Convulsions
- Headaches
- Loss of vision
- Diplopia (double vision)
- Deafness
- Tinnitus (ringing or roaring in the ears)
- Vertigo (a sense of movement of the environment or of the patient)
- Nausea and vomiting
- Dysphagia (difficulty in swallowing)
- Speech disorders (problems with articulation)

- Language disturbances (trouble with comprehension or execution of language)
- Weakness, stiffness, or paralysis of the limbs
- Gait imbalance and falls
- Tremors or other involuntary movements
- Pains and paresthesias
- Loss or decrease of sensation
- Disturbances in control of the bowel or bladder

Past Medical History

After you have completely explored the present illness, inquire about the patient's past medical history. The following list provides the major topics to be covered:

Major illnesses. Describe previous illnesses: age at onset, treatment, and resolution. Include childhood illnesses if indicated. Inquire about any trauma to the head, neck, or extremities.

Surgery. List all operative procedures, age at the time of the procedure, and outcome.

Allergies. List all allergic reactions to medications or intravenous dyes, particularly iodinated dyes. List allergies to food, pollens, and animals. Describe the symptoms of the allergic reactions.

Medications. List all medications currently used, with the doses and frequency of administration, including vitamins, herbal preparations, and nonprescription (over-the-counter) medicines.

System review. Inquire about the major organ systems, asking about symptoms referable to these systems. Include the head, ear, eyes, nose, throat, lungs, heart, upper gastrointestinal tract, lower gastrointestinal tract, urinary tract, menstrual function in women, bone and joint problems, and skin disorders.

Birth and developmental milestones. If appropriate in evaluating the current complaints, ask whether the birth was full term and natural or whether it required instrumentation or cesarean section. Ask about the age at which the patient held the head up, rolled over, stood independently, walked, and talked.

Family History

Ask whether the patient's parents are living, and if so, inquire about their ages and state of health. If they are no longer living, obtain the age of death and cause of death as well as any antecedent chronic illnesses, particularly neurologic disorders, in the mother and father. Make similar inquiries about siblings. Include inquiries about family members, immediate or remote, who had paralysis, gait or movement disorders, convulsions, or dementia. If a first-degree relative (mother, father, or sibling) had an illness similar to that of the patient, obtain as full a history of the illness as possible. Inquire about grandparents, aunts, uncles, and cousins who had similar illnesses as well. Inquire about the patient's children, including ages, genders, and any illnesses. If the family history includes several members of multiple generations with a similar illness, draw a full family tree.

Social History

Education. Record the years of education and diplomas or degrees received.

Occupation. List the work positions held and how the level of responsibility changed over time. Ask about occupational exposures to heavy metals, pesticides, and solvents.

Marriage. Inquire about the number of marriages and their duration as well as the patient's current marital state.

Sexual function. Ask about the level of desire for sexual intercourse and the frequency and level of satisfaction with intercourse. In men, ask about difficulty in achieving or maintaining an erection, premature ejaculation, or inability to ejaculate. If a man cannot achieve an erection, ask about the frequency of erections in the morning. In women, ask about painful intercourse and any difficulty in achieving orgasm.

Habits. Inquire about the frequency of use of alcohol, caffeine, tobacco, and "recreational" drugs. Estimate the number of packages of cigarettes smoked per day and the number of years at this level of smoking. Obtain details about alcohol consumption, including frequency of exposure, types of beverages used, morning drinking, binges, and effects of withdrawal from alcohol.

Living situation. Particularly in older people and those with cognitive disorders, determine whether the patient needs supervision or assistance with the activities of daily living.

Physical Examination

Obtain the patient's blood pressure, pulse, and respiratory rate. If you find hypertension when you take the blood pressure in one arm, take the blood pressure in the patient's other arm. Examine the heart, lungs, abdomen, extremities, joints, and skin, and listen for bruits over the carotid arteries in the neck.

Neurologic Examination

The neurologic examination usually requires only a few simple materials and pieces of equipment. For most examinations, you need a Snellen card or chart to test visual acuity, an ophthalmoscope, a tongue depressor, a small flashlight, a reflex hammer, a disposable safety pin, a small pledget of cotton wool, and both a 128 cycle per second (Hz) and a 256-Hz tuning fork. If the patient's history suggests a disorder of taste or smell, have available a scented substance such as coffee, mint, or cloves. For testing of higher cognitive functioning, you need a pencil or pen, a blank sheet of paper, and a paragraph of written material from a newspaper for testing reading. For testing cortical sensory function, you need a compass with two blunt tips that can be separated for measurable distances of millimeters, several small coins, and several small common objects such as nails, screws, bolts, and nuts.

The neurologic examination can be divided into five parts: mental status, cranial nerves, motor system, reflexes, and sensation.

Mental Status

- **Orientation.** Ask the patient to state the following: the date, including day, month, and year; the location (the name of the hospital or clinic); and the county, city, and state.
- **Attention and state of consciousness.** Determine by observation whether the patient remains alert, pays attention to you, and responds to your questions appropriately. If the patient displays an altered state of consciousness, use the following terms to describe the level of consciousness:
  1. Normal level of attention (alert, attentive, responsive).
  2. Confusional state (shortened attention span, difficulty following commands, minor disorientation, faulty memory).
  3. Delirium (disorientation, fear, irritability, hallucinations).
  4. Stupor (unresponsiveness, arousal only with vigorous and repeated stimuli).
  5. Coma (unarousable unresponsiveness).
- **Memory.** Test **remote memory** by asking the date of birth, date of marriage, dates that the patient's children were born, and any other personally important dates. For **intermediate memory,** ask for the events of the previous 5 years. For **recent memory,** ask about the present illness, events since the hospitalization, and events of the last 2 days. Test digit retention by reciting seven digits aloud, one per second, and asking the patient to repeat them in sequence, both forward and backward. Most people can remember seven digits forward and five backward. State a brief sentence or phrase and ask the patient to repeat it. Ask the patient to repeat three objects immediately and then again after 5 minutes. Examples include sailboat, basketball, and Webster Avenue. Tell the patient a brief story, and ask the patient to recall the story.
- **Calculations.** Ask the patient to subtract 7 from 100 in serial fashion, to compute 3×16, or to compute the interest on $200 at 10% annual rate for 18 months.
- **Grasp of general information.** Ask for the name of the president, vice president, secretary of state, mayor, and governor. Ask for the names of five of the largest cities in the United States. Ask for the dates of Washington's birthday or Christmas. Ask for the dates of the beginning and end of the World Wars.
- **Interpretation of proverbs and similarities.** Ask the patient to interpret a proverb such as, "People who live in glass houses shouldn't throw stones," or "Every cloud has a silver lining." The proverb should be interpreted in the abstract. Mentally retarded or demented people often give concrete interpretations. For example, in response to the proverb "People who live in glass houses

shouldn't throw stones,'' a neurologically normal person may say, ''Since everyone is vulnerable, people should not be critical of others,'' whereas a demented person may say, ''You will break the windows.'' Ask for the similarities between an apple and a lemon, a bicycle and an automobile, and a bird and an airplane. The interpretation should be abstract, such as, ''Apple and lemon are both fruit.'' If the patient gives a concrete interpretation such as ''Apple and lemon are round,'' suspect a cognitive disorder.

- **Insight and judgment.** Use the letter test and the fire test. In the **letter test,** describe a situation in which the patient is walking along a street and sees a stamped, addressed, sealed envelope on the ground. What should be done with it? The letter should be deposited in a mailbox or given to a postal employee. In the **fire test,** describe the patient as sitting in a theater and seeing a fire. Ask what the patient should do. The patient should stand up and walk slowly out and should not shout, ''fire!'' or run, because this may start a stampede. Abnormalities on tests of insight and judgment may result from a cognitive disorder.
- **Affect.** Observe for signs of anxiety, pressured speech, psychomotor retardation, melancholy, or lability of emotional responses. These findings can be particularly important in neurodegenerative disorders such as Alzheimer's disease, demyelinating diseases such as multiple sclerosis, and vascular disease. These findings are also important in people with multiple somatic complaints but few or no abnormal neurologic findings on physical and laboratory examination, because this may lead you to suspect a nonorganic disorder.
- **Special tests.** In evaluating suspected disorders of higher cerebral function, use the following tests:
  1. **Language.** Note the content of the patient's spontaneous speech and determine whether the speech is nonfluent (slow, effortful, hesitant speech) or fluent (rapid, facile, smooth speech). Nonfluent aphasia often results from a lesion in the anterior part of the dominant cerebral hemisphere, whereas fluent aphasia often results from a lesion in the posterior part of the dominant cerebral hemisphere. As you take the history, attempt to determine whether the patient responds directly to your questions or responds with tangential answers. The patient may have difficulty in understanding your questions or difficulty in expressing ongoing thoughts. Examine for dysarthria (difficulty articulating speech) as part of the cranial nerve evaluation.
  2. **Naming.** Ask the patient to name various objects (e.g., pen, thumb, watch, face, belt buckle, and colors).
  3. **Repetition.** Ask the patient to repeat a phrase such as ''no ifs, ands, or buts'' or ''the lawyer's closing argument convinced him.''
  4. **Comprehension.** Determine the patient's ability to follow commands such as ''Close your eyes'' or ''Pick up the paper, fold it in half, and hand it to me.''
  5. **Reading.** Test the patient's ability to read aloud and comprehend a paragraph from a newspaper. A disorder in comprehension of written material in an alert patient often results from disease in the posterior part of the dominant cerebral hemisphere.
  6. **Writing.** Ask the patient to write an original sentence and to copy a sentence. A disturbance of writing in an alert patient usually signifies a pathologic process in the posterior part of the dominant cerebral hemisphere.
  7. **Constructional ability.** Ask the patient to copy a cube or a complex figure. Ask the patient to draw a house or a flower. A disturbance of constructional ability in an alert, nonaphasic patient suggests a lesion in the nondominant (usually right) parietal lobe, particularly when the left parts of the drawings remain incomplete or have been ignored.
  8. **Praxis.** This refers to the motor integration used in the execution of complex learned movements. Give the patient commands such as ''Show me how to blow out a match,'' ''Show me how to use a toothbrush,'' ''Show me how to wave goodbye.'' Note the patient's perfor-

mance. Lesions of the prefrontal portions of the dominant hemisphere often cause apraxias.

Cranial Nerves

- **I. Olfactory nerve.** Test the patient's sense of smell with oil of lemon, cloves, or coffee. Do not use alcohol or other noxious vapors; these substances test cranial nerve V, not I. Most clinicians test olfactory sense only when indicated by the history.
- **II. Optic nerve.** Test visual acuity with a Snellen card for bedside use or a full-size Snellen chart. Visual acuity should be tested with and without the patient's corrective lenses. Record visual acuity as 20 (the distance to the Snellen chart) over the size of type read (20/20, for example, indicates excellent acuity; 20/200 indicates poor acuity). Test each eye independently. Test the visual fields with bedside confrontation by moving a finger in each of the four quadrants of the field of each eye. (See Chapter 19 for further details.) Test double simultaneous stimulation when the patient has both eyes open. If indicated, test the visual fields formally with a perimeter. Examine the optic fundi with an ophthalmoscope. (See Chapter 25.)
- **III, IV, and VI. Extraocular muscle function.** Examine the pupils and note the size, regularity, and equality. Test the reactions to light and accommodation. (See Chapter 19.) Look for strabismus (lack of parallel alignment of the eyes). Look for spontaneous nystagmus (beating movements of the eyes, either with the eyes looking straight ahead or on lateral or vertical gaze). Look for lid droop or retraction. Test extraocular movements to command and also to pursuit by having the patient follow an object through all four quadrants of movement. Test for ocular convergence. Oculocephalic maneuvers (see Chapter 19) and caloric stimulation of the external auditory canals to look for nystagmus (see Chapter 15) are useful in assessing supranuclear gaze disorders and abnormalities of vestibular function, respectively. These maneuvers are also useful in assessing unresponsive patients.
- **V. Trigeminal nerve.** Ask the patient to open and close the jaw against resistance. Test the jaw jerk reflex by asking the patient to open the jaw slightly, then tapping lightly over the chin and looking for reflex closure of the jaw. Compare the jaw jerk to the other deep tendon reflexes. Test sensation on the face with a light touch of a pin or a cold object such as one of the tines of a tuning fork. Test the corneal reflexes with a small wisp of cotton wool. (See the discussion of the sensory division of nerve V in Chapter 12.)
- **VII. Facial nerve.** Examine the face for asymmetry at rest, and examine facial movement with contraction during voluntary effort.
- **VIII. Auditory and vestibular nerves.** Whisper a different number in each of the patient's ears, and ask the patient to repeat each number. Perform the Rinne and Weber tests as described in Chapter 14. When indicated, use cold water to irrigate the external auditory canal and examine for nystagmus. Before performing this test, be certain that the eardrum is intact. (See Chapter 15.)
- **IX and X. Glossopharyngeal and vagus nerves.** Ask the patient to say "ah" while you look at the palate using a tongue depressor and a flashlight. Determine whether the palate elevates symmetrically with phonation to test the motor function of nerve X. Test the gag reflex on each side to test nerves IX (afferent) and X (efferent).
- **XI. Spinal accessory nerve.** Test the strength of contraction of the sternomastoid and trapezius muscles. Ask the patient to turn the head to the left and then to the right while you test the strength of muscle contraction by resisting the movement. Turning the head to the left requires contraction of the right sternomastoid, and vice versa. To test the strength of the trapezius muscles, ask the patient to shrug the shoulders against resistance.
- **XII. Hypoglossal nerve.** Ask the patient to protrude the tongue and to move it rapidly from side to side. Assess articulation to examine for dysarthria. If the patient has dysarthria, determine whether it is flaccid, hypokinetic, spastic, or ataxic.

Motor System

Posture. Inspect the patient's posture at rest, both seated and standing. Look for any asymmetry in the height of the shoulders and hips, for any deviation of the head, and for tremor or spasm. Ask the patient to extend the arms with the fingers spread apart, palms up, and eyes closed; then look for downward drift with pronation of either arm. This occurs with limb weakness and may be an early sign of hemiparesis.

Station and gait. Test the capacity of the patient to rise from a chair with arms crossed. Assess postural stability with the patient standing alone and the response to being pulled backward. To do this, stand behind the patient, and then forcefully pull the patient backward from both shoulders while being careful to prevent the patient from falling. Patients with Parkinson's disease cannot make compensating backward steps and tend to fall. Ask the patient to stand, feet together, eyes open, and determine whether the patient is stable. If the patient is stable, ask the patient to close the eyes, and determine whether this causes the patient to fall. Prevent the patient from falling by standing nearby during this test. If the person is stable at rest but falls with the eyes closed, you have demonstrated a positive Romberg sign. Previously used to determine whether position sense is impaired in the lower extremities, this test has been extended to include abnormalities of the motor system, and it tends to be positive in the ataxias and in parkinsonian syndromes. Ask the patient to walk normally down a long hall, then to walk on the heels, on the toes, and finally in tandem, touching the toes of one foot with the heel of the other foot. Look for broadening of the base (keeping the legs abnormally far apart), irregular size and directions of steps (ataxia of gait), asymmetries of arm swing, stooped posture, slowness or imbalance while turning, turning en bloc (with the head turning only when the rest of the body turns), and instability with walking on the heels, toes, or in tandem.

Strength. Examine the power of movement at the major joints in the neck, upper limbs, and lower limbs for flexion, extension, adduction, and abduction. Record strength on a scale of 0 to 5, as follows: 0, no contraction; 1, contraction insufficient for movement; 2, contraction sufficient for movement but insufficient to overcome gravity; 3, weak contraction able to overcome gravity; 4, fair but not full strength; 5, full power of contraction. Note the bulk of the muscles, and look for atrophy and fasciculations (twitching movements seen beneath the skin without movement of the limbs).

Resistance to passive manipulation of the limbs ("tone"). With the patient as relaxed as possible, test the resistance to passive manipulation of the limbs at the wrists, elbows, shoulders, hips, knees, and ankles. **Spasticity** consists of the "clasp-knife" phenomenon, in which the examiner feels a free interval, then a catch, and then a release of resistance. Spasticity characterizes the chronic upper motoneuron syndrome and usually occurs together with hyperreflexia and extensor plantar responses. **Rigidity** can be detected as increased resistance to passive manipulation of the limbs in three forms. In **cogwheel rigidity,** the examiner detects a succession of catches and releases during passive flexion or extension limb movements, usually best seen at the wrists and commonly found in Parkinson's disease and parkinsonian syndromes. In **plastic rigidity,** the examiner perceives a smooth, even resistance to passive limb manipulation. This commonly appears in the lower extremities in Parkinson's disease and parkinsonian syndromes. **Dystonic rigidity** consists of increasing resistance that mounts with passive manipulation as the movement continues, and, on release, the limb returns rapidly to its resting posture. Dystonic rigidity commonly appears in dystonias with fixed or relatively fixed limb postures such as cerebral palsy and dystonia musculorum deformans. **Hypotonia** consists of decreased resistance to manipulation and commonly occurs in motoneuron, peripheral nerve, and cerebellar diseases.

Coordination. Ask the patient to touch an index finger alternately to his or her nose and then to your finger, which you hold at a full arm's length away from the patient. Ask the patient to run his or her heel from the opposite knee straight down the shin to the foot, then elevate the leg in the air, and repeat the movement. Test rapid alternating movements by having the patient alternately pronate and supinate one hand, touching the palm of the opposite hand. Have the patient perform rhythmic tapping tests as well. Have the patient walk normally and also in tandem, heel to toe. Ask the patient to walk on the heels and then on the toes.

Involuntary movements. Look for involuntary movements, including tremor. **Parkinsonian tremor** consists of a 4- to 5-Hz distal tremor with flexion-extension movements of the fingers and wrists and, often, the feet. The tremor occurs at rest and decreases or stops with active movement, at least temporarily. **Essential (familial) tremor** also affects the distal parts of the limbs, but it does not occur at rest; it appears with a sustained posture (as with the arms outstretched, fingers extended) or with active movements such as writing. The tremor affects the fingers and, to some extent, the wrists, which usually move in flexion and extension, but the tremor may include adduction-abduction finger movements. Essential tremor often includes an involuntary flexion-extension tremor of the head, at times with a nodding tremor as well. When completely at rest, patients with essential tremor have no involuntary movements, whereas parkinsonian patients regularly do have tremor at rest. **Cerebellar tremor** consists of a proximal side-to-side tremor occurring only with movement, best shown on heel-knee-shin or finger-nose-finger testing. **Athetosis** consists of involuntary slow and writhing movements of the limbs and commonly occurs in cerebral palsy. **Chorea** consists of rapid movements that flow from limb to limb, with sweeping sideward movements of the head, wincing movements of the face, and ''piano-playing'' movements of the hands. **Hemiballismus** consists of rapid flinging movements of an arm and a leg on one side of the body. **Myoclonus** consists of lightning-like movements of segments of the extremities.

Reflexes

Examine the deep tendon (muscle stretch) reflexes, including the biceps reflex (innervated through the C5-6 reflex arc), triceps reflex (C7), brachioradialis reflex (C5-6), patellar reflex (L3), and ankle reflex (S1). Test the superficial reflexes, including the abdominal reflexes, the cremasteric reflexes in men, and the anal reflex. Examine the plantar response by moving a blunt object such as a key along the lateral border of the sole of the foot. An **extensor plantar response (Babinski's sign)** consists of a dorsal flexion movement of the great toe. A **flexor plantar response** consists of plantar flexion of the great toe.

Sensation

Test sensation first in areas where the patient has complaints and compare these responses with those in areas that are symptomatically unaffected. Compare the left and right sides of the body, and compare distal and proximal parts of the limbs. Compare the patient's face with the body, and check sensation on the trunk from the chest to the pelvis. Test the patient's response to pinprick, and use a new safety pin for each patient. Test light touch with a wisp of cotton wool, and test vibration sense using a 128-Hz tuning fork applied to bony prominences. Test position sense by moving up or down a distal joint such as the great toe, and ask the patient, with his or her eyes closed, to indicate which direction the toe has moved. Test thermal sensation with a tube of cold or warm water. As a screening test, one of the tines of a nonvibrating tuning fork can be used to examine cold sensation. To examine for cortical sensory loss, use a compass with two blunt points separated by approximately 1 mm on the fingers, and ask the patient, with his or her eyes closed, to determine whether you are touching with one or two tips. Gradually widen the distance between the tips until the patient detects two and record the separation distance, comparing the two sides of the body. Test stereognosis by asking the patient, with his or her eyes closed, to determine what size coin has been placed in the palm. Test tactile localization by asking the patient, with his or her eyes closed, to point to the part of the limb that the examiner touches. Test for the **Romberg sign** by having the patient stand with the feet together and the eyes open until the patient is stable; then ask the patient to close the eyes, to determine whether the patient can remain stable. The Romberg test is positive if the patient is steady with eyes open and sways or falls with eyes closed.

27

Neurologic Diagnostic Tests

Since the 1970s, advances in neurology and neurosurgery, aided by rapid progress in neuroscience, pharmacology, biochemistry, and molecular biology, have transformed the practice of neurology. Previously a field focused on diagnosis but offering relatively few opportunities for treatment, neurology has become a rapidly advancing, therapeutically focused field for clinical practice. Currently, treatments are available for many disorders that previously could only be diagnosed and followed. Among the diseases that can be managed with much greater efficacy are epilepsy, Parkinson's disease, stroke, multiple sclerosis, certain peripheral neuropathies, myasthenia gravis, multiple types of sleep disorders, and migraine headaches. A rapid pace of research on Alzheimer's disease in recent years has brought us to the point of ongoing clinical trials with therapeutic approaches that may prove effective in preventing or halting the progression of this dreadful disease.

In neurology, as in other fields of medicine, the formulation and diagnosis are key steps that must be taken before treatment can be prescribed. As indicated in Chapter 26, the most important methods of achieving a correct diagnosis include the history, physical examination, neurologic examination, and the thought processes that go into determining the localization of the lesion, the type of pathologic process, and the differential diagnosis. At this point in the formulation, specific laboratory tests can be used to complete or to verify the diagnosis. These tests are summarized in this chapter.

Cerebrospinal Fluid Analysis

Abnormalities of cerebrospinal fluid constituents occur in numerous disorders, including meningitis, encephalitis, syphilis affecting the nervous system, subarachnoid hemorrhage, peripheral neuropathy, brain tumors, stroke, and multiple sclerosis. Samples of cerebrospinal fluid for diagnostic tests can be obtained by inserting a needle designed for **lumbar puncture** between the vertebrae at the level of L3 and L4, L4 and L5, or L5 and S1. Advancing the needle slowly until it pierces the dura mater provides access to cerebrospinal fluid without the danger of striking the spinal cord, because the cord terminates rostral to level L2. This approach presents only a small chance of injuring the nerve roots of the cauda equina that are present at these levels. With the patient lying recumbent on one side and relaxed, the physician performing the tap records the pressure of the spinal fluid, which normally does not exceed 200 mm H_2O. Small oscillations of the fluid level in a manometer connected to the needle result from the transmission of cerebral arterial pulsations. These pulsations indicate that fluid in the manometer communicates freely with fluid in the cerebrospinal fluid spaces.

Lumbar puncture can be hazardous in the presence of elevated intracranial pressure resulting from an intracranial mass, especially a large mass in one cerebral hemisphere causing midline shift. In this situation, a sudden decrease of cerebrospinal fluid pressure from the lumbar puncture could promote downward herniation of the brain. This leads to herniation of the medial part of the temporal lobe (the uncus) through the tentorium cerebelli, which compresses the mesencephalon and results in coma with decerebrate rigidity. Lumbar puncture can also be hazardous in patients with a mass in the posterior fossa, because decompression can provoke herniation of the cerebellar tonsils through the foramen magnum and can cause medullary compression and consequent injury of neurons controlling cardiac and respiratory functions. Lumbar puncture can be dangerous in patients with tumors that fill the spinal canal because the change in cerebrospinal fluid pressure can impair spinal cord function by increasing compression from the tumor.

In addition to lumbar puncture, **cisternal puncture** or **lateral cervical puncture** can be employed to obtain cerebrospinal fluid. In performing a cisternal puncture, the physician passes a needle through the posterior cervical area at the base of the skull, then directly through the atlanto-occipital membrane into the cisterna magna. This approach avoids nervous system structures, except the medulla if the needle passes far beyond the cisterna magna. Lateral cervical puncture requires fluoroscopic guidance to pass a spinal needle laterally between the first and second cervical vertebrae. Physicians should perform these procedures only after full and appropriate training.

After collecting cerebrospinal fluid in four separate tubes, the physician describes the color, which normally should be clear and colorless, but can be xanthochromic (yellow) when the tap is bloody. The color should be examined again after centrifugation to determine whether the fluid remains xanthochromic. If it does, the patient may have had a pre-existent hemorrhage such as subarachnoid hemorrhage. The fluid can then be analyzed for cellular content in tubes number 1 and number 4, including white blood cells and red blood cells, and for glucose and protein concentrations. A blood glucose level should be obtained at the time of the spinal tap to compare with the cerebrospinal fluid glucose level. If the clinical history and examination suggest meningitis, a Gram stain and bacterial culture should be performed. The fluid should also be evaluated with smears and cultures for tubercle bacilli and for fungi.

If the clinical history suggests multiple sclerosis, additional helpful information can be obtained from tests for immunoglobulin G, oligoclonal bands, and myelin basic protein. The blood should be tested for oligoclonal bands at the same time as the cerebrospinal fluid studies. If the clinical history suggests neoplastic disease, particularly carcinomatous meningitis, but also metastatic disease, the cerebrospinal fluid should be centrifuged, and the spun-down cells should be examined microscopically.

Electroencephalography and Evoked-Potential Studies

Neuronal activity in the brain can be studied indirectly by recording electrical activity from the scalp surface with **electroencephalography (EEG).** This technique has proven useful in evaluating patients with epilepsy, coma, and other disturbances of the state of consciousness. Neuronal activity can also be recorded directly from the exposed cerebral cortical surface (**electrocorticography**) at the time of craniotomy by a neurosurgeon. The electrical responses of large aggregates of neurons can be recorded at sites distant from the origin of the responses because of **volume conduction,** which consists of the flow of current through the extracellular space. Changes in potential within neurons cause current to flow in the extracellular fluid. Although this fluid has low resistance, current flow across the resistance suffices to cause a potential change.

Clinical EEG recordings employ multiple active electrodes over the surface of the head with an indifferent electrode over one or both ears. The EEG records potential differences between adjacent active electrodes and also differences between each active electrode and an indifferent electrode. Although action potentials represent the largest signals that neurons generate, these potentials actually contribute little to EEG potentials because they do not occur simultaneously in large numbers of neurons. Most of the activity recorded in the EEG consists of extracellular current flow associated with summated postsynaptic potentials in synchronously active pyramidal cells of the cerebral cortex.

The frequencies of the potentials recorded from the surface of the scalp vary from 1 to 50 cycles per second (Hz), and the amplitudes typically range up to 300 μV. EEG potentials have complex frequency characteristics, but a few frequencies occur often. **Alpha rhythm** (8 to 13 Hz) can be recorded best from the parieto-occipital region and appears most prominently during relaxed wakefulness with the patient's eyes closed. **Beta activity** (14 to 30 Hz) normally appears over the frontal and central regions. **Theta** (4 to 7 Hz) and **delta** (0.5 to 4 Hz) activities develop during sleep in the adult.

Certain characteristic waveforms may suggest particular processes. Examples include sharp waves, which suggest epilepsy, and focal slowing, which can indicate dysfunction in the region of the brain showing this waveform.

Evoked potentials result from a change in the ongoing electrical activity of neurons in response to stimulation of a sensory organ or pathway. Specific for the sensory stimulus that evokes them, these potentials become time locked to the stimulus. Evoked potentials can be recorded from the scalp with electrodes and amplifiers similar to those used in EEG recordings, but they are too small in amplitude to be discerned in EEG tracings. Portraying and measuring these potentials require obtaining averaged responses from several hundred stimuli. Among the evoked potentials used clinically, **visual evoked potentials** can be elicited by having the patient view a checkerboard pattern that alternates colors, **brain stem auditory evoked potentials** can be elicited using clicking sounds, and **somatosensory evoked potentials** can be elicited using low-amplitude electrical stimuli on the extremities. Each of these techniques provides information concerning the conduction pathway of the modality activated. For example, multiple sclerosis tends to induce lesions in the visual system, often involving the optic nerves. At times, lesions that are not detectable on clinical examination can be detected through an abnormality of the visual evoked potential.

In **polysomnography,** multiple variables can be recorded during sleep, including EEG, eye movements, respirations, cardiac rate and rhythm, and muscle activity. Polysomnography has proven useful in the diagnosis of narcolepsy, sleep apnea, rapid-eye-movement behavior disorder, restless legs syndrome, and nocturnal myoclonus, among many other sleep disturbances.

Nerve Conduction Studies, Electromyography, and Muscle and Nerve Biopsy

Neurologists who specialize in peripheral nerve and muscle disorders frequently perform **nerve conduction studies and electromyography** together as a clinical diagnostic procedure to evaluate the function of peripheral nerves and muscles. **Nerve conduction studies** require the application of an electrical stimulus to the skin over a peripheral nerve while recording the electrical activity elsewhere over the nerve or in a muscle supplied by that nerve with an electrode placed on the skin surface. Nerve conduction studies permit assessment of the velocity of conduction through peripheral nerves and the amplitude of the response evoked in muscle. Demyelinating neuropathies (diseases of peripheral nerve that damage the myelin coating but leave the axons intact) usually cause conduction velocity to be slower than normal, whereas axonal neuropathies (diseases of peripheral nerve that damage the axons but leave the myelin intact) usually do not affect conduction velocity.

In **electromyography,** a neurologist inserts a needle electrode into muscle and uses an amplifier and an oscilloscope to display the electrical activity. Muscle activity can be evaluated at rest and during active contraction. Normal muscle shows no activity at rest. In denervated muscle, activity appears at rest, including **fibrillations** and **fasciculations.** Fibrillations consist of action potentials in single muscle fibers, probably occurring spontaneously as a result of denervation hypersensitivity of muscle receptor sites. Fasciculations represent action potentials involving entire motor units. Fasciculations commonly result from diseases of the anterior horn cells such as amyotrophic lateral sclerosis. During increasing muscular contraction, progressively larger numbers of motor units become recruited. In chronically denervated muscles, motor unit responses become unusually long in duration and large in amplitude, probably because with reinnervation each nerve fiber supplies an increased number of muscle fibers. In primary diseases of muscle, the responses of motor units become abnormally short in duration and small in amplitude, and the number of motor units becomes increased in relation to the force exerted.

Muscle tissue can be removed for study with a **biopsy** when the clinical evidence suggests a muscle disease. The tissue can be studied with conventional staining materials and also with special histochemical stains to detect specific biochemical abnormalities. In some diseases of peripheral nerves, biopsy of the sural nerve can be helpful diagnostically.

Anatomic Imaging Studies

Conventional x-ray studies of the head provide useful images of the skull but furnish little information about its contents. They can be helpful in detecting skull fractures and in screening for metal in the head or eyes of patients who need to be examined with magnetic resonance imaging. Most metals cannot be allowed in the same room with a magnetic resonance imaging machine, because the magnetic waves can cause rapid and large-amplitude movement of metals. Spine radiographs can be helpful in examining for a variety of conditions involving the vertebral column, including fractures, dislocations, congenital anomalies, and bone tumors, but they provide little information about the spinal cord.

X-ray computed tomography (CT) provides important diagnostic information about the brain or spinal cord. With CT, the machine passes x-rays through the patient from many different angles, and the computer determines the amount of beam attenuation at each point. The results can be displayed as cross-sectional layers through the brain, usually at an angle perpendicular to the axis of the body and spaced at 0.5- to 1.0-cm intervals. CT scans can be used to evaluate many different conditions, including subarachnoid and intracerebral hemorrhage, stroke, hydrocephalus, and brain atrophy, as well as abnormalities of the skull. CT scans can be performed both before and after intravenous infusion of a contrast agent. In regions where the blood-brain barrier has been disrupted, the contrast agent enters the brain and causes increased x-ray attenuation. Thus, contrast agent infusion increases the sensitivity of CT for detection of certain tumors and inflammatory conditions.

Magnetic resonance imaging (MRI) employs a strong magnetic field and radiofrequency (RF) waves. The magnetic field orients the spin of protons (hydrogen nuclei) parallel to the magnetic field. A brief RF current disturbs the orientation of the protons, and after the RF current stops, the protons reorient to the magnetic field and emit radio signals that can be detected. This results in an image of the anatomy of the structures under study. MRI portrays greater detail in the brain than CT and provides superior imaging for the diagnosis of certain conditions, including multiple sclerosis. MRI can also be used with and without a contrast agent to identify regions where the blood-brain barrier has been disrupted. It presents the advantage of being free of exposure to hazardous ionizing radiation, but it is more expensive and is less readily available than CT. Many newer sequence techniques such as diffusion-weighted imaging make MRI even more versatile than it was previously. MRI now appears poised to overcome CT scanning to become the procedure of choice for the diagnostic evaluation of many disorders, including the acute stroke.

Imaging the spine and spinal cord can be accomplished with MRI, CT scanning, and myelography. Currently, MRI constitutes the preferred method of imaging the vertebral column and spinal cord when clinical evidence suggests disorders of these structures. CT scanning also provides reliable information when MRI is contraindicated or is unavailable. CT scanning, coupled with myelography, presents the advantage of precisely delineating areas in the spinal cord involved by tumors, abscesses, and other mass lesions. **Myelography** consists of the injection of a small amount of an iodinated dye into the subarachnoid space by lumbar puncture or lateral cervical puncture. The patient lies on a table that can be tilted to cause the dye to move up and down the spinal canal. The dye can be visualized fluoroscopically, and permanent images can be made with conventional radiographs or CT images. Myelography can be extremely useful when the clinical problem requires additional information to supplement the results obtained by MRI or when MRI is contraindicated or is unavailable.

Imaging of the cerebral vessels can be performed with Doppler ultrasound, magnetic resonance angiography (MRA), and cerebral arteriography. **Doppler ultrasound** studies of the neck permit noninvasive imaging of the extracranial portions of the carotid arteries to detect surgically correctable stenosis (narrowing) caused by atherosclerosis. This condition occurs most commonly near the bifurcation of the common carotid artery into the internal and external carotid arteries. Transcranial Doppler ultrasound studies can be used to image the intracranial vessels as well. **MRA** provides another technique for noninvasive study of the cerebral vasculature, including both intracranial and extracranial vessels. Detection of the motion of hydrogen nuclei between the RF stimulus and the RF response permits imaging of the vessels. **Cerebral arteriography** continues to provide the optimal means of visual the cerebral vasculature. It involves injecting iodinated dye through a catheter passed from the femoral artery to the carotid and vertebral arteries while x-ray images are taken in rapid sequence. Cerebral arteriography offers better resolution and reliability than Doppler ultrasound and MRA, but it is an invasive procedure and entails a small risk of stroke. Frequently, cerebral arteriography studies are performed to confirm abnormalities of the extracranial vessels suggested by other techniques and to detect disorders of the intracranial vessels such as stenosis, aneurysms, and vasculitis.

Physiologic Imaging Studies

CT and MRI provide excellent information about brain structure, but **positron emission tomography (PET), single photon emission computed tomography (SPECT),** and **functional MRI** can provide quantitative information about brain function. For **PET,** a physicist uses a cyclotron to produce a positron (a positively charged electron)–emitting nuclide of fluorine, carbon, nitrogen, or oxygen. A radiochemist radiopharmacist then incorporates this nuclide into metabolic substrates and pharmaceuticals. The resulting radiopharmaceuticals can be injected intravenously. Decay of the radionuclides releases positrons, which react with electrons present in tissue (a matter-antimatter reaction) to produce two gamma rays. The gamma rays can be detected with a scanner that portrays the distribution of the radionuclide through the brain. Neurologists use PET most commonly to display images of local metabolic rate for glucose throughout the brain, but they can also use it to evaluate cerebral blood flow, oxygen metabolism, and neurotransmitter receptor density. Recently developed radiopharmaceuticals have made it possible to visualize and to measure quantitatively dopaminergic, cholinergic, and adrenergic neurotransmitters and neurotransmitter receptors. PET has been used also to visualize opioid and gamma-aminobutyric acid type A (benzodiazepine) neurotransmitter receptors. It has proven useful for detection of epileptic foci in the brain and for the diagnosis of degenerative conditions such as Alzheimer's disease, Parkinson's disease, multiple system atrophy, and progressive supranuclear palsy, among others. It has also been useful in elucidating neurochemical changes in many psychiatric disorders, including schizophrenia.

Activation scans permit the mapping of brain regions that develop enhanced activity during cognitive tasks, motor tasks, or sensory stimulation. In PET activation scans, injection of a blood-flow tracer during the activation permits comparisons of the resulting scan with a scan performed before activation. Brain regions participating in the neural processing appear as areas of increased blood flow.

SPECT is similar to PET in requiring the intravenous injection of a radionuclide and recording the distribution of the tracer in brain. SPECT presents the advantages of using radioactive tracers with long half-lives, so commercially available nuclides can be purchased and used. This saves the expenses associated with maintaining a cyclotron and permits even smaller hospitals to be able to use this technology. In addition, SPECT has been used effectively to evaluate cerebral blood flow, although precise measurements cannot be made. SPECT has also been used to evaluate some neurotransmitter substances, notably dopamine. SPECT has the disadvantages that the nuclide distributions cannot be measured quantitatively, it provides less detail than PET, and the available nuclides, including technetium and iodine, have less biologic interest than the nuclides available for PET.

Functional MRI uses MRI machines equipped with special software that permits visualization of changes in local cerebral blood flow without injection of radioactive substances. The technique depends on the change in magnetization that occurs when oxygenated hemoglobin becomes deoxygenated. Functional MRI has been used extensively to study brain activation and has done a great deal to elucidate the central nervous structures involved in sensory perceptual, motor planning and execution, cognitive processing, and emotional activities in the normal nervous system.

Suggested Readings

Adams, HP, Jr, et al: Ischemic Cerebrovascular Disease. Oxford University Press, New York, 2001.

Alheid, GF, et al: Basal ganglia. In Paxinos, G (ed): The Human Nervous System. Academic Press, San Diego, 1990, p 483.

Baloh, RW, and Honrubia, V: Clinical Neurophysiology of the Vestibular System, ed 3. Oxford University Press, New York, 2001.

Büttner-Ennever, JA: A review of otolith pathways to brainstem and cerebellum. Ann NY Acad Sci 871:51, 1999.

Cooper, JR, et al: Biochemical Basis of Neuropharmacology, ed 7. Oxford University Press, New York, 1996.

Darlison, MG, and Richter, D: Multiple genes for neuropeptides and their receptors: Co-evolution and physiology. Trends Neurosci 22:81, 1999.

Fuster, JM: The Prefrontal Cortex, ed 3. Lippincott–Raven, Philadelphia, 1997.

Gilman, S: Clinical Examination of the Nervous System, McGraw–Hill, New York, 1999.

Goetz, CG, and Pappert, EJ: Textbook of Clinical Neurology. WB Saunders, Philadelphia, 1999.

Gloor, P: The Temporal Lobe and Limbic System. Oxford University Press, New York, 1997.

Hardman, JG, et al: Goodman & Gilman's The Pharmacological Basis of Therapeutics, ed 9. McGraw–Hill, New York, 1996.

Hildebrand, JG, and Shepherd, GM: Mechanisms of olfactory discrimination: Converging evidence for common principles across phyla. Annu Rev Neurosci 20:595, 1997.

Kandel, ER, et al: Principles of Neural Science, ed 4. McGraw–Hill, New York, 2000.

Klockgether, T: Handbook of Ataxia Disorders. Marcel Dekker, New York, 2000.

Leigh, RJ, and Zee, DS: The Neurobiology of Eye Movements, ed 3. Oxford University Press, New York, 1999.

Mesulam, MM: Principles of Behavioral and Cognitive Neurology, ed 2. Oxford University Press, New York, 2000.

Nieuwenhuys, R, et al: The Human Central Nervous System: A Synopsis and Atlas, ed 3. Springer-Verlag, Berlin, 1988.

Nobili, R, et al: How well do we understand the cochlea? Trends Neurosci 21:159, 1998.

Parent, A: Carpenter's Human Neuroanatomy, ed 9. Williams & Wilkins, Baltimore, 1996.

Rowland, LP: Merritt's Neurology, ed 10. Lippincott Williams & Wilkins, Philadelphia, 2000.

Saper, CB: Hypothalamus. In Paxinos, G (ed): The Human Nervous System. Academic Press, San Diego, 1990, p 389.

Saper, CB: Cholinergic system. In Paxinos, G (ed): The Human Nervous System. Academic Press, San Diego, 1990, p 1095.

Shepherd, GM: The Synaptic Organization of the Brain, ed 4. Oxford University Press, New York, 1998.

Siegel, GJ, et al: Basic Neurochemistry. Lippincott Williams & Wilkins, Philadelphia, 1998.

Taylor, EW, et al: Central control of the cardiovascular and respiratory systems and their interactions in vertebrates. Physiol Rev 79:855, 1999.

Toga, AW, and Mazziota, JC: Brain Mapping: The Systems. Academic Press, San Diego, 2000.

Trobe, JD: The Neurology of Vision. Oxford University Press, New York, 2001.

Victor, M, and Ropper, AH: Adams and Victor's Principles of Neurology, ed 7. McGraw–Hill, New York, 2001.

Voogd J, et al: Mammals. In Nieuwenhuys, R, et al (eds): The Central Nervous System of Vertebrates, Vol 3. Springer-Verlag, Berlin, 1998, p 1753.

Watts RL, and Koller, WC: Movement Disorders: Neurologic Principles and Practice. McGraw–Hill, New York, 1997.

Winn, P: Frontal syndrome as a consequence of lesions in the pedunculopontine tegmental nucleus: A short theoretical review. Brain Res Bull 47:551, 1998.

Index

An "f" following a page number indicates a figure; a "t" following a page number indicates a table.

A fiber(s), 25–26, 25t
  Aα fiber, 26, 42, 52, 66f, 74f
  Aβ fiber, 26, 42, 52, 66f
  Aγ fiber, 26
  Aδ fiber, 42, 46–47, 66f, 74f
  mechanoreceptor reflexes and, 52
  pain sensation and, 42, 46–47
  temperature sense and, 47
Abdominal reflex(es), 73
Abdominal viscera
  sympathetic innervation of, 35
  vagus nerve and, 36, 100, 102
Abdominal wall muscle(s), vagal system and, 103
Abducens nerve. *See* Cranial nerve VI
Abducens nucleus, 64, 80, 84, 84f, 91f, 92, 104, 129f, 131, 169–170, 172
Abducens palsy, 105, 114
Absolute refractory period, 19
Acalculia, 188
Accessory cuneate nucleus, 53, 53f, 88–89, 89f, 140
Accessory nerve. *See* Cranial nerve XI
Accessory nucleus. *See* Spinal accessory nucleus
Accessory optic system, 173
Accommodation, 105, 163, 168–169
Acetylcholine (ACh), 4, 19, 87, 139, 154, 161, 196, 207–209, 209f
  in autonomic nervous system, 34
  in pain sensation, 42
  interneurons of the striatum and, 151, 209
  neuromuscular junction and, 21
  production of, 208
Acetylcholine cell groups, 189, 208–209, 209f
Acetylcholine receptor(s), 208
Acetylcholinesterase, 208
Acetylcoenzyme A, 208
ACh. *See* Acetylcholine
Acoustic nerve. *See* Cranial nerve VIII
Acoustic neuroma, 115, 126
Action current, 2f, 18
Action potential, 1, 2f, 16–18, 17f–18f, 20, 160
  compound, 25, 26f
  synapses and, 20
Activation scan(s), 245
Active zone, postsynaptic membrane, 19
Acuity, visual. *See* Visual acuity
Addiction, 154
Adenohypophysis. *See* Anterior pituitary
Adenoma, 165
Adenosine triphosphate (ATP), energy for sodium-potassium pump, 16
Adenyl cyclase, 210
Adie's tonic pupil, 168–169
Adipose tissue (fat), 4
Adrenal gland, sympathetic innervation of, 35
Adrenergic neuron(s). *See* Epinephrine
Adrenergic receptor(s), 212–213
Adrenocorticotropic hormone, 201, 215, 218
Affect, 143, 154, 189, 197, 202. *See also* Emotion(s)
  clinical evaluation of, 237
Affective disorder(s), 144, 188
Afferent fiber(s), 1, 4, 23, 24f. *See also* C fiber(s); General somatic afferent fiber(s); General visceral afferent fiber(s); Special somatic afferent fiber(s); Special visceral afferent fiber(s)
  of cranial nerves, 83–85
  of spinal nerves, 23, 24f
Afterpotential, 18–19, 18f
Aggressiveness, 197, 200, 206
Agnosia, 189–190, 234. *See also* *specific types*
Agraphia, 187, 192
Air conduction, of sound, 124–125
Air sinus, parasympathetic innervation of, 36
Alar plate, 14, 83
Alcoholic cerebellar degeneration, 146
Alcoholism, 69, 118, 135, 146
Alexia, 187, 192
Allergy, 235
Allocortex, 154, 175, 177, 189, 193, 199, 206
Alpha-adrenergic receptors. *See* Adrenergic receptors
Alpha motoneuron(s), 11, 28f, 29–31, 62f. *See* also Aα fiber; Anterior horn cell(s); General somatic efferent (GSE) fiber(s); Lower motoneuron(s); Motoneuron(s)
  acetylcholine and, 208
  innervation of extrafusal muscle fibers, 29
  muscle spindles and, 29
  spasticity and, 72
Alpha rhythm, 242
ALS. *See* Amyotrophic lateral sclerosis
Alternating hemiplegia. *See* Hemiplegia
Alzheimer's disease, 208, 234, 237, 245
Amacrine cell(s), retinal, 160, 160f
Amaurosis fugax, 222
Ambient cistern, 227
Amino acid neurotransmitter(s), 207, 217f, 218–219

Ammon's horn, 194
Amnesia, anterograde, 195
Ampulla, 120f, 128. *See also* Semicircular canal(s)
Ampullary crest, 128, 130
Amygdala, 64, 150f, 162f, 177, 189, 193, 194f, 195–197, 196f, 205f, 211f, 212f, 217f
  basolateral, 195–196, 208
  central nucleus of, 196, 216f
  corticomedial, 196, 204, 206, 216f
  extended, 196–197
  functions of, 100–101, 197, 202
  intra-amygdalar connections, 196
  lesions of, 197
  sexual behavior and, 201
  visceral function network and, 100–101
Amyotrophic lateral sclerosis (ALS), 75, 219, 243
Analgesia, endogenous, 49
Androgen, 201
Anemia, pernicious, 75, 206
Anesthesia
  brain stem lesions and, 115, 116f
  dorsal root irritation and, 49
  dorsal root lesions and, 73
  gamma-aminobutyric acid receptors and, 218
  trigeminal system lesions and, 110
Aneurysm, 105, 117
Angular gyrus, 5f
  lesions of, 187, 192
Anhidrosis, Horner's syndrome and, 35
Ankle reflex, 27, 32, 240
Anomia, 145, 187
Anosmia, 206
ANS. *See* Autonomic nervous system
Anterior aphasia. *See* Nonfluent aphasia
Anterior cerebral artery, 221, 222f, 223, 224f, 225, 225f
  occlusion of, 223
Anterior choroidal artery, 225f, 226
Anterior cingulate gyrus, 154, 179f
Anterior circulation, 221
Anterior cochlear nucleus. *See* Ventral cochlear nucleus
Anterior commissure, 5f, 6f, 198f, 204, 205f
Anterior communicating artery, 225, 225f
Anterior femoral cutaneous nerve, 43f
Anterior horn cell(s), 29, 70, 70f. *See also* Alpha motoneuron(s); Lower motoneuron(s); Motoneuron(s); Ventral horn cell column(s)
  trophic effect on muscle, 69–70
Anterior hypothalamus, 88, 201, 216f, 225
  anterior hypothalamic nucleus, 198f, 199
Anterior inferior cerebellar artery, 95, 95f, 225f
  occlusion of, 115
Anterior lobe of cerebellum, 53f, 54, 129f, 130, 137, 137f, 142
Anterior medullary velum, 80, 80f, 92f, 93, 137f
Anterior neuropore, 11
Anterior nuclear group, of thalamus, 177, 179f, 180, 189, 194f, 195, 200
Anterior olfactory nucleus, 204, 205f
Anterior perforated substance, 7f, 149, 149t, 154, 205, 205f, 225
Anterior pituitary, 199, 201
Anterior spinal artery, 76f, 95, 95f
  disease of, 113
  thrombosis of, 75–76, 76f
Anterior thalamic nucleus. *See* Anterior nuclear group, of thalamus
Anterolateral funiculus. *See* Anterolateral system
Anterolateral system, 11f, 42, 46, 94. *See also* Spinoreticular tract; Spinothalamic tract
  at transition from spinal cord to brain stem, 81f, 82
Antidiuretic hormone. *See* Vasopressin
Antigravity muscle(s), 130
Antipsychotic drug(s), 211
Anton's syndrome, 185–186
Aorticorenal ganglion, 35. *See also* Prevertebral ganglion
Aphasia, 174, 187, 190–192, 191f, 222, 223, 234, 237. *See also* specific types
Aphonia, 190
Apraxia, 190, 234, 238
Aqueduct. *See* Cerebral aqueduct
Arachidonic acid cascade, 42
Arachnoid, 7
Arachnoid villi, 227–228, 228f, 230
Arbor vitae, 5f, 6
Archicerebellum, 137. *See also* Flocculonodular lobe
Arcuate fiber(s). *See* Internal arcuate fiber(s)
Arcuate nucleus of hypothalamus, 197, 198f, 199, 201–202, 210, 216f
Area postrema, 103, 230
Argyll Robertson pupil, 169
Arousal, 86–87, 154, 199, 208–209, 213
Arteriosclerosis, 39
Artery(ies). *See* Blood supply; Cerebral arteries
Ascending reticular activating system, 86–87, 91, 182, 208–209
Aspartate. *See* Glutamate/aspartate
Aspastic paralysis, 113
Association area(s), of cerebral cortex, 175. *See also* Cerebral cortex, heteromodal association areas of; Cerebral cortex, unimodal association areas of
Association fiber(s), of cerebral cortex, 175
Associative memory, 197
Astereognosis, 58
Astrocyte(s), 3, 202, 229
Asynergia. *See* Cerebellar ataxia
Ataxia, 77, 96, 239. *See also* specific types
  brain stem lesions and, 111, 113 115, 117
  cerebellar disease and,
    expanded triplet repeats, 145
    Friedreich's ataxia, 145–146
    spinocerebellar ataxia, 145
    sporadic olivopontocerebellar atrophy, 146
Athetosis, 155–157, 240
Atonic bladder, 38
ATP. *See* Adenosine triphosphate

Atrophy
brain, 244
muscle, 21, 69, 75, 97
Atropine, pupillary reaction to, 169
Attention, 174, 177, 193, 208
evaluation of, 236
Audiofrequency analyzer, 122
Audiometer, 125
Audiomotor reflex, 125
Auditory agnosia, 190
Auditory association area of cerebral cortex, 175, 179f, 185
lesions of, 185
Auditory cortex, processing in, 122–124, 179f. *See also* Primary auditory cortex; Transverse temporal gyri
Auditory evoked potential(s), 125, 185, 243
Auditory nerve. *See* Cranial nerve VIII
Auditory pathways, 122–124, 123f
binaural, 122
monaural, 122
Auditory radiation, 122
Auditory reflex(es), 125
auditory-oculogyric, 125
auditory-palpebral, 125
Auditory tube, sensory innervation of, 100
Auricle, 119–121, 120f
facial nerve and, 106
sensory innervation of
auricular branch of X, 101
spinal nucleus of V, 99
superior ganglion of IX, 101
superior ganglion of X, 101
Auricular branch, of vagus nerve, 101
Automatic bladder, 38
Autonomic nervous system (ANS), 33–39, 193
amygdala regulation of, 196
corticoreticular and reticulospinal tract, control of, 65
divisions of, 33–34
ganglia, 35, 208. *See also* Chain ganglia; Paravertebral ganglia; Prevertebral ganglia; Terminal ganglia
hypothalamic control of, 199-200
innervation of genitourinary tract, 36–38, 37f
neurotransmitters of, 34
parasympathetic division of, 34, 36
reflexes mediated by, 38
sympathetic division of, 34–36
Autoreceptor(s), 20, 210, 211
Axillary nerve, 43f, 44f
Axon(s), 1, 2f
Axon cylinder. *See* Axon(s)
Axon sprouting, 68–69
Axonal neuropathy, 243

B fiber(s), 25, 25t, 34
Babinski sign (extensor plantar response), 70, 72–73, 75, 113-116, 146, 182, 240
Balance, 127, 128, 142. *See also* Posture
Balint's syndrome, 188
Ballism, 155–156
Barbiturate(s), 218
Baroreceptor(s), 100, 102
Basal ganglia, 147–157
blood supply, 224f, 226
cognition and, 147, 155
connections of pallidum with brain stem, 154
connections with cerebral cortex, 150–154, 182,184
connections with midline and intralaminar thalamic nuclei, 181–182
control of gamma motoneurons, 30
degeneration of, 145
diseases of, 31, 155–157
functions of, 147
lesions of, 145, 171
motor function and, 147, 155, 182, 184
physiologic properties of neurons, 155
rigidity and, 31
structure of, 148–149, 148f, 149f
ventral striatum and pallidum, 154, 181. *See also* Ventral pallidum; Ventral striatum
Basal ganglia loop(s), 147, 151–152
direct loop, 151-152, 151f, 153f
indirect loop, 152f, 153, 153f
modulation of function of cerebral cortex, 147, 152–153
Basal nucleus of Meynert, 87, 154, 189, 199, 208, 209f
Basal plate, 14
Basal sulcus, 78f, 80
Basilar artery, 95, 95f, 222f, 223, 225, 225f. *See also* Basal sulcus
aneurysm of, 117
occlusion of, 117–118
Basilar membrane, 120f, 121–122
Basket cell(s), of cerebellum, 137, 139
Basolateral amygdala, 195–196, 208, 209f. *See also* Amygdala
Bed nucleus of the stria terminalis, 196, 216f
Behavior. *See also* specific types
homeostatic, 193, 200
planning complex behavior, 174
Bell's palsy, 107, 110
Benedikt's syndrome, 117
Benign intracranial hypertension. *See* Idiopathic intracranial hypertension
Benzodiazepine(s), 218
Beta activity, electroencephalography, 242
Beta-adrenergic receptors. *See* Adrenergic receptors
Beta motoneuron(s), 11, 29–30
acetylcholine and, 208
innervation of intrafusal muscle fibers, 29–30
muscle spindles and, 29
Beta-endorphin, 215, 216f. *See also* Endorphin(s)
Betz cell(s), 61, 63
Biceps reflex, 240
Binaural central auditory pathway, 122
Biogenic amine(s). *See* Monoamine(s)
Biopsy
muscle, 243
nerve, 243
Bipolar cell(s), retinal, 160–161, 160f
Bipolar neuron(s), of olfactory epithelium, 204
Bitemporal hemianopia, 165–166
Bladder. *See* Urinary bladder
Blind spot, 164
Blindness, 165, 222. *See also* Cortical blindness
Blood clot. *See* Thrombosis
Blood pressure, 102, 202, 213. *See also* Hypertension

Blood supply
brain stem, 95, 95f
cerebellum, 95, 95f
forebrain, 221–226, 222f, 224f, 225f
imaging studies of, 244–245
spinal cord, 75-76, 76f
Blood-brain barrier, 229
Blood-cerebrospinal fluid barrier, 229
Blood vessels, sympathetic innervation of, 34
Blurred vision, 173
Body image disturbance, 190
Body position, 41
Body temperature, 201, 213. *See also* Thermoregulation
Body weight, 201–202
Bone conduction, of sound, 124–125
Bony labyrinth, 120f, 121, 127
Botulinum toxin, 21, 157
Bowel function, spinal cord transection and, 73
Brachia conjunctiva. *See* Superior cerebellar peduncle
Brachia pontis. *See* Middle cerebellar peduncle
Brachioradialis reflex, 240
Brachium, 3
of inferior colliculus, 80f, 94f, 122, 123f
of superior colliculus, 80f
Bradykinesia, 155
Bradykinin, 42
Brain
atrophy of, 244
development of, 11–14, 13f
lateral view of, 5f
midsagittal section of, 5f, 6f
ventral surface of, 7f
vesicles of, 12–13, 13f
weight of, 4
Brain edema, 69; 229
Brain stem, 4. *See also* Cerebellopontine angle; Medulla oblongata; Midbrain; Pons
amygdala and, 196
anatomy of, 5f, 6
dorsal surface, 80f, 84f
internal, 82–94
lateral surface, 79f
surface, 77–82
transverse section(s), 88–94, 88f–94f
ventral surface, 78f
connections with pallidum, 154
cranial nerves of, 83–86
descending fibers influencing motor activity, 61–66
development of, 14, 83
habenula and, 203
hypothalamus and, 199–200
lesions of, 72, 111–118, 133
coma and, 112, 118
localization of, 111–112, 233–234
locked-in syndrome and, 118
medulla, 112–114, 112f
midbrain, 116–118, 117f
pons, 114–116, 114f, 116f
transection of, 131
transition to spinal cord, 81f, 82–83
tumor of, 112, 230
Brain stem auditory evoked potential(s), 125, 243
Branchiomeric muscle(s), 61, 83, 85, 90, 92, 97, 99, 106, 107
Bridged junction, 19
Broca's aphasia. *See* Nonfluent aphasia
Broca's area, 183, 191, 191f
lesions of, 174, 191–192
Brodmann's area(s), 175, 176f, 182–191.
area 1, 150, 184
area 2, 150, 184, 186
area 3, 150, 184, 186
area 4, 143, 150, 182
area 6, 150, 152, 169, 182, 183
area 8, 169, 182, 188
area 17, 162f, 163, 170f, 185–186
area 18, 162f, 163, 170f, 185–186
area 19, 162f, 163, 170f
area 22, 185–186, 187, 190, 191
area 41, 122
area 42, 122
area 43, 100, 186
Bronchial branch, of vagus nerve, 102
Bronchi
parasympathetic innervation of, 99
sensory innervation of, 100
Brown-Séquard syndrome, 73–76, 74f, 76
Buccinator muscle, 106
Bulbar nerve(s). *See* Cranial nerve(s)
Bulbocavernosus
muscle, 38
reflex, 38
Bulk flow, cerebrospinal fluid, 228

C fiber(s), 25–26, 25t, 34
drC fiber, 26, 42, 66f, 74f
pain perception and, 42, 46–47
sC fiber, 26
temperature sense and, 47
Calcarine artery, 222f, 223
Calcarine fissure, 5f, 159f, 162f, 163, 185
Calcitonin gene-related peptide, 46
Calcium, synaptic transmission and, 20
Calcium channel(s), 20, 208
blocker(s), 20
Calculations, testing ability to do, 236
Callosomarginal artery, 222f, 223
Caloric test, of nystagmus, 132, 238
Capacitance, 16
Capillary endothelium, 228
Carbidopa, 156–157
Cardiac branch, of vagus nerve, 102
Cardiac muscle, 4
autonomic nervous system and, 33
cranial nerve XI innervation of, 36
parasympathetic innervation of, cranial nerve X, 36, 99, 102
reflex regulation, 102
sensory innervation of, cranial nerve X, 100, 102
spinal nerves and, 25
sympathetic innervation of, 35
Cardiac nerve(s) of the cervical sympathetic ganglia, 35, 102
Cardiac plexus, 35, 102
Cardiovascular regulation, 35
Carotid artery, 221, 244
Carotid body, 100–102
Carotid body reflex, 102
Carotid branch, of glossopharyngeal nerve, 101
Carotid plexus, 35
Carotid sinus, 100–102
Carotid sinus reflex, 99, 102

Catecholamine(s). *See* Dopamine; Epinephrine; Norepinephrine
Catechol-*O*-methyl transferase, 210
Cauda equina, 8f, 9
  lesions of, 38
Caudal orbitofrontal cortex. *See* Orbitofrontal cortex
Caudate nucleus, 80f, 148f–150f, 149–150, 149t, 151f, 152f, 153, 169, 179f, 180f, 182, 196f, 211f, 214f, 218
  body of, 149
  excitatory input from isocortex, 150, 151f
  head of, 148f, 149, 149f, 169, 170f, 180f, 188, 189
  tail of, 149, 180f
Cavernosus sinus, 104, 105
Celiac ganglion, 35. *See also* Prevertebral ganglion
Cell body(ies), neuronal, 1, 2f. *See also* Neuron(s)
Cell column
  brain stem, 84, 84f
  spinal cord, 9–11
Cell death, synaptic contacts and, 14
Cell layers
  cerebellum, 137
  cerebral cortex, 174
Cell migration, in development, 14
Cellular edema, 229
Central artery(ies), of circle of Willis, 225
  anterior lateral group of, 226
  anterior medial group of, 225
  posterior lateral group of, 226
  posterior medial group of, 225–226
Central canal, 5f, 9f, 77, 82, 88, 88f
Central nervous system (CNS), 3
Central nucleus, of amygdala, 196. *See also* Amygdala
Central pain, 49–50, 224
Central pontine myelinolysis, 118
Central scotoma, 165
Central sulcus of Rolando, 4, 5f, 6f
Central tegmental tract, 91, 91f, 93f, 109, 143, 212
Cephalic flexure, 13f
Centromedian thalamic nucleus, 151, 181–182
Cerebellar ataxia, brain stem lesions and, 113, 115
Cerebellar cortex, 3, 6, 135–140, 138f, 140f, 217f
  afferents to, 132, 141–142
    aminergic, 138–139, 212f, 214f
    cholinergic, 209f
    glutamatergic, 217f
    serotonergic, 214f
  basket cells of, 137, 138f, 139
  cell layers of, 137, 138, 138f
  climbing fibers of, 138, 138f, 139
  Golgi II cells of, 137, 138f, 139
  glomerulus(i) of, 137, 138f
  granule cells of, 137, 138, 138f, 139
  information processing in, 139–140
  mossy fibers of, 138, 138f, 139
  parallel fibers of, 137, 138f, 139
  patterns of excitation in, 139
  Purkinje cells of, 137, 138, 138f, 139
  somatotopic organization of, 145
  stellate cells of, 137, 138f, 139
  synaptic organization of, 138–139
Cerebellar nuclei. *See* Deep cerebellar nuclei
Cerebellar peduncle(s), 79f, 80f, 135, 136f 139–141, 140f. *See also* Inferior cerebellar peduncle; Middle cerebellar peduncle; Superior cerebellar peduncle
Cerebellar tonsils, 137
  herniation of, 137, 241
Cerebellar tremor, 225, 240
Cerebellar vermis. *See* Cerebellum, vermal zone of
Cerebellopontine angle, 80, 106, 107
  lesions at, 114, 115, 126
Cerebellum, 4, 135–147. *See also* Anterior lobe of cerebellum; Deep cerebellar nuclei; Flocculonodular lobe; Posterior lobe of cerebellum
  anatomy of, 5f, 6, 7f, 135–140, 136f, 137f
  arbor vitae of, 5f, 6
  cerebro-olivocerebellar pathway, 142
  cerebroreticulocerebellar pathway, 142
  control of gamma motoneurons, 30
  development of, 12
  diseases of, 31, 133, 144–146, 171
  dysfunction of,
    lateral zone dysfunction, 144–145
    midline zone dysfunction, 144
  function(s) of, 135, 139, 143–144, 182
  hemispheres of, 136, 142–144
  lobes of, 135–137, 136f. *See also* Anterior lobe of cerebellum; Flocculonodular lobe; Posterior lobe of cerebellum
  lobules I – X of, 136f, 137
  longitudinal sagittal zonal patterns of, 136f, 137, 142
  pathways from lower limb to, 52–53, 53f
  pathways from upper limb to, 53–54, 53f
  posterolateral fissure of, 136, 137f
  primary fissure of, 137, 137f
  tumor of, 230
  vision and, 161
  zones of, 136f, 137
    lateral, 143, 144–145
    intermediate (paravermal), 54, 136, 142–143
    vermal, 54, 136, 142, 144
Cerebral aqueduct, 6f, 82, 93f, 94f, 162f, 186f, 227, 228f, 230
Cerebral arteriography, 244–245
Cerebral artery(ies), 221–226
  occlusion of, 221
Cerebral cortex, 3–4, 5f, 174–192
  allocortex, 154, 175, 177, 189, 193, 199. *See also* Limbic lobe
  cell layers of, 174, 175, 177. *See also* Isocortex
  column(s) of. *See* Cortical column
  connections with basal ganglia, 150–154

Cerebral cortex *(Continued)*
connections with cerebellum, 141–142
corticoid areas. *See* Corticoid area(s)
descending fibers influencing motor activity, 61–66
development of, 14
disorders of cortical networks, 189–192
functional regions of, 175, 177, 182–189
heteromodal association areas of, 175–177, 178f, 187–189, 195
hypothalamus and, 202
information processing in, 177, 178f
isocortex, 175–177, 199. *See* Isocortex
limbic areas of. *See* Limbic lobe
mesocortex, 175, 177
motor areas of, 60–61, 182–184, 183f
networks of, 177
in movement and cognition, 143–144
paralimbic areas of, 189
pathways of, 54–57, 55f–56f
relationships of cortical areas, 174–177, 176f
sensory areas of, 184–186
thalamocortical connections, 180
unimodal association areas of, 175, 177, 178f, 182–186
vestibular areas of, 186–187
Cerebral dominance. *See* Lateralization of function of cerebral cortex
Cerebral hemisphere(s), 5f
development of, 12
dominant, 190–191
lobes of, 4–6
Cerebral palsy, 157, 239–240
Cerebral peduncle(s), 7f, 62f, 82, 93–94, 162f
ischemic infarction of, 118
lesions of, 116, 117f
Cerebral vessels, 221–226
imaging of, 244
Cerebrospinal fluid (CSF), 6–7, 227–231
analysis of, 241–242
blood-cerebrospinal fluid barrier, 229
cellular content of, 242
circulation of, 79, 227–228, 228f
color of, 242
composition of, 228–229
formation of, 7, 227–228
function of, 228–229
glucose and protein in, 242
intracranial pressure and, 229–231
volume of, 227
Cerebrospinal fluid rhinorrhea, 206
Cerebrovascular disease, 67, 96. *See also* Stroke
Cerebrum. *See* Cerebral *entries*
Cervical chain ganglia, 35
Cervical flexure, 13f
Cervical spinal cord, 7, 10f
Cervical spinal nerve(s), 7, 34
Cervicothoracic ganglion, 34
Chain ganglia, 24f, 34. *See also* Sympathetic trunk
Check and rebound, impaired, 145
Chemical synapse, 19, 207–219
Chemoreceptors
stimuli for, 42
in carotid body, 100, 102
pain and, 42
Chiasmatic cistern, 227
Chickenpox, 50
Chief complaint, 234
Chloride
resting membrane potential and, 15–16
synaptic transmission and, 20
Chloride channel(s), 20, 208, 218
Cholecystokinin, 20, 202, 215, 218
Choline, 208
Choline acetyltransferase, 208–209
Cholinergic neuron(s). *See* Acetylcholine
Cholinergic receptor(s), 208
Cholinergic terminal(s), 34
Chorda tympani nerve, 100–101
Chordoma, 103
Chorea, 155–157, 240
Choreic movement(s), brain stem lesions and, 117
Choroid plexus, 7, 78, 227, 228f
Chromaffin cell(s), 35
Chromatolysis, 68
Cilia, of olfactory receptors. *See* Olfactory cilia
Ciliary ganglion, 36, 159f, 161, 167-168
lesions of, 167–169
preganglionic parasympathetic fibers to, 105
Ciliary muscle(s), 36, 105, 161, 168
Cingulate gyrus, 5f, 6, 6f, 47, 149f, 177, 179f, 189, 193, 211f, 212f
Cingulate sulcus, 5f
Cingulotomy, 47
Circadian rhythm, 161, 199, 203
Circle of Willis, 105, 221, 225–226, 225f
Circumferential arteries, 95f
Cisterna magna, 227, 228f, 242
Cisternal puncture, 242
Clarke's nucleus. *See* Nucleus dorsalis
Clasp-knife phenomenon, 31, 72, 113, 239
Claustrum, 148f
Clava, 78–79, 80f
Climbing fiber(s), 138–139
Clinical evaluation, 233–245
Clivus, tumor of, 103
Clonus, 70, 72–73
Cluneal nerves, 44f
CNS. *See* Central nervous system
Coactivation, 30
Cocaine, pupillary reaction to, 169
Coccygeal spinal cord, 7
Coccygeal spinal nerve, 7
Cochlea, 120f, 121
bilateral representation in each temporal lobe, 123f, 124
damage to, 124
Cochlear duct. *See* Scala media
Cochlear nerve. *See* Cranial nerve VIII
Cochlear nucleus(i), 122
Cochleopupillary reflex, 125
Cognition, 174
basal ganglia and, 147, 152, 155
cognitive maps, 195
deficits with lesions, 177
heteromodal association areas and, 187, 188
integration of cerebellum and cerebral cortex in, 135, 143–144
Cogwheel phenomenon, 31, 156, 239. *See also* Basal ganglia, lesions of; Rigidity

Collateral sulcus, 205f
Collateral ganglion. *See* Prevertebral ganglion
Colliculus. *See* Facial colliculus; Inferior colliculus; Superior colliculus
Color vision, 158, 161, 164–165, 186
Column of cerebral cortex. *See* Cortical column(s)
Column of fibers, 3. *See also* Dorsal column(s)
Coma, 236, 241, 242
  brain stem lesions and, 112, 118
  oculocephalic response in, 172
Combined systems disease. *See* Subacute degeneration of the spinal cord
Common carotid artery, 221
Common cold, 206
Communicating arteries, 221
  anterior, 225
  posterior, 225
Communicating hydrocephalus, 230
Comportment, 177, 193
Compound action potential, 25, 26f
Comprehension, 189
  testing of, 237
Computed tomography (CT), 231, 234, 244
Conductance, 16, 17f
Conduction aphasia, 188, 192
Conduction velocity, of action potential, 18, 25, 25t
Conductive deafness, 124
  diagnosis of, 124–125
Cones, 158–161, 160f, 167
  hyperpolarization by light, 158–160
  influence on ganglion cells through bipolar cells, 160–161, 160f
Confluent sinus, 228f
Confrontation method, testing visual fields, 164
Confusional state, 236
Conjugate eye movement(s). *See* Eye movement(s)
Consciousness, state of, 236, 242
Consensual corneal reflex, 110
Consensual light reflex, 167–168
Constructional ability, evaluation of, 237
Constructional apraxia, 187–188
Contrast, in visual processing, 161, 163
Conus medullaris, 7, 8f
  lesions of causing urinary incontinence, 38
Convergence of the eyes, 118, 163, 168, 169, 173, 238. *See also* Vergence
Convergence of somatosensory information, 57
Conversion disorder, 165, 206, 224
Coordination, 135, 142, 143, 145
  assessment of, 239–240
Cornea, 158, 159f
  pain sensation from, 109
Corneal reflex, 106, 110
  consensual, 110
  direct, 110
  loss of, 104, 113, 115–116
  testing of, 238
Corona radiata, 79f–80f, 180
Coronary heart disease, pain of, 48
Corpora arenacea, 203
Corpora quadrigemina, 82. *See also* Inferior colliculus; Superior colliculus; Tectum
Corpus callosum, 4, 5f, 6f, 149f, 151f, 152f, 175, 179f, 180f, 190, 223.
  development of, 14
  lesions of, 190
Cortical blindness, 167, 185, 223–224
Cortical column(s)
  of isocortex, 175
  of somatosensory cortex, 58
  of visual cortex, 164
Cortical deafness, 185
Corticobulbar tract, 62f, 63, 78, 88, 88f–94f, 93, 148, 180f, 181, 182
  lesions of, 31, 67, 70, 75, 116, 118
  motor activity and, 63, 182
Corticoid area(s), 175, 177, 189, 193
Corticomedial amygdala, 196, 204, 206. *See also* Amygdala
Corticomesencephalic tract. *See* Corticotectal tract
Corticopontine fiber(s), 92–93, 93f, 94f, 141f, 142, 172, 180f, 184, 217f
Corticopontocerebellar pathway, 142. *See also* Corticopontine fibers
Corticoreticular tract, 64–65
Corticorubral tract, 64
Corticospinal tract, 28f, 29, 61, 62f, 66f, 78, 82, 88, 88f-94f, 90, 92–93, 111, 141f, 143, 148, 180f, 181, 182, 184, 217f. *See also* Pyramid
  control of urination and, 37f, 38
  decussation of, 81f, 88, 88f. *See also* Decussation of the pyramids
  degeneration of, 59, 146
  lesions of, 31, 67, 70–73, 71f, 75, 112-113, 113f, 114, 114f, 115, 116f, 117f, 118, 145
  motor activity and, 61–63, 182, 184
  at transition from spinal cord to brain stem, 81f, 82, 88f
Corticosteroid(s), for spinal cord injury, 74–75
Corticotectal tract
  extraocular motor activity and, 63–64
  lesions of, 116
Corticothalamic projection(s), 174, 178, 182, 217f
Corticotropin-releasing hormone, 202, 218
Cough reflex, 103
Cranial division, of parasympathetic nervous system, 36
Cranial nerve(s), 3–4. *See also* specific nerves
  afferent fibers of, 83
  classification by function, 83
  disorders of, 71f
  efferent fibers of, 83–84
  functional components of, 84–86
  hypothalamus and, 199
  of medulla, 97–103
  of midbrain, 104–110
  neurologic examination and, 238
  nuclei of, 83, 84f, 85f
    classification by function, 83
    relation to alar plate and basal plate, 83
  organization of, 77–96
  of pons, 104–110

Cranial nerve I (olfactory nerve), 204
examination of, 238
Cranial nerve II (optic nerve), 7f, 78f, 79f, 82, 149f, 159f, 161–163, 198f
examination of, 238
lesions of, 165, 167–168, 173
swelling of, 229
head of, 161
Cranial nerve III (oculomotor nerve), 5f, 7f, 78f, 79f, 82, 84, 94, 94f, 129f, 131, 159f 167. *See also* Ciliary ganglion; Edinger Westphal nucleus
corticobulbar influence on, 63
course of, 94, 105
examination of, 238
functional components of, 84–85
lesions of, 61f, 105, 106, 116–117, 117f, 118, 167
oculomotor nucleus of. *See* Oculomotor nuclear complex
pursuit movements and, 172. *See also* Pursuit eye movements
saccades and, 169–170. *See also* Saccade(s)
vergence and, 173. *See also* Vergence eye movements
Cranial nerve IV (trochlear nerve), 7f, 78f, 79f, 80f, 82, 84, 105, 131
corticobulbar influence on, 63
course of, 105
examination of, 238
functional components of, 84–85
lesions of, 105
nucleus of, 94, 105. *See also* Trochlear nucleus
Cranial nerve V (trigeminal nerve), 7f, 46, 78f, 79f, 80f, 90, 93. *See also* Mandibular nerve; Maxillary nerve; Mesencephalic nucleus of; Ophthalmic nerve; Principal sensory nucleus of; Spinal nucleus of; Spinal tract of; Trigeminal ganglion
auditory reflexes and, 125
corneal blink reflex, 110
corticobulbar tract control of, 63
examination of, 108-109, 238
functional components of, 84–86
lesions of, 95–96, 110, 115, 116f
mesencephalic nucleus of, 93, 108–109, 108f
motor division of, 107–109, 108f
motor nucleus of, 62f, 63, 85–86, 93, 107, 108f
pathway to cerebral cortex, 108f, 109–110
pons and, 107–110
principal sensory nucleus of, 84f, 92-93, 108f, 109
root of, 92f
sensory division of, 108f, 109
spinal nucleus of, 45f, 47, 84f, 88f, 89-90, 88f–91f, 95, 99, 108f, 109, 110, 216f, 217f
spinal tract of, 45f, 46–47, 88f–91f, 89-90, 95, 101, 108f, 109, 110, 112f, 113
Cranial nerve VI (abducens nerve), 7f, 78f, 79f, 80, 84, 91f, 92,104-105, 129f, 131
corticobulbar influence on, 63
course of, 91f, 92, 104
examination of, 238
functional components of, 83–85
lesions of, 104–105, 114
nucleus of, 63, 104
paralysis and, 105
pursuit movements and, 172
saccades and, 169
vergence and, 173
Cranial nerve VII (facial nerve), 7f, 78f, 79f, 80, 90, 106-107, 110. *See also* Geniculate ganglion; Nervus intermedius; Pterygopalatine ganglion; Submandibular ganglion; Vagal system
auditory reflexes and, 125
corticobulbar tract control of, 63
damage to, 107
course and distribution of, 91-92, 91f, 106
examination of, 238
functional components of, 84–86, 106
internal genu of, 91–92, 91f
lesions of, 106–107, 110, 114-115
motor nucleus of, 63, 91, 91f, 106. *See also* Facial nucleus
nervus intermedius of, 98-103, 98f, 106
pons and, 106–107
Cranial nerve VIII (vestibulocochlear nerve), 7f, 78f, 79f, 80, 129–130, 129f, 140. *See also* Spiral ganglion; Vestibular ganglion
cochlear division of, 119, 121-122, 123f
deafness and, 124
examination of, 132, 238
functional components of, 84–86
lesions of, 124–126, 132–133
surgical section of, 133
tumor of, 115, 126
vestibular division of, 89, 119, 128
Cranial nerve IX (glossopharyngeal nerve), 7f, 78, 78f, 79f, 90, 98f. *See also* Otic ganglion; Vagal system
corticobulbar tract, control of, 63
course and distribution of, 101
examination of, 238
functional components of, 84–86
inferior ganglion of, 101
general visceral sensory function of, 100
taste (special visceral sensory) function of, 100
reflexes of, 102, 103
superior ganglion of, 101
vagal system and, 98-103, 98f
Cranial nerve X (vagus nerve), 7f, 36,78f, 79f, 90, 90f, 199. *See also* Terminal ganglia; Vagal system
corticobulbar control of, 63
course and distribution of, 101–102
dorsal motor nucleus of, 79, 84f, 85, 85f, 89, 98–99, 102

examination of, 238
functional components of, 84–86
inferior (nodose) ganglion of, 101
general visceral sensory function of, 100
taste (special visceral sensory) function of, 100
lesions of, 99, 112f
reflexes of, 102, 103
superior (jugular) ganglion of, 101
vagal system and, 98-103, 98f
Cranial nerve XI (accessory nerve), 36, 102. *See also* Vagal system
corticobulbar tract control of, 63
cranial portion of, 78, 78f, 79f, 83, 90, 97–103, 98f
external nucleus of the nucleus ambiguus and, 99
examination of, 238
functional components of, 84–85
spinal portion of, 7f, 78, 78f, 79f, 83, 97, 98f
Cranial nerve XII (hypoglossal nerve), 7f, 78, 78f, 79f
corticobulbar tract control of, 63
examination of, 238
functional components of, 84–85
lesions of, 97, 103, 112, 112f
nucleus of, 62f, 63, 79, 84, 84f, 85f, 89, 89f, 90f
rootlets of, 78, 78f, 90f, 97
Craniopharyngioma, 165
Cremasteric reflex, 73
Cribriform plate, 204
fracture of, 206
Cricothyroid muscle(s), 102
Crista ampullaris. *See* Ampullary crest
Crossed extensor reflex, 27, 31
Crus cerebri. *See* Cerebral peduncle(s)
CSF. *See* Cerebrospinal fluid
CT. *See* Computed tomography
Cuneate tubercle, 79, 80f
Cuneocerebellar tract, 52–54, 53f, 89, 138, 140, 142
Cuneus, 5f, 159f, 162f, 163, 165, 185
Cupula, 128
Cutaneous nerves
branches of peripheral nerves, 42
patern of distribution to body surface, 43f, 44f
Cutaneous reflexes, 31
Cyanosis, 39
Cyclic AMP, 218
Cystometry, 38
Cytotoxic edema, 229

Deafness, 115, 124, 133, 185. *See also* Hearing loss; Conductive deafness; Sensorineural deafness
Decerebrate rigidity, 131
Decibel, 119
Declarative memory, 195, 197
Decussation
of the pyramids, 62f, 63, 71f, 78, 78f, 81f, 82, 88, 88f. *See also* Corticospinal tracts
of the spinal (medial) lemniscus, 54, 82, 88, 89f. *See also* Internal arcuate fibers
Deep cerebellar nuclei, 92, 135, 137, 138-139, 209f, 217f
efferents of, 139, 142–143, 143f
in thalamic fasciculus, 151
Deep pain, 47
Deep peroneal nerve, 43f
Deep tendon reflex(es), 27, 30, 32, 52,113-115, 240. *See also* Stretch reflex
absence of, 59, 69-70, 168
decreased, 70
increased, 72
Defecation reflex, 38
Degeneration
of nerve cells and fibers, 68–69
wallerian, 68
Delirium, 236
Delta activity, electroencephalography, 242
Delta opioid receptor(s), 215
Dementia, 156, 208, 230. *See also* Alzheimer's disease
Demyelinating diseases, 234, 243. *See also* Multiple sclerosis
Dendrite(s), 1, 2f
Denervation
of striated muscle, 21
supersensitivity, 168
Dentate gyrus, 194–195, 194f, 216f
Dentate nucleus, 92, 135, 137, 140f–141f, 141–145
Denticulate ligament, 7
Depolarization, 15–16, 17f, 19–20
Depression, 156, 213
Depth perception, 186
Dermatome(s)
pain and, 42, 50
sympathetic innervation of, 34
Dermatomyositis, 39
Descending vestibular nucleus, 129f, 130
Detrusor muscle, 36–38, 37f
Diabetes mellitus, 36, 67, 69, 106, 111, 133, 169, 229
Diagnostic test(s), 241–245
Diagonal band of Broca, 189, 208, 209f
Dichotic listening task(s), 185
Diencephalon, 4, 177, 197
development of, 12
Differential diagnosis, 233–234
Digastric muscle
anterior belly, 107
posterior belly, 106
Dilation of the pupil. *See* Mydriasis
Diplopia, 105–106, 168
Direct corneal reflex, 110
Direct light reflex, 167–168
Direct loop of basal ganglia, 151–154, 151f
Direct optokinetic pathway, 173
Disinhibition, 152
of thalamocortical neurons, 152, 156–157
Dissociated sensory loss, 112
Distal feedback inhibition. *See* Inhibition, distal feedback
Divergence of the eyes, 169, 173. *See also* Vergence
Divergence of somatosensory information, 57
Dizziness, 133
Doll's eye test, 172
Doll's head test, 172
Dominance. *See* Hemispheric dominance
Dopamine, 19, 153–154, 161, 201, 209–211, 211f
analgesia and, 49
depletion of, 155–156

Dopamine *(Continued)*
nigrostriatal connections and, 153-154
synthesis of, 210
Dopamine beta-hydroxylase, 210
Dopamine receptor(s), 153-154, 153f, 210
in Parkinson's disease, 155
Dopaminergic cell group(s), 87, 210–211, 211f
Dopaminergic fiber(s), 87, 138–139
Doppler ultrasound, 244
Dorsal acoustic stria, 122, 123f
Dorsal cochlear nucleus, 122, 123f
Dorsal column(s), 82
lesions of, 58
Dorsal column nuclei, 54. *See also* Spinal lemniscal system
Dorsal column pathway(s), 54. *See also* Spinal lemniscal system
lesions of, 58, 59, 59f, 75
Dorsal funiculus, 9, 10f
lesions of, 75
Dorsal horn(s), 9, 10f, 24f, 216f
Dorsal intermediate sulcus, 10, 80f
Dorsal longitudinal fasciculus, 200, 212
Dorsal median sulcus, 9, 10f, 80f
Dorsal motor nucleus, of X, 79, 84f, 85, 85f, 89, 89f, 90f, 98, 98f, 99, 102, 112f, 199. *See also* Cranial nerve X
Dorsal pallidum, 149, 149t
Dorsal root(s), 7, 10f, 24f
irritation of, 49, 50
lesions of, 69–70, 70f, 73
pain and, 42–46
pattern of innervation of dermatomes, 42, 43f–44f
radicular pain, 49
Dorsal root entry zone, 9, 42
Dorsal root ganglia, 7, 23, 24f, 42, 45f, 217, 217f
degeneration of, 59
herpes zoster and, 50
Dorsal spinocerebellar tract, 11f, 52, 53f, 54, 88f, 89f, 138, 140, 140f
Dorsal striatum, 148f, 149–150, 149f–150f, 149t, 216f, 217f, 218
connections with cerebral cortex, 150–154
excitatory input from isocortex, 150, 151f
inhibition of substantia nigra reticulata and globus pallidus, 150
Dorsal tegmental decussation, 64, 94, 94f
Dorsal tegmentum, 213
Dorsal trigeminothalamic tract, 109
Dorsolateral fasciculus, 49
Dorsolateral pathway, 54, 59f
Dorsolateral pontine nuclei, 171f, 172
Dorsolateral prefrontal cortex, 152, 179f
Dorsolateral sulcus, 9, 78, 79f, 80f
Dorsomedial hypothalamic nucleus, 198f, 199, 202
Dorsomedial thalamic nucleus. *See* Mediodorsal thalamic nucleus
Double athetosis, 157
Double vision. *See* Diplopia
Dreaming, 209
Dressing apraxia, 188
Drinking behavior, 200
Drug(s)
effect on synaptic transmission, 20
entry into central nervous system, 228
hearing loss and, 124–125
intracranial pressure and, 230
Dura mater, 7
sensory innervation of, 107, 109
Dural sac, 8f
Dural venous sinus, 227
thrombosis of, 230
Dynorphin, 49, 215
Dysarthria, 144–145, 190, 237
Dysdiadochokinesis, 144
Dysexecutive syndrome, 189
Dyskinesia, 156
Dysmetria, 144–145, 170
Dysphagia, 99, 114
Dysphonia, 99, 113
Dysprosody, 145
Dysrhythmokinesis, 144
Dyssynergia. *See* Cerebellar ataxia
Dystonia, 155, 157
botulinum treatment and, 21
musculorum deformans, 157, 239
Dystonic rigidity, 239
Ear, 119–126, 120f. *See also* Auditory entries; Hearing
Eating behavior, 199-202
Ectodermal placode(s), 12
nasal placode, 12
otic placode, 12
Edema, 69, 229
Edinger-Westphal nucleus, 84f, 85, 94f, 105, 159f, 161, 167
EEG. *See* Electroencephalography
Efferent fiber(s), 1, 3, 23. *See also* C fiber(s); General somatic efferent fiber(s); General visceral efferent fiber(s); Special visceral efferent fiber(s)
of cranial nerves, 83–84
of motor nuclei, 85
of spinal nerves, 23, 24f
Ejaculation, 36
premature, 36
Electrical stimulation, analgesia produced by, 49
Electrical synapse(s), 19, 160
Electrocorticography, 242
Electroencephalography (EEG), 242–243
Electromotive force, 16
Electromyography, 243
Emboliform nucleus, 92, 135, 141, 141f
Embolus, 221–222
Emission, 36
Emotion(s), 65, 100-101, 107, 152, 154, 187, 193, 197, 200, 202. *See also* Emotional behavior
disturbance of, 188
memory and, 197
processing of, 188
Encephalitis, 234, 241
Endocrine activity, 193, 196, 200–201
Endogenous analgesia, 49
Endolymph, 121, 127, 131–132
Endolymphatic hydrops, 133
Endorphin(s), 20, 49, 215, 216f
Enkephalin(s), 20, 49, 151, 215, 216f, 217
Enophthalmos, 35
Entorhinal cortex, 193, 194, 194f, 195, 204, 205f, 206, 216f, 219
Enzymatic degradation of neurotransmitters, 210

Ependyma, 11, 213, 228
Ependymoma, 230
Epilepsy, 219, 242
Epinephrine, 34–35, 209–210, 213, 216f. *See also* Adrenergic receptors
Epiphysis. *See* Epithalamus
Epithalamus, 177, 202–203
EPSP. *See* Excitatory postsynaptic potential(s)
Equilibrium potential, 15
Erection, 36
Erector pili muscles, 34
Esophageal branch, of vagus nerve, 102
Essential tremor, 240
Estrogen, 201
Evoked potential(s). *See* Auditory evoked potential(s); Visual evoked potential(s); Somatosensory evoked potentials
Evoked-potential study, 242–243
  recording of potentials, 243
Examination. *See* Clinical evaluation; Diagnostic test(s); Neurologic examination
Excitatory amino acid(s), 219. *See also* Glutamate/aspartate
Excitatory neurotransmitter(s), 19
Excitatory postsynaptic potential(s) (EPSP), 20, 65, 150
Excitotoxins, 219
Executive functioning, 142–143, 152
  basal ganglia loop and, 152
  cerebellum and, 142-143
  disturbances of, 145
Explicit memory. *See* Declarative memory
Extended amygdala, 196-197
Extensor plantar reflex. *See* Babinski sign
External auditory meatus, 119, 120f, 125
  facial nerve and, 106
  sensory innervation of, 101
External carotid artery, 221
External ear, 119. *See also* Auricle
External granular layer, of isocortex, 175
External pyramidal layer, of isocortex, 175
External strabismus, 106
Exteroceptive receptor(s), 23, 41
Extrafusal muscle fiber(s), 26, 28, 28f
  innervation by alpha motor neurons, 29
Extraocular muscle(s), 64, 104-106
  testing of, 238
  yoked pairs of, 172
Extrapyramidal system, 148
Extremity(ies)
  distal muscles of, 61–63
  paralysis of, 112–113
  peripheral neuropathy and, 69
  resistance to passive manipulation of limbs, 239
Eye(s)
  Benedikt's syndrome, 117
  blood supply to, 221–222
  brain stem lesions and, 116
  corneal blink reflex, 110
  frontal eye field, 60, 63, 152, 169, 183–184, 188
  parasympathetic innervation of, 36
  parietal eye field, 169
  pontine lesions and, 114–115
  sympathetic innervation of, 35
  vision, 158–166
  Weber's syndrome, 111, 116–118
Eye movement(s), 64, 66, 127, 130–133, 142, 154, 161, 163, 184. *See also* Cranial nerve III; Cranial nerve IV; Cranial nerve VI; Diplopia; Extraocular muscles; Nystagmus; Strabismus
  abnormal, 128, 144-145
  basal ganglia and, 152, 154, 155
  optokinetics, 169, 173
  pursuit, 169, 171–173, 171f
  saccades, 169–171, 170f
  testing of, 238
  vergence, 169, 173
  vestibulo-ocular subsystem, 131, 169, 172–173
Eyelid(s)
  closure of, 110
  drooping of, 106
    Horner's syndrome and, 35
  examination of, 238
  muscles of, 94
Face, sensory innervation of, 107. *See also* Cranial nerve V
Face-object recognition, 177. *See also* Object recognition
Facial canal, 101, 106, 107
Facial colliculus, 80f
Facial expression, 61, 92, 106
  masked face, 155
  muscles of,
    innervation by lower motor neurons vs. upper motor neurons, 107
    paralysis of, 106, 110, 114-115
Facial nerve. *See* Cranial nerve VII
Facial nucleus, 63, 84f, 85, 91, 91f, 106
Familial tremor, 240
Family history, 235
Fasciculation(s), 69, 107, 243
  amyotrophic lateral sclerosis and, 75
  thrombosis of anterior spinal artery and, 75
Fasciculus, 3. *See also* Medial longitudinal fasciculus
Fasciculus cuneatus, 11f, 53–54, 53f, 55f, 78, 80f, 81f, 82, 88, 88f, 89f
Fasciculus gracilis, 11f, 52, 53f, 54, 55f, 78, 80f, 81f, 82, 88, 88f, 89f
Fasciculus mammillary princeps, 200
Fasciculus retroflexus. *See* Habenulopeduncular tract
Fast pain, 47
Fastigial nucleus, 92, 130, 135, 137, 140f, 142, 144, 171f
Fastigiobulbar tract, 130, 140
Fauces, 101
Feeding behavior, 199-202
Festinating gait, 155–156
Fibrillation(s), 69, 243
Fifth nerve palsy, 115
Fight or flight phenomenon, 35
Filum terminale, 7, 8f
Finely controlled movement(s). *See* Movement, fine control of
Finger agnosia, 188
Fire test, 237
Fissure, 4
Flaccid paralysis. *See* Paralysis
Flavor recognition, 206

Flexor plantar response, 240
Flexor reflex, 27, 31
Flocculonodular lobe, 129f, 130, 136, 137, 137f, 142, 144, 171f, 172
Fluent aphasia, 187, 192, 237
Flutter-vibration, sense of, 51, 55f, 57
Folium(a), 6, 135
Follicle-stimulating hormone, 201
Food intake, 199–202
Foramen magnum, 77, 97, 137
Foramen of Magendie. *See* Median ventricular foramen
Foramina of Luschka. *See* Lateral ventricular foramina
Foramina of Monro. *See* Interventricular foramina
Forebrain, arteries to, 221–226
Fornix, 5f, 6f, 148f, 150f, 180f, 186f, 194–195, 194f, 197, 198f, 199, 205f
Fourth ventricle, 5f, 6f, 77, 79–80, 82, 90f, 91f, 92f, 93, 137f, 227, 228f
Fovea centralis, 158, 169
Foville's syndrome, 115
Free nerve ending(s), 52
  hair follicles and, 52
  pain and, 42, 45f
  temperature sensation and, 45f, 47f
  touch and, 52
Friedreich's ataxia, 59, 145–146
Frontal eye field, 60, 63, 150, 152, 169, 170f, 171f, 179f, 183–184, 188
  lesions of, 184
Frontal lobe, 4, 7f, 148f. *See also* Frontal eye field; Motor areas; Orbital cortex; Prefrontal cortex
  lesions of, 190
Frontal lobe syndrome, 189
Frontopontine fibers. *See* Corticopontine fibers
Funiculi, of spinal cord, 9
Functional magnetic resonance imaging, 245
Fusiform layer. *See* Multiform layer
Fusimotor neuron(s). *See* Gamma motoneuron(s)
GABA. *See* Gamma-aminobutyric acid
Gag reflex, 103, 238
Gait
  assessment of, 239
  disorders of, 144-146, 155–156, 190, 230
    festinating gait, 156
    gait apraxia, 190
Galanin neuron(s), 202
Gamma motoneuron(s), 11, 28f, 29–30
  acetylcholine release, 208
  decerebrate rigidity and, 131
  dynamic, 30
  innervation of intrafusal muscle fibers, 29–30
  muscle spindles and, 29
  plate endings of, 28f, 29
  spasticity and, 72
  static, 30
  supraspinal control of, 30
  trail endings of, 28f, 29
Gamma-aminobutyric acid (GABA), 19, 88, 161, 182, 217–219, 217f, 218-219
  amygdala and, 195–196
  basal ganglia and, 150–153, 218
  cerebellum and, 139
  synthesis of, 218
Gamma-aminobutyric acid (GABA) neuron(s), 88, 196, 217, 218
Gamma-aminobutyric acid (GABA) receptor(s), 218
Ganglion(a), 3. *See also* specific ganglia
Ganglion cell(s) of the retina, 160–163, 160f
  classes of, 164
  receptive field characteristics of, 163
Gap junction at electrical synapse, 19
Gasserian ganglion. *See* Trigeminal ganglion
Gastrointestinal tract
  parasympathetic innervation of, 99, 101
  pelvic splanchnic nerves and, 36
  sensory innervation of, 100
Gaze, 130
  paralysis of, 115–116, 172
General acoustic muscle reflex, 125
General afferent fiber(s), 23, 83–84
General efferent fiber(s), 23–25
General nerve fiber(s), 23
General sensory visceral portion, of vagal system, 100–101
General somatic afferent (GSA) fiber(s), 23
  cranial nerves and, 83, 86
  spinal nerves and, 23, 24f
General somatic afferent cell column, 84, 84f, 85, 85f, 99
General somatic efferent (GSE) fiber(s)
  cranial nerves and, 83
  spinal nerves and, 24f, 25
General somatic efferent cell column, 84, 84f, 85, 85f
General somatic sensation, 101
General visceral afferent (GVA) fiber(s)
  autonomic nervous system and, 33
  cranial nerves and, 83–84, 86
  pain sensation and, 48
  spinal nerves and, 23, 24f
  of vagal system, 100–101
General visceral afferent (GVA) cell column, 84, 84f, 85–86, 85f, 98-99, 98f
General visceral efferent (GVE) fiber(s)
  autonomic nervous system and, 33
  cranial nerves and, 83–86
  spinal nerves and, 24f, 25
General visceral efferent (GVE) cell column, 98. *See also* Parasympathetic nervous system; Sympathetic nervous system
  cranial nerves and, 84–86, 84f, 85f
Geniculate ganglion, 100–101
Geniculocalcarine tract. *See* Optic radiation(s)
Genioglossus muscle, 97, 103
Genitofemoral nerve, 43f
Genitourinary tract, 64
  autonomic innervation of, 36–38, 37f
  pelvic splanchnic nerves and, 36

Genu of internal capsule, 181. *See also* Internal capsule
Gerstmann syndrome, 188
Gland(s), 4. *See also* specific glands
  autonomic nervous system and, 33
  spinal nerves and, 25
  vagal system and, 99
Glial cell(s), 3, 19, 218
  cerebellar glomeruli and, 138
  gap junctions of, 19
  types of, 3
Glioblast, 11
Glioma, 206
Globose nucleus, 92, 135, 141, 141f
Globus pallidus, 148–150, 148f, 149f, 150f, 153, 181, 184, 217, 217f, 218
  input to thalamus, 151, 152f
  externa, 150, 151f, 152f, 153, 216f
  inhibition by dorsal striatum, 150
  interna, 150, 151, 151f, 152f, 153, 153f, 154, 217, 217f
Glomeruli, 137
Glossopharyngeal nerve. *See* Cranial nerve IX
Glove-and-stocking sensory loss, 69
Glucose, blood, 202
Glucose receptor(s), 202
Glutamate/aspartate, 19, 46, 63, 87, 138–139, 150–151, 153, 153f, 160, 195–196, 217, 217f, 219
Glutamate receptor(s), 219
Glutamic acid decarboxylase, 218
Glutaminase, 218
Glutamine, 218
Glycine, 19, 63, 218–219
Golgi tendon organ(s), 30–31, 52
Golgi type II cell(s), 137, 138f, 139
Gonadal hormone, 201
Gonadal regulation, 201
Gonadotropin-releasing hormone, 201, 218
Goose-pimpling, 202
G-protein-coupled receptor(s), 20–21, 208, 210, 212–214, 218–219
Gracile nucleus. *See* Nucleus gracilis
Graded potential(s), 160
Granular cell layer, of cerebellar cortex, 137–138, 138f
Gray matter, 3
  of spinal cord, 9–11
    division into horns, 9
    division into nuclei, 9, 11f
    division into laminae, 9, 11f
Gray ramus(i) communicans(tes), 24f, 34
Great auricular nerve, 43f, 44f
Greater occipital nerve, 43f
Greater splanchnic nerve, 35. *See also* Thoracic splanchnic nerves
Greater superficial petrosal nerve, 101
Growth hormone, 201
Growth hormone-releasing hormone, 218
GSA fiber(s). *See* General somatic afferent fiber(s)
GSE fiber(s). *See* General somatic efferent fiber(s)
Guillain-Barré syndrome, 69, 230
Gustation. *See* Taste entries
Gustatory cortex, 179f, 184, 189
Gut-brain peptide(s), 202, 215–218
GVA fiber(s). *See* General visceral afferent fiber(s)
GVE fiber(s). *See* General visceral efferent fiber(s)
Gyri of Heschl. *See* Transverse temporal gyri
Gyrus(i), 4
Gyrus rectus, 7f, 162f, 204, 205f

Habenular commissure, 202–203
Habenular nucleus(i), 202–203, 209, 217f
Habenulopeduncular tract, 203
Hair cell(s)
  cochlear, 121–122, 124
  vestibular, 127, 128
Hamstring muscle, 30
Handedness, 190
Head
  pain sensations from, 46–47
  sympathetic innervation of, 34–35
Head movement, 64, 66, 130–133, 161. *See also* Tectospinal tract
  acceleration, 127–128
  angular motion, 127
  linear motion, 127
  medial longitudinal fasciculus and, 66
  in response to sound, 125
  tectospinal tract and, 64, 161
Head position (tilt), 127–128, 130, 133
  rotated or tilted postures, 144
Head shaking acuity test, 172
Headache, 230
Hearing, 119–126, 185. *See also* Auditory entries; Ear
  central auditory pathways, 122–124, 123f
Hearing loss, 119, 124–126, 185
  from conductive defects, 124–125
  diagnosis of, 124–125
  from nerve damage, 124–125
Heart. *See* Cardiac entries
Heart rate, 99, 202
Helicotrema, 120f, 121
Hemianopia, 165
Hemiataxia, 225
Hemiballismus, 156, 224, 240
Hemichorea, 157, 224
Hemiplegia, 70, 71f, 72, 192, 222–223, 234
  alternating, 113
  brain stem lesions and, 111–117
Hemispheric dominance, 190-191. *See also* Lateralization of function, cerebral cortex and
Hemorrhage, 223
  brain stem, 112
Herniation
  of cerebellar tonsils, 241
  of intervertebral disc, 32, 69
  of temporal lobe, 241
Herpes zoster, 50
Hertz, 119
Heschl's gyrus. *See* Transverse temporal gyri
Heteromodal association area(s), 175–177, 178f, 187–189, 195
Hippocampal formation, 177, 189, 193–195, 193f, 209f, 212f, 216f, 217f, 219
  connections of, 194–195
  in learning and memory, 195
  lesions of, 195
  structure of, 193–194
Hippocampus, 143f, 148f, 186f, 189, 194–195

Histamine, 209
in pain sensation, 42
synthesis of, 210
in wakefulness, 87–88, 199
Histaminergic neuron(s), 199
Histidine, 210
Histogenesis, nervous system and, 14
Hoarseness, 99, 113
Hoffmann sign, 72
Homeostasis, 189, 193, 197
of the nervous system, 229
Homeostatic behavior, 193, 200
Homonymous hemianopia, 165, 223
Homotypic isocortex, 175
Homunculus, 60, 183f. *See also* Somatotopic organization
Hook bundle, 130
Horizontal cell(s), retinal, 160–161, 160f
Horizontal diplopia, 105
Horizontal nystagmus, 133
Horizontal saccade(s), 169–170, 170f
Hormone(s). *See* specific hormones
Horn(s), spinal cord, 9, 10f
nuclei, cell columns, and laminae within, 9–11, 11f
Horner's syndrome, 35, 113
5-HT. *See* Serotonin
Hue discrimination threshold, 186
Huntington's disease, 156–157, 218–219
Hydrocephalic edema, 229
Hydrocephalus, 230, 244
5-Hydroxytryptamine. *See* Serotonin
Hyperactive reflex. *See* Hyperreflexia
Hyperacusis, 107
Hyperesthesia, 49
Hyperkinetic movement disorder(s), 155, 156–157
Hypermetria, 144
Hyperosmia, 206
Hyperpolarization, 15, 19–20, 160
Hyperpolarizing afterpotential, 18–19
Hyperreflexia, 70, 73, 113-116
Hypertension, 67, 96, 111, 133
Hypertensive encephalopathy, 230
Hyperthermia, chronic, 201
Hypertonia, 31, 70, 72. *See also* Rigidity; Spasticity
Hypesthesia, 49, 223
Hypogastric ganglion, 35. *See also* Prevertebral ganglion
Hypogastric plexus, 37–38
Hypoglossal nerve. *See* Cranial nerve XII
Hypoglossal nucleus, 62f, 63, 79, 84, 84f, 85f, 89, 89f, 90f, 97, 98f, 112f
injury to, 97
Hypoglossal trigone, 79, 80f
Hypometria, 144, 170
Hypophyseal portal system, 201
Hypophysiotrophic peptide(s), 218
Hypophysis. *See* Pituitary
Hypothalamic sulcus, 197
Hypothalamohypophyseal tract, 200
Hypothalamus, 177, 194f, 195, 196f, 197–202, 198f, 209f, 212f, 216f. *See also* specific entries
afferents to cerebellar cortex, 142
amygdala and, 196
anterior, 88, 197–199, 201
blood supply, 225-226
cerebral cortex and, 202
fiber connections of, 199–200
functions of, 200–202
hippocampal formation and, 195
hypothalamic-pituitary relationships, 200–201
lateral zone of, 197
lesions of, 201
mammillary region of, 194f, 195, 197, 199
medial zone of, 197
nuclei of, 65, 197–199
pain and, 45f, 46–47
periventricular zone of, 197
posterior, 88, 199
posterior lateral, 209
preoptic area of, 197, 198
reticular formation control, 65
subdivisions of, 197–199, 198f
tuberal region of, 197, 199
visceral sensory pathway to, 100
Hypothermia, 201
Hypotonia, 31, 69–70, 144, 182, 239
brain stem lesions and, 113-115
of spastic type, 70
Hypotonic hemiplegia, 222
Hypotonic paralysis, 69
Hypoxia, 229
Ideational apraxia, 190
Ideomotor apraxia, 190
Idiopathic intracranial hypertension, 230
Idiotypic isocortex, 175
Iliohypogastric nerve, 43f, 44f
Ilioinguinal nerve, 43f
Image slip, 172
Imaging study(ies)
anatomic, 244–245
physiologic, 245
Impedance matching, 121
Impotence, 36
Incertohypothalamic projection(s), 210
Incontinence, urinary, 38, 230
Incus, 119, 120f
Indirect loop, 153–154, 153f
Indirect optokinetic pathway, 173
Indolamine. *See* Serotonin
Infarction, 222
Inferior cerebellar peduncle, 53f, 54, 79f, 80f, 81f, 82, 89, 90f, 112f, 123f, 140–141
Inferior colliculus, 5f, 79f, 80f, 82, 93f, 94, 122, 123f, 124, 217f
brachium of, 122, 123f
commissural connections, 124
nucleus of, 93f, 94
Inferior frontal gyrus, 5f, 191
Inferior frontal sulcus, 5f
Inferior ganglion
of glossopharyngeal nerve, 101
of vagus nerve, 101
Inferior mesenteric ganglion, 35, 37, 37f. *See also* Prevertebral ganglion
Inferior oblique muscle, 105, 172
Inferior olivary nuclear complex, 78, 89, 89f, 90f, 139-140, 140f, 143, 217f, 219
degeneration of, 145
Inferior parietal lobule, 5f
Inferior rectus muscle, 105, 172
Inferior salivatory nucleus, 84f, 85, 98–99, 98f, 102
Inferior temporal gyrus, 5f, 7f, 186
Inferior vestibular nucleus, 89, 90f. *See also* Descending vestibular nucleus
Information processing
in cerebellar cortex, 139–140
in cerebral cortex, 177, 178f

parallel processing in
large-scale functional networks, 177
in visual pathways, 163–164
Infundibular recess, 6f, 197
Infundibulum, 197, 201. *See also* Pituitary
Inherited disorders
Dystonia musculorum deformans, 157
Friedreich's ataxia, 145-146
Spinocerebellar ataxias, 145
Huntington's disease, 156-157
Inhibition
distal feedback, 57
local feedback 57, 210
of motoneurons, 63. *See also* Renshaw cell
Inhibitory interneuron(s), 57, 63, 139
Inhibitory neurotransmitter(s), 19
Inhibitory postsynaptic potential(s) (IPSP), 20, 150
Inhibitory surround, 57–58, 163
Inner ear, 119, 120f, 121–122
vestibular portion of, 127–128
Inner hair cell(s), 120f, 121–122
Innervation. *See* specific nerves; specific sites
Insight, evaluation of, 237
Insular cortex, 148f, 179f, 184, 186, 187, 189, 193, 196f
visceral sensory pathway to, 100
Insular lobe, 6, 177, 195
Intercostal nerve, 43f, 102
Intercostobrachial nerve, 44f
Intermediate acoustic stria, 122, 123f
Intermediate memory, 236
Intermediolateral cell column, 11, 11f, 25, 33–34
Intermediomedial cell column, 11, 11f, 48
Internal anal sphincter reflex, 38
Internal arcuate fiber(s), 54, 81f, 82, 88, 89f
Internal auditory artery, 225f
occlusion of, 125
thrombosis of, 115
Internal auditory canal, 101, 106, 107, 129
Internal capsule, 67, 149f, 152f, 180f
anterior limb of, 148f, 149, 180–181, 180f, 181f
blood supply of, 223
genu of, 180f, 181
lesion of, 70-72, 71f
posterior limb of, 62f, 70–72, 71f, 148f, 150f, 180–181, 180f, 181f
retrolenticular portion of, 180f, 181
sublenticular part of, 181
thalamus and, 180–181
Internal carotid artery, 221–223, 222f, 225, 225f
occlusion of, 223, 225
Internal genu of facial nerve, 91–92
Internal granular layer of isocortex, 175
Internal medullary lamina, of thalamus, 177
Internal pyramidal layer of isocortex, 175
Internal strabismus, 105
Interneuron(s), 24f, 27, 57, 63, 139
of cerebellum, 138
of reticular formation, 86
of striatum, 208
Internuclear ophthalmoplegia, 66, 115
Interoceptive
information, 23
receptor(s), 41
Interpeduncular cistern, 227
Interpeduncular fossa, 78f, 82, 94, 105, 143f
Interpeduncular nucleus, 203, 209, 216f, 217f
Interposed nuclei. *See* Nucleus interpositus
Intersegmental reflex, 27
gamma motoneurons and, 29
Interstitial edema, 229
Interstitial nucleus of Cajal, 64–65, 67, 118, 131, 170. *See also* Interstitiospinal tract
Interstitiospinal tract, 65, 66f, 67, 90–91
Interthalamic adhesion. *See* Massa intermedia
Interventricular foramen(ina) of Monro, 6f, 227, 228f, 230
Intervertebral disc, herniation of, 32, 69
Intervertebral foramina, 9
Intracerebral hemorrhage, 244
Intracranial pressure, 229–231
elevated, 103–104, 223, 230, 241
Intrafusal muscle fiber(s), 26, 28–29, 28f
innervation by gamma and beta motor neurons, 29–30
Intralaminar nuclei, of thalamus, 45f, 46–47, 87, 142, 143, 151, 152, 178, 179f, 181
Intraparietal sulcus, 5f
Involuntary movement(s) 155. *See also* Chorea; Movements; Tremor
assessment of, 240
Iodopsin, 158
Ion channel(s), 15–16, 208
ligand-gated, 16
membrane potential and, 16
voltage-gated, 16
Ionotropic receptor(s), 20, 208, 219
IPSP. *See* Inhibitory postsynaptic potential(s)
Iris, muscles of. *See also* Horner's syndrome; Miosis; Mydriasis; Pupillary constrictor muscle
lesions of, 167-169
radial muscle of, 106
sphincter muscle of, 36, 105, 167
Ischemic vascular disease, 96, 118
Isocortex, 175–177, 178f, 199
cell layers of, 175
functional regions of, 175–177, 176f
Itching sensation, 42, 51

Jaw jerk, 93, 108–109, 238
Jaw muscle(s). *See* Mastication, muscles of
Jaw reflex. *See* Jaw jerk
Joint movement(s), 186
Joint receptor(s), 52
Judgment, evaluation of, 237
Jugular foramen, 97, 101
Juxtarestiform body, 130, 140

Kappa opioid receptor(s), 215
Kinesthesia, 41, 51–52, 56
Kinetic apraxia, 182, 190
Kinetic tremor, 145
Kinocilium, 128
Kluver-Bucy syndrome, 197

Laboratory test(s). *See* Diagnostic test(s)
Labyrinth. *See* Inner ear
Lacrimal gland
  facial nerve and, 106
  lacrimation
    associated with corneal blink reflex, 110
    loss of, 107
  parasympathetic innervation of, 36, 99
  sympathetic innervation from carotid plexus, 35
Lacunar stroke, 223
Lamina(ae), of spinal cord, 9-11
  pain sensation and, 46
Lamina terminalis, 5f, 198f
Language, 174, 177, 187, 190, 191f, 192. *See also* Aphasia
  evaluation of language ability, 237
  production/speech, 142-145
Larynx
  cough reflex and, 103
  motor innervation from
    nucleus ambiguus, 99
    vagus nerve branches, 102
    cranial accessory nerve XI, 102
  muscles of, 61
  paralysis of, 113–114
  sensory innervation from
    inferior ganglion of X, 100
    vagus nerve branches, 102
Lateral antebrachial cutaneous nerve, 43f, 44f
Lateral brachial cutaneous nerve, 43f, 44f
Lateral brain stem system, to spinal cord, 66–67
Lateral cervical nucleus, 56f, 57
Lateral cervical puncture, 242
Lateral cervical system, 52, 54, 56f, 57, 59
Lateral corticospinal tract, 11f, 62f, 63, 66, 66f, 74, 81f, 82
  blood supply to, 75, 76f
  lesions of, 75, 76
Lateral cuneate nucleus. *See* Accessory cuneate nucleus
Lateral dorsal nucleus of thalamus, 179f, 189
Lateral fissure (of Sylvius), 4, 5f
  floor of, 6
  opercula of, 6
Lateral foramen(ina), 227
Lateral funiculus(i), 9, 10f
  lesions of, 75
Lateral gaze, paralysis of, 115. *See also* Paramedian pontine reticular formation
Lateral geniculate nucleus (body) (LGN), 78f, 79f, 80f, 159f, 161, 163–164, 170f, 171f, 179f, 185, 186f
  monocular input to, 161
  receptive field characteristics, cells of, 163
  retinotopically organized input to, 161
Lateral horn, 9, 10f, 24f, 25
Lateral hypothalamic nucleus (area), 198f, 202, 203, 208, 209
Lateral inhibition. *See* Inhibition, local feedback
Lateralization of function, cerebral cortex and, 187–188, 190–191, 202
Lateral lemniscus, 91f, 92f, 93f, 94, 122, 123f, 124
  lesions of, 124
  nuclei of, 122, 123f, 124
Lateral nuclear group, of thalamus, 177, 180. *See also* Lateral dorsal nucleus; Lateral posterior thalamic nucleus; Pulvinar
Lateral occipital gyri, 5f
Lateral olfactory stria. *See* Lateral olfactory tract
Lateral olfactory tract, 204–205
Lateral orbitofrontal cortex, 152, 187, 206. *See also* Orbitofrontal cortex
Lateral plantar nerve, 44f
Lateral posterior thalamic nucleus, 179f, 185, 187
Lateral preoptic area, 198
Lateral recess, 79–80, 80f, 227. *See also* Lateral ventricular foramen
Lateral rectus muscle, 92, 104, 106, 129f, 131, 169, 170f, 171f, 172
Lateral reticular nucleus, 213
Lateral reticulospinal tract. *See* Medullary reticulospinal tract
Lateral striate artery(ies), 224f, 225f, 226
  occlusion of, 223
Lateral sural cutaneous nerve, 43f, 44f
Lateral tegmental norepinephrine cell group(s), 212
Lateral tuberal nucleus(i), 197, 199
Lateral ventricle, 148f, 186f, 227, 228f
  anterior horn, 148f, 180f
  inferior (temporal) horn, 148f, 162f, 194, 196f, 228f
  posterior horn, 180f
Lateral ventricular foramina, 79, 227
Lateral vestibular nucleus, 91f, 129f, 130
Lateral vestibulospinal tract, 11f, 29, 65, 66f, 67, 129f, 130
Laterodorsal tegmental nucleus, 208–209, 209f
Laterodorsal thalamic nucleus. *See* Lateral dorsal thalamic nucleus
Learning, 177, 189, 208
  motor, 143, 155
  hippocampus and, 193, 195
  amygdala and, 193
Least splanchnic nerve, 35. *See also* Thoracic splanchnic nerve
Lemniscus, 3. *See also* Lateral lemniscus; Medial lemniscus; Spinal lemniscal system
Lens, of eye, 158, 159f, 163
Lenticular nucleus. *See* Lentiform nucleus
Lenticulostriate artery(ies), 222–223, 226
Lentiform nucleus, 79f, 148f, 149, 149t
Leptin, 202
Lesion(s). *See* specific location
Lesser occipital nerve, 43f
Lesser splanchnic nerve, 35. *See also* Thoracic splanchnic nerve
Lesser superficial petrosal nerve, 101
Letter test, 237

Leu-enkephalin, 215. *See also* Enkephalin(s)
Levator palpebrae superioris muscle, 35, 105
 general somatic efferent innervation, 105
 Horner's syndrome and, 35
 sympathetic innervation, 35
 paralysis of, 106, 116
Levodopa, 155–157
Lewy bodies, 155
LGN. *See* Lateral geniculate nucleus
Libido, 36
Ligand-gated channel(s), 16, 19–20
Light perception, 158
Light reflex(es), 167–168
Light touch, 51, 109
 spinal cord lesions and, 58
 testing of, 51, 240
Limb(s). *See* Extremity(ies)
Limb movement, sensation of. *See* Kinesthesia
Limb position, sensation of, 51–52, 56
 inability to recognize, 58
Limbic cortex, 154, 193. *See also* Allocortex; Limbic lobe
Limbic lobe, 4–6, 64, 154, 177, 189. *See also* Allocortex
Limbic system, 107, 177, 193–203
 epithalamus, 202–203
 functions of, 193
 hypothalamus. *See* Hypothalamus
 pain and, 46–47
 telencephalic, 177, 178f, 181, 193–197, 194f
Line of Gennari, 163
Lingual branch, of glossopharyngeal nerve, 101
Lingual gyrus, 5f, 159f, 162f, 163, 185
 lesions of, 165
Lipid bilayer, 15–16
Lissauer's tract. *See* Posterolateral fasciculus
Literal paraphasia, 192
Lobes
 of cerebellum, 136-137
 of cerebral hemisphere, 4-6
Local feedback inhibition. *See* Inhibition, local feedback
Localization of lesions, 111, 233, 234
Locked-in syndrome, 118
Locomotion, 61, 64, 130, 142, 200, 201. *See also* Walking
Locus ceruleus, 87–88, 139, 212–213, 212f, 216f
 degeneration of, 155
 projections to spinal cord, 65
Longitudinal sagittal zonal patterns, of cerebellum, 136f, 137
Lou Gehrig's disease. *See* Amyotrophic lateral sclerosis
Lower facial nucleus, 63. *See also* Facial nucleus
Lower motoneuron(s). *See also* Alpha motoneuron(s); Anterior horn cells; General somatic efferent fiber(s)
 innervation of muscles by, 61
 lesions of, 69, 107
 regulation by upper motoneurons, 61
Lumbar puncture, 241–242
Lumbar spinal cord, 7, 10f
Lumbar spinal nerve(s), 7, 9
Lumbar splanchnic nerve, 35, 37, 37f
Lungs, vagal system and, 36, 100
Luteinizing hormone, 201

MI. *See* Primary motor cortex
Macrosmatic vertebrate, 204, 206
Macula(ae)
 of inner ear, 128, 130
 of eye, 158
Macular sparing, 165, 223-224
Magnesium, 20
Magnetic resonance angiography (MRA), 244
Magnetic resonance imaging (MRI), 6f, 67, 96, 126, 143f, 149f–150f, 162f, 173, 181f, 186f, 196f, 205f, 230, 244
 diagnostic, 234
 functional, 245
 problems with metal, 244
Magnocellular neurosecretory cell(s), 199
Magnocellular red nucleus, 66, 142. *See also* Red nucleus
Magnocellular stream. *See* Visual pathway
Main sensory nucleus of V. *See* Principal sensory nucleus of trigeminal nerve
Malingering, 165
Malleus, 119, 120f
Malnutrition, 69, 75, 146
Mammillary body, 5f, 7f, 78f, 148f, 194f, 195, 197, 198f, 199
Mammillary peduncle, 200
Mammillotegmental tract, 200
Mammillothalamic tract, 194f, 198f, 200
Mandibular nerve, 43f, 101, 107. *See also* Cranial nerve V
Massa intermedia, 5f, 6f, 177
Masseter muscle, 107, 109
Mastication, muscles of, 61, 93, 107-108. *See also* Jaw jerk
 denervation of, 107–109, 115
 upper motoneuron innervation, 108
Maxillary nerve, 43f, 107. *See also* Cranial nerve V
Mechanoreceptor(s), 52
Medial antebrachial cutaneous nerve, 43f, 44f
Medial brachial cutaneous nerve, 43f, 44f
Medial femoral cutaneous nerve, 44f
Medial forebrain bundle (MFB), 199–200, 212–213
Medial geniculate nucleus (body), 79f, 80f, 94, 94f, 122, 123f, 124, 179f, 185
Medial lemniscus, 55f, 56f, 59f, 81f, 89f, 90–91, 90f-94f, 93–94, 111, 184
 decussation of, 54, 88. *See also* Internal arcuate fibers
 lesions of, 58, 112f, 113, 114f, 115, 116–117, 116f, 117f
Medial longitudinal fasciculus (MLF), 11f, 64–66, 90–91, 90f-94f, 94, 129f, 130, 131, 132, 169, 170f, 171f
 rostral interstitial nucleus of, 118, 170
 lesions of, 115
Medial nuclear group, of thalamus, 177, 180
Medial olfactory stria, 204–205

Medial orbitofrontal gyrus, 154. *See also* Orbitofrontal cortex
Medial plantar nerve, 44f
Medial preoptic area, 198, 201
Medial rectus muscle, 104–105, 129f, 132, 168, 170f, 171f, 172
Medial reticulospinal tract. *See* Pontine reticulospinal tract
Medial septal nucleus, 189, 208, 209f
Medial striate artery, 223, 224f, 225f, 226
Medial sural cutaneous nerve, 44f
Medial thalamic nuclei, 47, 177, 180, 189. *See also* Mediodorsal thalamic nucleus
Medial vestibular nucleus, 89, 90f, 91f, 129f, 130–131, 171f, 172
Medial vestibulospinal tract, 65, 90, 129f, 130
Median eminence, 197, 201
Median nerve, 43f, 44f
Median ventricular foramen, 79, 227, 228f
Medical history, 235
Mediodorsal thalamic nucleus, 151, 154, 179f, 196, 206. *See also* Medial thalamic nuclei
  lateral part, 188
  medial part, 187, 189
Medulla oblongata, 5f, 6. *See also* Brain stem
  anatomy of, 77–79, 78f, 80f
    anterior (ventral) aspect, 78
    internal structures, 88–89, 88f–90f
    lateral aspect, 78
    posterior (dorsal) aspect, 78–79
    rostral half, 89–90, 90f
    transverse section, 81f, 88f–90f
    ventral surface, 78f
  blood supply to, 95f
  cranial nerves of, 97–103
  development of, 12
  disorders in, 95–96
  lesions of, 112–114, 112f
    lateral sector, 112f, 113
    Wallenberg's syndrome, 112f, 113–114
  motor (pyramidal) decussation of, 88
  pyramid of, 61–63
  respiratory center of, 102
  sensory decussation of, 82. *See also* Decussation of the medial lemniscus; Internal arcuate fibers
Medullary reticulospinal tract, 11f, 64–65, 66f, 67
Meissner's corpuscle, 52
Melanin, 93, 202, 210
Melanin concentrating hormone, 202
Melanocyte-stimulating hormone, 210, 218
Melatonin, 199, 203
Membrane potential. *See also* Action potential
  ion channels and, 16
  resting. *See* Resting membrane potential
Membranous labyrinth, 120f, 121, 127–128, 133
Memory, 174, 177, 185, 189, 193, 195, 208, 219
  associative, 189, 197
  declarative, 195, 197
  disorders of, 145, 146, 189
  emotions and, 189, 197
  explicit, 189, 195
  testing of, 236
Ménière's disease, 125, 127, 133
Meninges, 6–7
Meningioma, 206
  cerebellopontine angle, 115
Meningitis, 206, 230, 234, 241–242
Mental status examination, 236–238
Mesencephalic nucleus of V, 84f, 86, 92f, 93, 108, 109. *See also* Cranial nerve V
Mesencephalic tract, 92f, 93. *See also* Cranial nerve V
Mesencephalon, 12, 13f
Mesocortex, 175, 177, 178f, 189, 193
Mesocortical dopaminergic system, 154. *See also* Mesotelencephalic system
Mesolimbic system, 211
Mesotelencephalic system, 211
Metabotropic receptor(s). *See* G-protein-coupled receptor(s)
Metencephalon, 12, 13f
Met-enkephalin, 215. *See also* Enkephalin(s)
1-Methyl-4-phenyl-1,2,3,6-tetrahydropyridine (MPTP), 156
MFB. *See* Medial forebrain bundle
Microglia, 3
Microsmatic vertebrate, 204, 206
Micturition, 64. *See also* Urination
Midbrain, 5f, 6. *See also* Brain stem
  anatomy of, 78f, 80–82, 80f
    anterior (ventral) aspect, 82
    caudal half, 93–94, 93f
    internal structures, 93–94, 93f, 94f
    posterior (dorsal) aspect, 82
    rostral half, 94, 94f
    transverse section, 93f, 94f
    ventral surface, 78f
  blood supply to, 95f
  cranial nerves of, 104–110
  development of, 12
  lesions of, 116–118, 117f
    Benedikt's syndrome, 117, 117f
    Parinaud's syndrome, 117f, 118
    Weber's syndrome, 111, 116–118, 117f
Middle cerebellar peduncle, 79f, 80, 80f, 91, 91f, 92f, 140–142, 141f
Middle cerebral artery, 221–223, 222f, 224f, 225f
  occlusion of, 222
Middle cervical ganglion, 34
Middle ear, 119–121, 120f, 122
  lesions of, 124
  sensory innervation of, 100-101
Middle frontal gyrus, 5f, 184
Middle temporal cortex, 172
Middle temporal gyrus, 5f, 186
Middle temporal sulcus, 5f
Midline thalamic nucleus(i), 178, 179f, 180–181, 189, 196
Milk ejection, 200
Millard-Gubler syndrome, 115
Mimetic muscle(s), 106. *See also* Facial expression
Miniature end-plate potential(s), 20
Miosis, 35, 168. *See also* Horner's syndrome
Mitral cell(s), 204–206
MLF. *See* Medial longitudinal fasciculus

Modiolus, 121
Molecular layer
of cerebellar cortex, 137
of cerebral cortex, 175
Monaural central auditory pathway, 122
Monoamine(s), 207, 209–214
reuptake and degradation of, 210
Monoamine oxidase, 210
Monoamine neurons, 87, 207, 209-213
in reticular formation, 87
functions, 87
Monoplegia, 72
Monosynaptic reflex, 27
Mood, 154, 187
changes in, 188
Mossy fiber(s), 138-139, 138f
Motion sickness, 133
Motivation, 143, 154–155, 177, 187–188, 197, 206
Motoneuron(s), 2f, 11, 24f, 25. *See also* Alpha motoneuron(s); Anterior horn cell(s); General somatic efferent (GSE) fibers; Lower motoneuron(s); Upper motoneuron(s)
responsiveness of, 65
Motor activity. *See* Movement(s)
Motor aphasia. *See* Nonfluent aphasia
Motor apraxia. *See* Kinetic apraxia
Motor area(s), of cerebral cortex, 60–61, 182. *See also* Motor association cortex; Primary motor cortex
Motor association area(s) of cerebral cortex, 60, 143, 175, 178f, 179f, 182–183. *See also* Premotor area; Supplementary motor area
Motor cell column, of brain stem, 82–85, 84f
Motor decussation. *See* Decussation, of the pyramids
Motor end plate, 2f, 4. *See also* Neuromuscular junction
Motor loop, of basal ganglia, 152
Motor nerve fiber(s), 25, 25t. *See also* Efferent fiber(s)
Motor neuron(s). *See* Motoneuron(s)
Motor nucleus of V, 84f, 85, 92f, 93. *See also* Cranial nerve V
Motor system, in neurologic examination, 238–240
Motor unit, 29. *See also* Fasciculations
brief contractions of, 69
Movement(s), 64, 182
apraxia. *See* Apraxia
basal ganglia neuronal activity related to, 155
decomposition of, 144
descending fibers from cerebral cortex and brain stem and, 61–66, 182
direction of, 61
disorders of, 144-146, 155-157, 184, 190
eye. *See* Eye movement(s)
fine control of, 29, 66, 135, 142, 182
force of, 61
integration of cerebellum and cerebral cortex in, 143–144
involuntary, 155
planning of, 143–144, 183
repetitive movements, 135, 157
sequencing of, 135, 155, 183
skilled, 155. *See also* Learning, motor
visually-guided, 184
MPTP. *See* 1-Methyl-4-phenyl-1,2,3,6-tetrahydropyridine
MRA. *See* Magnetic resonance angiography
MRI. *See* Magnetic resonance imaging
Mu opioid receptor(s), 215
Multiform layer, of isocortex, 175
Multiple sclerosis, 112, 115, 125, 167, 173, 234, 237, 241–243
Multiple system atrophy, 156, 245
Multipolar neuron(s), 1
Muscarinic receptor(s), 208
Muscle(s). *See also* Paralysis; Smooth muscle(s)
atrophy of, 21, 69
lower motoneuron lesions and, 69
motor unit and, 29
upper motoneuron lesions and, 70–72
Muscle biopsy, 243
Muscle spindle, 52, 184, 186. *See also* Gamma motoneuron
anatomy of, 28–29, 28f
function, size, and distribution of, 27–28
innervation of, 29
sensory function of, 30
Muscle stretch reflex. *See* Stretch reflex
Muscle tone, 31, 130, 131, 155. *See also* Hypertonia; Hypotonia; Rigidity; Spasticity
examination of, 239
Mydriasis, 106, 117, 168
Myelencephalon, 12, 13f
Myelin sheath, 1, 2f, 3, 18, 25
Myelinated fiber(s), 1–3, 25
conduction velocity of, 18, 25t
staining of, 88
Myelography, 244
Mylohyoid muscle, 107
Myoclonus, 240
Myotatic reflex. *See* Stretch reflex
Myotome, 85

Naked nerve endings. *See* Free nerve ending(s)
Naming test, 237
Narcolepsy, 243
Nasal cavity
pain sensation from, 109
parasympathetic innervation of, 36
sensory innervation of, 107. *See also* Cranial nerve V
Nasal septum, 204
Nausea and vomiting, 95, 100, 128, 230
vomiting reflex, 103
Neck muscle(s), 64–65
Negative afterpotential, 19
Neocerebellum, 137
Neologism, 192
Neospinothalamic tract, 46–47
Nernst equation, 15, 17f
Nerve(s), 3. *See also* specific nerves
Nerve biopsy, 243
Nerve cell(s), 1–3. *See also* Neuron(s)
degeneration and regeneration of, 68–69
Nerve conduction study, 243
Nerve cord, 3

Nerve fiber(s), 1–3
degeneration and regeneration of, 68–69
diameter of, 25–26
functional classification of, 23, 25, 25t
physiologic classification of, 25–26, 25t
Nerve impulse. *See* Action potential
Nerve trunk, 3
Nervi erigentes. *See* Pelvic splanchnic nerve(s)
Nervous system. *See also* Autonomic nervous system; Central nervous system; Peripheral nervous system
development of, 11–14, 12f–13f
Nervus intermedius, 36, 78f, 79f, 98-101, 98f, 106, 107, 110. *See also* Cranial nerve VII; Geniculate ganglion; Pterygopalatine ganglion
damage to, 107
course and distribution of, 101
Networks, of cerebral cortex, 177
Neural crest, 12, 12f
derivatives, 35
Neural fold(s), 11,12f
Neural groove, 11,12f
Neural tube, 11,12f
Neuroblast(s), 11
Neurodegenerative diseases. *See* Alzheimer's disease; Huntington's disease; Multiple system atrophy; Parkinson's disease; Progressive supranuclear palsy; Sporadic olivopontocerebellar atrophy
Neurohypophysis. *See* Posterior pituitary
Neurokinin(s), 215
Neurokinin receptor(s), 218
Neurolemma, 1–2, 2f
Neurologic disorder(s). *See also* specific disorders
clinical evaluation of, 233–240
localization of, 233
Neurologic evaluation, 233–240
Neurologic examination, 234, 236–240
cranial nerves and, 238
equipment for, 236
lemniscal pathway, 58–59
mental status examination, 236–238
motor system exam, 238–240
reflexes, 240
sensation, 240
Neurologic history, 233–235
Neuroma, acoustic, 115, 126
Neuromediator(s), 207
Neuromuscular junction, 2f, 4, 21, 61, 208
Neuron(s), 1, 2f. *See also* specific types
Neuropeptide(s), 19, 161, 207, 214–218, 216f, 217f
Neuropeptide Y, 202, 218
Neurophysin, 200
Neuropil, 3, 207, 213
Neurotensin, 215
Neurotransmitter(s), 1, 19–20, 207–219. *See also* specific compounds
astrocytes and, 3
autonomic nervous system and, 34
characteristics of, 207
imaging studies on, 245
Neurotransmitter receptor(s), 20–21. *See also* specific neurotransmitters; specific receptors
functional characterization of, 207–208
imaging studies of, 245
Nicotinic receptor(s), 208
Nigrostriatal dopamine system, 151f, 153f, 211
Nissl bodies, 68
Nociceptin. *See* Orphanin FQ
Nocturnal vision, 158
Node(s) of Ranvier, 2, 2f, 18
Nodose ganglion. *See* Cranial nerve X, inferior ganglion
Nodulus of the cerebellum. *See* Flocculonodular lobe
Noncommunicating hydrocephalus, 230
Nonfluent aphasia, 191–192, 222, 237
Nonmyelinated postganglionic fiber(s). *See* C fiber(s)
Noradrenaline. *See* Norepinephrine
Noradrenergic fiber(s), 138–139. *See also* Norepinephrine
Norepinephrine, 19, 34, 138-139, 209–213, 212f
analgesia and, 49
influence on motoneurons, 65
synthesis of, 210
Norepinephrine cell(s), 65, 87, 211–212
Norepinephrine receptor(s), 212–213
Normal-pressure hydrocephalus, 230–231
Nuclear bag fiber(s), 28f, 29–30
Nuclear chain fiber(s), 28f, 29-30
Nucleus(i), 3, 9–11
Nucleus accumbens, 148f–149f, 149, 149t, 154, 196, 211f
Nucleus ambiguus, 62f, 84f, 85, 85f, 89–90, 90f, 97–99, 98f, 102–103, 199
external subnucleus of, 98–99, 102
lesions of, 112f, 113
Nucleus basalis of Meynert. *See* Basal nucleus of Meynert
Nucleus cuneatus, 54, 55f, 63, 79, 81f, 82, 88f, 89f
lesion of, 58
Nucleus dorsalis, 11, 11f, 52
Nucleus gracilis, 54, 55f, 59f, 63, 79, 81f, 82, 88f, 89f
lesion of, 58
Nucleus interpositus, 130, 135, 137,141-144, 141f. *See also* Globose nucleus; Emboliform nucleus
Nucleus locus ceruleus. *See* Locus ceruleus
Nucleus of Darkschewitsch, 64
Nucleus of the accessory optic system, 173
Nucleus of the diagonal band, 208, 209f
Nucleus of the optic tract, 173
Nucleus prepositus hypoglossi, 170, 170f, 171f, 172
Nucleus proprius, 11f
Nucleus raphe magnus, 65
Nucleus raphe obscurus, 65
Nucleus raphe pallidus, 65
Nucleus reticularis pontis oralis, 87–88
Nucleus solitarius, 63, 84f, 85f, 86, 88f, 89f, 100, 103, 199, 216f, 217f
general visceral, 86
special visceral (taste), 86

Nucleus subceruleus, 65
Nutrient metabolism, 199
Nutritional deficiency. *See* Malnutrition
Nystagmus, 77, 95, 113, 115, 132, 173, 238. *See also* Horizontal nystagmus; Rotatory nystagmus; Vertical nystagmus
  clinical testing to elicit, 132
  spontaneous, 132–133, 144-145, 238

Obdurator nerve, 43f, 44f
Obex, 77, 79, 80f
Object recognition, 164, 174, 186, 187, 189
Obsessive-compulsive disorder, 213
Occipital lobe, 4, 185. *See also* Primary visual cortex; Striate cortex
  lesions of, 165
  vision and, 163
Occipital pole, 162f, 163, 185
Occipitotemporal gyrus, 7f, 205f
Ocular dominance column, 164
Ocular pursuit, 163
Oculocephalic maneuver, 238
Oculocephalic test, 172
Oculomotor nerve. *See* Cranial nerve III
Oculomotor nuclear complex, 61f, 62f, 64, 84, 84f, 94, 94f, 105, 117f, 129f, 131, 132, 167, 169, 170
  lesions of, 167
Oculomotor palsy, 117, 224
Oculomotor system. *See* Eye movement(s)
Off-center ganglion cell(s), 163
Olfaction, 186–187, 204–206
  deficits in, 206
Olfactory bulb, 7f, 186, 195–196, 204–206, 205f, 210, 211f, 212f, 214f, 216f
Olfactory cilia, 204
Olfactory cortical area(s), 206. *See also* Piriform cortex; Primary olfactory cortex
Olfactory discrimination, 187
Olfactory epithelium, 204
Olfactory nerve. *See* Cranial nerve I
Olfactory receptor(s), 204
Olfactory stalk, 204, 205f
Olfactory stria, 204-205
Olfactory sulcus, 204, 205f
Olfactory system, 204–206, 205f
Olfactory tract, 7f. *See also* Lateral olfactory tract; Olfactory stria
Olfactory trigone, 205f
Olfactory tubercle, 204, 205
Oligodendrocyte(s), 2f, 3
Olive, 7f, 78, 78f, 79f
Olivocochlear bundle, 121, 124
On-center ganglion cell(s), 163
Ophthalmic artery, 221–222
  occlusion of, 222
Ophthalmic nerve, 43f, 107. *See also* Cranial nerve V
Ophthalmoscope, 238
Opioid peptide(s), 214–215. *See also* Beta-endorphin; Dynorphin; Enkephalin
  analgesia and, 49
Opioid receptor(s), 49, 215
Opioid-receptor-like protein, 215
Optic chiasm, 5f, 6f, 7f, 78f, 159f, 161, 197–198, 198f, 205f
  lesions of, 165–166
Optic disc. *See* Optic nerve head
Optic nerve. *See* Cranial nerve II
Optic nerve head, 161, 223, 229
Optic radiation(s), 159f, 163, 180f, 181
  lesions of, 165
Optic reflex(es)
  Adie's tonic pupil, 168–169
  Argyll Robertson pupil, 169
  light reflexes, 167–168
  near-point reaction and, 168
Optic tract, 7f, 78f, 82, 150f, 159f, 161
  lesions of, 165
  nucleus of, 173
Optic vesicles, 158
Optokinetic eye movement(s), 169, 173
Optokinetic nystagmus, 173
Optokinetic pathways
  direct, 173
  indirect, 173
Orbicularis oculi muscle, 106, 110
Orbit
  muscles of, 94
    motor innervation of, 104-106
  sensory innervation of, 107
Orbital cortex, 188
Orbitofrontal cortex, 189, 193, 195, 204. *See also* Orbital cortex
  caudal, 177, 179f, 189, 193
  lateral, 152, 187, 206
  medial, 154, 202
Orbital gyri, 7f
Organ of Corti, 120f, 121–122, 124
Organic anion(s), resting membrane potential and, 15
Orientation, evaluation of, 236
Orphanin FQ, 215
Oscillopsia, 172
Ossicle(s), 119, 120f, 121
Otic ganglion, 36, 99, 101–102
Otitis media, 125
Otoconia, 128
Otosclerosis, 125
Outer hair cell(s), 120f, 121. *See also* Hair cell(s)
Oval window, 119, 120f, 121
Oxytocin, 199–200, 218

Pacchionian granulation. *See* Arachnoid villi
Pacinian corpuscle(s), 52
Pain sensation, 41–50, 109
  central pain, 49–50, 224
  chemicals implicated in, 42
  dorsal root lesions and, 69–70
  emotional responses to, 47. *See also* Cingulate gyrus; Cingulotomy
  endogenous analgesia, 49, 65
  fast pain, 47
  from cranial cavity, 109
  from head, 46–47, 86, 109
  loss of, 69-70, 75, 76, 113, 115–117
  opioids and, 215
  pathways for, 42–48
  receptors for, 42,48
  referred pain, 48
  serotonin and, 213
  slow pain, 47
  spatial localization of, 47
  spinal cord lesions and, 58, 59f, 73
  spinal cord tumor and, 76
  substance P and, 217
  syringomyelia and, 75
  visceral pain, 47-48

Palate, parasympathetic innervation of, 36, 99. *See also* Soft palate
Palatine tonsil, 101
Paleocerebellum, 137. *See also* Anterior lobe of cerebellum
Paleospinothalamic tract, 46–47
Pallidum, 154
connections with brain stem, 154
connections with cerebral cortex, 150–154
Pallor, 39
Palsy. *See* specific types
Papilledema, 229–230
Parabrachial nucleus, 100
Paracentral lobule, 5f, 46, 60, 223
Paracentral scotoma, 165
Parafascicular thalamic nucleus, 181–182
Parahippocampal gyrus, 5f, 6, 7f, 177, 179f, 189, 193, 194, 194f, 204, 205f
Paralimbic area(s), 177, 178f, 189, 193, 195, 197
connections with thalamus, 181, 189
lesions of, 189
Parallel processing, 177
Paralysis, 222
agitans. *See* Parkinsonism
amyotrophic lateral sclerosis and, 75
brain stem lesions and, 112-117
botulism and, 21
of facial muscles, 106–107
flaccid, 69, 75
hypotonic, 69
lesions of cranial nerve XII and, 103
lesions of lateral corticospinal tract and, 75, 76
localization of lesions producing, 72
lower motoneuron lesions and, 69
occlusion of middle cerebral artery and, 222
peripheral nerve lesions and, 69
spinal cord lesions and, 73
spinal cord tumor and, 76
syringomyelia and, 75
of the tongue, 103
thrombosis of anterior spinal artery and, 75
upper motoneuron lesions and, 70, 72
Paralysis agitans. *See* Parkinsonism
Paramedian arteries to brainstem, 95f
Paramedian pontine reticular formation (PPRF), 161, 169–170, 170f
lesions of, 115, 116
Paraparesis, 146, 234
Paraplegia, 72
thrombosis of anterior spinal artery and, 75
Parasympathetic nervous system (PNS), 34, 36. *See also* Autonomic nervous system
acetylcholine and, 208
cranial division (outflow) of, 34, 36, 85
innervation of eye, 105
innervation of urinary bladder by, 36–37, 37f
innervation of viscera by, 99
neurotransmitters of, 34
sacral division (outflow) of, 34, 36
terminal ganglia of, 36
Paraterminal gyrus, 5f, 6, 177, 193
Paraventricular hypothalamic nucleus, 197–200, 198f, 202, 209, 209f
Paravertebral ganglion, 24f, 34. *See also* Chain ganglion; Sympathetic trunk
Parental behavior, 200, 206
Paresis, 72, 182, 223–224
Paresthesia
dorsal root irritation and, 49
dorsal root lesions and, 69–70, 73
Parietal eye field, 169, 170f
Parietal lobe, 4, 45f, 54, 55f, 56f, 61,185. *See also* Heteromodal association area; Primary somatosensory cortex; Somatosensory association area; Temporoparietal association area
lesions of, 190
Parietal operculum, 184, 186, 191
Parieto-occipital fissure, 4, 5f, 6f
Parieto-temporo-occipito-pontine fibers. *See* Corticopontine fibers
Parinaud's syndrome, 117f, 118
Parkinson's disease, 147, 155–157, 211, 239, 245
treatment of, 156
Parkinsonian tremor, 156, 240
Parkinsonism, 146, 155–156, 209, 239
Parotid gland
parasympathetic innervation of, 36, 99
Parvocellular division, of red nucleus, 143. *See also* Red nucleus
Parvocellular stream. *See* Visual pathway
Past medical history, 235
Patellar reflex, 30, 240
Patient history, 234–236
Peduncle(s), 3. *See also* specific peduncles
Pedunculopontine tegmental nucleus, 138, 152f, 154, 208–209, 209f
Pelvic splanchnic nerve(s), 36, 37f, 38
Pelvic viscera, sympathetic innervation of, 35
Penis, dorsal nerve of, 43f
Peptides. *See* Neuropeptides
Peptidase, 214
Peptide-releasing hormone(s), 201
Peptide release-inhibiting hormones, 201
Perforant pathway, 194–195, 194f
Perforating cutaneous nerve, 44f
Periaqueductal gray matter, 93f, 94, 94f, 100, 216f, 217f
Pericallosal artery, 222f, 223
Pericardial branch, of vagus nerve, 102
Perikaryon, 1. *See also* Cell body
Perilymph, 121, 127
Perimeter, 238
Peripheral nerve(s)
afferent fibers of, 4
efferent fibers of, 4
formation of, 42
lesions of, 68–76, 70f, 145
clinical consequences of, 69
pattern of innervation of body surface, 43f–44f
Peripheral nervous system (PNS), 3
acetylcholine neurons in, 208–209
functional fibers types in, 23, 25t

peripheral nerve lesions, 68–76
regeneration of damaged nerves, 68–69
Peripheral neuropathy, 241
pernicious anemia and, 75
Peristriate cortex, 164, 173, 186. *See also* Visual association area
Peritoneum, inflammation of, 48
Perivascular spaces, 228
Periventricular hypothalamic nuclei. *See* Periventricular zone of hypothalamus
Periventricular zone, of hypothalamus, 197, 201, 210
Pernicious anemia, 75, 206
Personal/extrapersonal space, 185, 187–188
Personality change, 145
PET. *See* Positron emission tomography
Petrosal ganglion. *See* Cranial nerve IX, inferior ganglion
Petrotympanic fissure, 101
Pharyngeal branch
of glossopharyngeal nerve, 101
of vagus nerve, 102
Pharynx
motor innervation
from nucleus ambiguus, 99
from vagus nerve, 102
muscles of, 61
paralysis of, 113–114
parasympathetic innervation of, 36
sensory innervation of, 100, 101
Phenylethanolamine-N-methyl-transferase (PNMT), 210
Phrenic nerve, 102
Physical examination, 234, 236
Pia mater, 7, 228
Pill-rolling movement, 156
Pilocarpine, 168
Pineal, 5f, 80f, 118, 199, 202–203
tumor of, 118
Pineal recess, of third ventricle, 6f
Pinealocyte(s), 202–203
Piriform (pyriform) cortex, 177, 184, 189, 204–206. *See also* Primary olfactory cortex
Pitch of sound, 119–121
Pituitary, 5f, 7f, 78f, 79f, 159f, 161
amygdala modulation of, 196
anterior lobe of, 198f, 199, 201
hypothalamic-pituitary relationships, 197, 200–201
infundibulum (stalk) of, 197, 201
posterior lobe of, 198f, 200
tumor of, 165–166
Plantar response. *See* Babinski sign
Planum temporale, 122, 185
Plastic resistance, 31
Plastic rigidity, 239
Plasticity, of central nervous system, 145
Plate ending(s), 28f, 29. *See also* Gamma motoneuron(s)
Platysma muscle, 106
PNMT. *See* Phenylethanolamine-N-methyl-transferase
PNS. *See* Peripheral nervous system
Polyneuropathy, 69
Polysomnography, 243
Polysynaptic reflex, 27, 31
Pons, 5f, 6, 7f, 143f. *See also* Brain stem
anatomy of, 78f, 79–80, 80f, 90–93
anterior (ventral) aspect, 79–80
basilar portion, 90
caudal portion, 90–92, 91f
internal structures, 90–93, 91f, 92f
lateral aspect, 80
middle portion, 92–93, 92f
posterior (dorsal) aspect, 80
transverse section, 91f, 92f
ventral surface, 78f
blood supply to, 95f
cranial nerves of, 104–110
degeneration of, 146
development of, 12
lesions of, 114–116, 114f, 116f, 145, 171
cerebellopontine angle, 112f, 115
medial sector of caudal part, 114–115, 114f
middle region, 115–116, 116f
Pontine cistern, 227
Pontine fibers. *See* Pontocerebellar projections
Pontine nuclei, 90–92, 91f, 92f, 141, 141f
cerebral cortex fibers to, 184. *See also* Corticopontine fibers
Pontine reticulospinal tract, 64–65, 66f, 67, 90–91
Pontocerebellar projection(s), 91, 141, 142
Pontomedullary junction, 80
Portal veins. *See* Hypophyseal portal system
Position sense, 41, 109. *See also* Head position
loss of, 58, 113, 115–116, 146, 184
spinal cord lesions and, 73
testing of, 240
Positive afterpotential, 19
Positive feedback, 16
sodium channels and, 16
Positron emission tomography (PET), 245
activation scan, 245
Postcentral gyrus, 5f, 46, 54, 60–61
lesions of, 58
of parietal lobe, 54, 61
Postcentral sulcus, 5f
Posterior aphasia. *See* Fluent aphasia
Posterior antebrachial cutaneous nerve, 44f
Posterior brachial cutaneous nerve, 44f
Posterior cerebral artery, 95 95f, 222f, 223–225, 224f, 225f
occlusion of, 223–224
perforating branches of, 224
Posterior choroidal artery, 225f, 226
Posterior circulation, 221
Posterior cochlear nucleus. *See* Dorsal cochlear nucleus
Posterior commissure, 118, 202–203
Posterior communicating artery(ies), 225, 225f
Posterior femoral cutaneous nerve, 44f
Posterior hypothalamic nucleus, 88, 198f, 199
Posterior inferior cerebellar artery, 95, 95f, 225f
thrombosis of, 113

Posterior lobe, of cerebellum, 53f, 54, 129f, 137, 137f 142
Posterior neuropore, 11, 12f
Posterior perforated substance, 225
Posterior pituitary, 200
Posterior spinal artery, 75, 76f, 95f
Posterolateral fasciculus, 10f, 11f, 45f, 46, 66f
Posterolateral fissure. *See* Cerebellum, posterolateral fissure.
Posteromarginal nucleus, 11f, 46
Postganglionic neuron(s) of the autonomic nervous system, 33. *See also* Chain ganglia; Sympathetic trunk; Terminal ganglia of parasympathetic nervous system
Postganglionic parasympathetic neuron(s), 208. *See also* Terminal ganglia of parasympathetic nervous system
Postrotatory nystagmus, 132
Postsynaptic membrane, 2f, 19
Postsynaptic neuron(s), 19–21
Posture, 29, 64–65, 67, 130, 135, 142, 155
  assessment of, 238–239
  head, 144
  imbalance, 128
Potassium
  action potential and, 16, 17f
  astrocytes and, 3
  channels, 16, 18, 20, 208
  conductance, 17f
  efflux, 17f
  pain stimulus, 42
  resting membrane potential and, 15–16
  synaptic transmission and, 20
Potassium channel(s), 208
PPRF. *See* Paramedian pontine reticular formation
Praxis, 237–238
Precallosal region, 189
Precentral gyrus, 5f, 60
Precentral sulcus, 5f
Precuneus, 5f
Prefrontal cortex, 143, 173, 180, 185, 188–189, 197, 202, 211f
  lesions of, 188–189
Prefrontal leukotomy, 47
Preganglionic neuron(s) of the autonomic nervous system, 33, 208
Preganglionic parasympathetic cell body(ies), 25, 36, 37f, 83–86
Preganglionic sympathetic cell body(ies), 24f, 25, 37f
  acetylcholine and, 208
Premature ejaculation, 36
Premotor area, of cerebral cortex, 60–61, 150, 152, 183–184
  lesions of, 184
Preoccipital notch, 4, 5f
Preoptic recess, 6f
Preoptic region, 197, 198f, 201. *See also* Medial preoptic area; Lateral preoptic area
Present illness, 234–235
Pressure sensation, 109. *See also* Touch
Presynaptic ending, 2f, 19
  calcium channels of, 20
Presynaptic inhibition. *See* Inhibition, distal feedback
Presynaptic membrane, 2f
Presynaptic neuron(s), 19–21
Pretectal area, 159f, 161–163, 167, 203
Prevertebral ganglion, 24f, 34–35
Primary auditory cortex, 122, 123f,124, 185, 191
  bilateral representation of cochlea, 123f, 124, 185
  Brodmann's areas 41 and 42, 122, 185
  descending auditory pathway and, 124
  function(s)
    language interpretation, 124
    precise localization of sound, 124
    temporal analysis of sound, 122
  lesions of, 124, 185
  transverse temporal gyri, 122
Primary ending, muscle spindle and, 29
Primary fissure, of cerebellum, 137
Primary motor cortex (MI), 60–61, 71f, 150, 152, 175, 179f, 182, 183f, 184
  connections with thalamus, 179f, 182
  descending projections of, 60-63, 62f, 182
  lesions of, 182
  somatotopic organization of, 60, 182, 183f
Primary olfactory cortex, 177, 184, 186-187, 189, 193, 195–196, 204-206, 205f. *See also* Piriform cortex
Primary somatosensory cortex, 45f, 46–47, 54–56, 55f, 56f, 58, 60, 133, 150, 152, 175, 179f, 184–186
  columns of, 58
Primary taste area, 186
Primary vestibular area, 186
Primary visual cortex, 163-164, 185–186, 213. *See also* Striate cortex
  columns of, 164
  lesions of, 165
  retinotopic organization of, 163
Principal sensory nucleus of trigeminal nerve, 84f, 86, 92f, 93, 108f, 109. *See also* Cranial nerve V
Prodynorphin, 215
Proenkephalin, 215
Progesterone, 201
Prognosis, in neurologic disorder, 233
Progressive supranuclear palsy, 156, 245
Prohormone, 200
Prolactin, 201, 210
Prolactin-releasing hormone, 201
Pro-opiomelanocortin, 215
Proprioception, 23, 51–59, 55f
  loss of, 58
  pathways of, 51–57
  spinal cord lesions and, 58, 76
  testing of, 51
Proprioceptive receptor(s), 37, 41
Propriospinal pathway, 66f, 67
Prosencephalon, 12, 13f, 158
Prosopagnosia, 190
Protrusion of the tongue, 97
Proverbs, ability to interpret, 236–237
Pseudotumor cerebri. *See* Idiopathic intracranial hypertension
Pseudounipolar cell(s), 1, 23, 24f, 42
Pterygoid muscles, 101, 107–108

Pterygopalatine ganglion, 36, 99, 101
Ptosis, 35, 106, 116–117, 118
Pudendal nerve, 37, 37f
Pulvinar, 79f, 80f, 186f
  inferior and lateral parts of, 179f, 186
  medial part of, 179f, 187, 189
Pupil. *See also* Optic reflex(es); Pupillary reflex(es)
  Adie's tonic, 168–169
  Argyll Robertson, 169
  constriction of, 167–168
    in Horner's syndrome, 35
  dilatation of, 106, 117, 125, 168, 169
  fixed and unreactive, 118
  pupillary response, 167, 173
Pupillary constrictor muscle(s), 159f, 161, 167, 168. *See also* Sphincter muscle of pupil
Pupillary reflex(es)
  consensual light reflex, 167–168, 223
  direct light reflex, 167-168, 185, 223
  neural pathways for, 161–163, 167
  pupillary constriction accompanying accommodation, 168
Pure word deafness, 185
Purkinje cell(s), 137–138, 142, 218
Pursuit eye movement(s), 163, 169, 171–173, 171f, 184
Putamen, 148f–152f, 149–150, 149t, 153, 169, 179f, 180f, 211f, 214f, 218
  excitatory input from isocortex, 150, 151f
Pyramid, 7f, 61, 62f, 78, 78f, 79f, 81f, 82, 88, 88f, 89f, 90f, 112, 112f
Pyramidal cells of cerebral cortex
  in layer III, 175
  in layer V, 175
Pyramidal system, 148
Pyramidal tract, 61. *See* Corticobulbar tract; Corticospinal tract
  decussation of, 62f, 63, 78
Pyrogens, 201

Quadriceps femoris muscle, 30
Quadrigeminal plate. *See* Corpora quadrigemina
Quadriplegia, 72
Quadrantanopia, 165
Quanta, 20

Radial muscle of iris, 106. *See also* Sympathetic nervous system, innervation of eye
Radial nerve, 43f, 44f
Radicular pain, 49
  root lesions and, 73, 76
Ramus(i), 3
  ramus(i) communicans(tes), 24f, 34
Raphe nuclei, 49, 65, 87–88, 139, 203, 213, 216f, 217f
Raphe spinal tract, 29, 65
Rapid-eye movement (REM) sleep, 87–88, 154, 209
Raynaud's disease, 39
Raynaud's phenomenon, 38–39
Reactive hyperemia, 39
Reading test, 237
Recent memory, 236
Receptive field, 57–58, 163–164, 184
Receptor(s), *See also* specific types; Autoreceptors
  androgen, 201
  estrogen, 201
  hypothalamic, 200
    core body temperature, 201
    glucose, 202
  neurotransmitter, 1, 19, 20, 207–219
  sensory. *See* Sensory receptors
Rectal reflex, 38
Recurrent artery of Huebner. *See* Medial striate artery
Recurrent laryngeal nerve, 99, 102
Red nucleus, 64, 71f, 94, 94f, 142–143, 143f, 182, 217f
  lesions of, 117, 117f
  magnocellular division of, 66, 140f, 141f, 142
  parvocellular division of, 140f, 141f, 143
Referred pain, 48
Reflex(es), 27. *See also specific reflexes*
  corticospinal tract influence on, 63
  cutaneous, 31
  motor pathway lesions affecting, 72–73
  neurologic examination and, 240
  of pelvic parasympathetic nervous system, 38
  pupillary, 161, 167–169
  of vagal system, 102–103
Reflex arcs, 24f
Reflexive saccade(s), 169
Reflexive visually guided saccade(s), 169
Refractory period, 18–19
Regeneration, of nerve cells and fibers, 68–69
Relative refractory period, 19
REM sleep. *See* Rapid-eye movement sleep
Remote memory, 236
Renshaw cell(s), 28f, 29, 208
Repetition test, 237
Repolarization, 16, 17f
Reproductive system, 201
  pelvic splanchnic nerves and, 36
Resistance, 16, 239
Respiration, 103
  center, of medulla, 102
  rate, vagal system and, 102
  reticulospinal tract influence, 65, 102
Restiform body. *See* Inferior cerebellar peduncle
Resting membrane potential, 15–16
Reticular activating system. *See* Ascending reticular activating system
Reticular formation, 45f, 46–48, 64–65, 86–88, 88f, 89f, 90f, 92f, 93f, 94f, 182. *See also* Raphe nuclei; Reticulospinal tracts; Vagal system, reflexes
  ascending projections from, 86–87, 91, 100, 182
  cholinergic neurons in, 87
  connections with cerebellum, 140, 142
  control of gamma motoneurons, 30
  functions of, 86
  hypothalamus and, 86, 199
  lateral zone of, 86
  lesions of, 112, 113
  medial zone of, 86

Reticular formation *(Continued)*
noradrenergic cell groups of, 87, 211–212
pain and, 45f, 46–48
serotonergic cell groups of, 87
sleep and, 87
ventrolateral, 102
vestibular connections and, 130
visceral reflexes and, 100
visceral network, 100–101
Reticular nucleus, of thalamus, 178, 179f, 182, 218
Reticulocerebellar fiber(s), 140
Reticulohypothalamic pathway, 46, 201
Reticulospinal tract(s), 29, 74f, 90–91, 103. *See also* Medullary reticulospinal tract; Pontine reticulospinal tract
decerebrate rigidity and, 131
lesions of, 70
motor activity and, 64–65
Retina, 158–161, 159f, 163, 210
bipolar cells of, 160–161, 160f
hyperpolarization of rods and cones by light, 158–160
lesions of, 167–168
Retinal slip, 172–173
Retinal vein, 229
Retinotopic projections in visual pathway
lateral geniculate nucleus, 161
superior colliculus, 161
visual cortex, 162f, 163
Retrosplenial area, 177, 189
Reuptake, of monoamines, 210
Rhinal sulcus, 205f
Rhodopsin, 158
Rhombencephalon, 12
Rigidity, 31, 155–156
assessment of, 239
cogwheel, 156
decerebrate, 131
Rinne test, 124–125, 238
Rods, 158–161, 160f, 167
hyperpolarization by light, 158–160
influence on ganglion cells through bipolar cells, 160–161, 160f
Romberg sign, 58–59, 75, 239–240
Rostral interstitial nucleus of the medial longitudinal fasciculus, 131, 170
Rostral spinocerebellar tract, 52–54, 53f, 140, 141
Rotation test, 132
Rotatory nystagmus, 133
Round window, 120f, 122
Rubor, 39
Rubro-olivary tract, 91, 143
Rubrospinal tract, 11f, 64, 66, 66f, 71f, 74f, 88f, 89f, 90f, 92f, 93f, 94, 141f, 142
lesions of, 70

Saccade(s), 154, 163, 169–170, 170f, 184. *See also* Eye movements
lesions of saccadic pathway, 170–171
Saccadic intrusion(s), 171
Saccadic palsy, 170
Saccadic pursuit, 172
Saccule, 120f, 127–128, 130
Sacral division, of parasympathetic nervous system, 36
Sacral outflow, of parasympathetic nervous system, 34
Sacral sparing, 74
Sacral spinal cord, 7
Sacral spinal nerve(s), 7, 9
Salivary gland(s)
parasympathetic innervation of, 36, 99, 102, 106
branches of VII and IX innervating, 101
Salivary-taste reflex, 102
Salivatory nucleus(i), 84f, 85, 98, 98f, 99, 102
Saltatory conduction, 18
Saphenous nerve, 43f, 44f
Satellite cell(s), 3
Scala media, 120f, 121–122
Scala tympani, 120f, 121–122
Scala vestibuli, 120f, 121–122
Scalp, sensory innervation of, 107
Schizophrenia, 211, 245
Schwann cell(s), 2–3, 2f, 68
Scotoma, 164–165
Scrotal branch of perineal nerve, 43f
Second messenger system, 16, 208
Secondary auditory area, 122, 185
Secondary ending(s), muscle spindle and, 29
Secondary motor area, 60
Secondary somatosensory cortex (SII), 45f, 47, 60, 184–185, 186
Secondary visual cortex, 185
Segmental reflex(es), 27
Seizure, 229
Semicircular canal(s), 120f, 121, 127–128, 130, 131, 172
Semilunar ganglion. *See* Trigeminal ganglion
Semilunar nucleus. *See* Ventral posteromedial nucleus
Sensation
development of sense organs, 12
neurologic examination and, 240
Sensorimotor cortex, 61, 63, 151f, 152
Sensorineural deafness, 124–126
diagnosis of, 124–125
Sensory aphasia. *See* Fluent aphasia
Sensory area(s), of cerebral cortex, 184–186
Sensory cell column, in medulla oblongata, 82–83
Sensory decussation. *See* Decussation of the spinal lemniscus
Sensory dissociation, 75
Sensory ganglia. *See also* Dorsal root ganglia
afferent fibers of cranial nerves originating in, 85
Sensory loss, dissociated, 112
Sensory neglect, 188, 222–223
Sensory nerve fiber(s), 25
Sensory receptor(s), 4, 41, 193. *See also specific receptors*
Septal region 149f, 177, 189, 193, 195, 203, 208, 211f, 216f. *See also* Medial septal nucleus
Septum pellucidum, 5f, 180f
Serotonergic fiber(s), 65, 87, 138–139
Serotonin, 19, 209, 213, 214f
analgesia and, 49, 65
in pain sensation, 42, 65, 213
synthesis of, 210
Serotonin cell(s), in raphe nuclei, 65, 87, 213
Serotonin receptor(s), 213
Serotonin reuptake inhibitor(s), 213
Sexual behavior, 197–201, 206, 210
Sexual function, 36
drugs affecting, 36

Sheath of Schwann, 1–2
Shunt for cerebrospinal fluid, 231
Signal transduction, 16
Similarities, ability to interpret, 236–237
Simple spike. *See* Spike
Single photon emission computed tomography (SPECT), 245
Skeletal muscle(s), 4. *See also* Muscle(s); Somatic muscle fiber(s); Voluntary muscle fiber
Skin, sensory receptors in, 31
Sleep, 87–88. *See also* Rapid eye movement sleep; Slow wave sleep
  polysomnography, 243
Sleep disturbance, 243
Sleep-waking cycle, 65, 87-88, 198–200
Slow pain, 47
Slow-wave sleep, 87–88, 218
Smell, sense of. *See* Olfactory *entries*
Smooth muscle(s), 4
  autonomic nervous system and, 33
  spinal nerves and, 25
  vagal system and, 99
Smooth-pursuit eye movement(s), 135
Snellen card, 236
Social behavior, 100–101, 154, 188-189, 193, 196, 200, 206, 210
Social history, 235–236
Sodium
  action potential and, 16, 17f
  channels, 16, 18
  conductance, 17f, 160
  influx, 16, 17f
  resting membrane potential and, 15–16
  synaptic transmission and, 20
Sodium-potassium pump, 16
Soft palate
  in gag reflex, 103
  motor innervation of,
    from nucleus ambiguus, 99
    from vagus nerve 102
  paralysis of, 113-114
  sensory innervation of, 100
  vagal system and, 99–100, 102–103
Solitary tract, 63, 90, 90f, 100, 103, 112f
  nucleus of, 88f, 89f, 90, 90f, 98, 98f, 100, 102–103, 112f. *See also* Nucleus solitarius
Somatic fiber(s), 23. *See also* General somatic afferent fiber(s); General somatic efferent fiber(s); Special somatic afferent fiber(s)
Somatic motor fiber(s), 4
  of pudendal nerve, 37
Somatic muscle fiber(s), 61
Somatic sensation(s), 41
Somatic sensory fiber(s), 4. *See also* General somatic afferent fiber(s); Special somatic afferent fiber(s)
Somatosensory association area(s), 175, 184-185
Somatosensory cortex. *See* Primary somato-sensory cortex
Somatosensory evoked potential(s), 243
Somatostatin, 201, 215, 218
Somatostatin receptor(s), 218
Somatotopic organization, 46, 54, 182, 184. *See also* Homunculus
Sound, 119. *See also* Hearing
  amplitude of, 119
  decoding pattern of complex sounds, 124
  frequency of, 119, 122, 185
  localization of, 122, 124, 185
  loudness of, 119
  pitch of, 119, 121, 122
  temporal patterns of, 122, 185
Spasmodic torticollis, 157
Spastic hemiplegia, 222
Spastic paralysis, 70–72
Spasticity, 31, 76, 182
  assessment of, 239
  brain stem lesions and, 113-115
  spinal cord lesions and, 73
  upper motoneuron lesions and, 72, 75
Spatial processing, 142, 143
  impaired, 145
  neglect, 188
  orientation, 186
  relationships, 187
  in visual system, 164
Special fiber(s), 23
Special somatic afferent (SSA) fiber(s), 83, 86
Special somatic afferent (SSA) cell column, 84, 84f, 85f, 86
Special visceral afferent (SVA) fiber(s), cranial nerves and, 83, 86
Special visceral afferent (SVA) cell column, 84, 84f, 85f, 86, 98f, 99
Special visceral efferent (SVE) fiber(s)
  cranial nerves and, 84–86
  facial nerve, 106
  trigeminal nerve, 107
Special visceral efferent (SVE) cell column, 84–86, 84f, 85f, 98
Special visceral motor column, 98
SPECT. *See* Single photon emission computed tomography
Speech, 90, 190–192. *See also* Aphasia
Sphincter muscle of pupil, 36, 105. *See also* Pupillary constrictor muscle
Spike. *See also* Action potential
  complex spike, 139
  simple spike, 139
Spike potential, 19
Spina bifida, 11
Spinal accessory nerve. *See* Cranial nerve XI
Spinal accessory nucleus, 64, 78, 84f, 97. *See also* Cranial nerve XI
Spinal arachnoid villi, 227
Spinal cord
  afferents to cerebellar cortex, 142
  anatomy of, 7–9, 8f
  cell columns of, 9
  cross section of, 10f, 11f
  development of, 11–14, 13f
  enlargements of, 7
  function of lateral, medial, and propriospinal pathways in, 66–67, 66f
  funiculi of, 9, 10f
  ganglia of, 13f. *See* Dorsal root ganglia
  hemisection of, 73–75, 74f
  hypothalamus and, 199–200
  imaging of, 244
  internal anatomy of, 9–11

Spinal cord *(Continued)*
laminae of, 9–11
lesions of, 38, 68–76
effect on touch sensation, 58–59, 59f
nuclei of, 9
regions of, 7, 8f
subacute degeneration of, 75
transection of, 73
transition to brain stem, 82–83
transverse sections of, 9, 10f, 11f
tumor of, 69, 76
extramedullary, 76, 242
white matter to gray matter ratio, 9
Spinal lemniscal system, 52, 54–57, 55f, 81f
lesions of, 58-59, 59f
at transition from spinal cord to brain stem, 82
Spinal nerve(s), 3–4, 7–9, 8f. *See also specific nerves*
fibers of, 23–26
formation of peripheral nerves, 42
functional components of, 24f
Spinal nerve root, 7–9. *See also* Dorsal root(s); Ventral root(s)
lesions of, 68–76
Spinal nucleus of V, 45f, 47, 84f, 85f, 86, 88-90, 88f-91f, 95, 99, 101, 110, 112f, 216f, 217f. *See also* Cranial nerve V
Spinal reflex(es), 27–32. *See also* Muscle tone
Spinal shock, 73
Spinal tract of V, 45f, 89–90, 88f-91f, 95, 101, 110, 112f, 113. *See also* Cranial nerve V
Spinal vestibular nucleus. *See* Descending vestibular nucleus
Spinocerebellar ataxia, 145–146
Spinocerebellar tract, 52, 137, 142. *See also* Cuneocerebellar tact, Dorsal spinocerebellar tract, Rostral spinocerebellar, tract, Ventral spinocerebellar tract
lesions of, 59
at transition from spinal cord to brain stem, 81f, 82
Spinocervicothalamic pathway. *See* Lateral cervical system
Spinoreticular tract, 45f, 46–47, 201
control of urination and, 38
somatic and visceral sensations and, 42
Spinothalamic tract, 45f, 46, 52, 54, 82, 88f–94f, 94, 184
blood supply to, 75, 76f
lesions of, 48, 49, 58–59, 59f, 74f, 76 112f, 113, 116
somatic sensations and, 42
syringomyelia and, 75
thrombosis of anterior spinal artery and, 75–76
at transition from spinal cord to brain stem, 82
Spinothalamic tractotomy, 48
Spiral ganglion, 121
cells of, 120f, 122, 123f
Spiral lamina, 121
Splanchnic nerve, 24f, 34, 35, 36, 48. *See also* Lumbar splanchnic nerves; Pelvic splanchnic nerves; Thoracic splanchnic nerves
Spontaneous nystagmus, 132–133, 144
Sporadic olivopontocerebellar atrophy, 146
Squint, 105
Stance, disorders of, 144
Stapedius muscle, 106, 107, 110, 125
Stapes, 119, 120f, 121
Startle reflex, 125
Static tremor, 145
Station, assessment of, 239. *See also* Posture
Stellate cell(s)
of cerebellar cortex, 137, 139
of cerebral cortex, 175
Stellate ganglion. *See* Cervicothoracic ganglion
Stereocilia
of cochlear hair cells, 121
of vestibular hair cells, 128
Stereognosis, 51, 184, 240
Sternomastoid muscle, 97, 238
Strabismus, 105–106, 116, 118, 238. *See also specific types*
Straight sinus, 228f
Strength, assessment of, 239
Stress, response to, 199, 215
Stretch reflex, 27, 30, 52, 130, 146, 182, 240. *See also* Deep tendon reflex(es)
loss of, 146
Striae medullaris, 79, 80f, 202–203
Stria terminalis, 80f, 194f, 196–197, 199
Striate cortex, 163, 185. *See also* Cuneus; Lingual gyrus; Primary visual cortex
lesions of, 165, 185
receptive field characteristics of cells of, 163–164
Striatum. *See* Dorsal striatum; Ventral striatum
Striola, 128
Stroke, 49, 67, 112, 125, 145, 174, 192, 219, 221, 229, 233, 241, 244. *See also* Cerebrovascular disease; Hemorrhage; Infarction; Ischemic vascular disease
Stupor, 236
Stylohyoid muscle, 106
Stylomastoid foramen, 106
Stylopharyngeal branch, of glossopharyngeal nerve, 101
Stylopharyngeus muscle, 101
Subacute degeneration of the spinal cord, 75
Subarachnoid hemorrhage, 230, 241–242, 244
Subarachnoid space, 7, 8f, 227–230, 228f
Subcallosal region, 177, 189
Subcutaneous tissue, sensory receptors in, 31
Subiculum, 194–195, 194f
Submandibular ganglion, 36, 99, 101–102
Substance P, 20, 42, 46, 151, 215–218, 217f
Substantia gelatinosa, 9, 11f, 45f, 46, 86, 217, 217f
Substantia innominata, 177, 189, 193, 196
Substantia nigra, 93–94, 93f, 94f, 139, 143, 143f, 149, 149t, 211, 211f, 216f, 217f, 218
degeneration of, 155
effect on thalamus, 151, 152f, 153, 153f
pars compacta, 149t, 151f, 152f, 153–154, 153f, 209f

pars reticulata, 149t, 150, 151, 151f, 152f, 153–154, 153f, 169, 170f, 184, 217
Subthalamic nucleus, 148f, 149, 149t, 152f, 153, 153f, 224
decreased activity in hyperkinetic movement disorders, 156–157
Subthalamus, 151, 177
Sulci, 4. *See also specific sulci*
Sulcus limitans, 80f, 89
Superficial peroneal nerve, 43f
Superficial petrosal nerve, 101
Superficial reflex(es), 72–73, 113
Superior cerebellar artery, 95, 95f, 225f
Superior cerebellar peduncle, 53f, 54, 79f, 80, 80f, 91f, 93–94, 141–142, 141f, 151f
decussation of, 92f, 93, 93f
lesions of, 117, 225
Superior cervical cardiac rami, 102. *See also* Cardiac nerves of the cervical sympathetic ganglia
Superior cervical ganglion, 34–35
Superior colliculus, 5f, 46, 64, 67, 79f, 80f, 82, 94f, 117f, 118, 152f, 154, 161, 169, 170f, 217f
Superior concha, 204
Superior frontal gyrus, 5f, 184
Superior frontal sulcus, 5f
Superior ganglion
of glossopharyngeal nerve, 101
of vagus nerve, 101
Superior laryngeal internal branch, of vagus nerve, 102
Superior mesenteric ganglion, 35. *See also* Prevertebral ganglion
Superior oblique muscle, 105, 172
Superior olivary nuclear complex, 91, 91f, 121, 122, 123f, 124
Superior orbital fissure, 104–105
Superior parietal lobule, 5f
Superior rectus muscle, 105, 172
Superior sagittal sinus, 228, 228f
Superior salivatory nucleus, 84f, 85, 98–99, 98f, 102
Superior temporal gyrus, 5f, 133, 171f, 172, 185, 187, 190
Superior temporal sulcus, 5f
Superior vestibular nucleus, 91f, 129f, 130–131
Supplementary motor area (MII), 60–61, 143, 150, 152, 183
lesions of, 184
Suprachiasmatic nucleus, 161, 197–199, 198f
Supraclavicular nerve, 43f, 44f
Supramarginal gyrus, 5f, 188, 190
Supranuclear gaze palsy, 172
Supraoptic nucleus, 198–200, 198f, 209, 209f
Supraspinal reflex(es), 27
Sural nerve, 43f, 44f
SVA fiber(s). *See* Special visceral afferent fiber(s)
SVE fiber(s). *See* Special visceral afferent fiber(s)
Swallowing, 75, 90, 99, 113
Sweat gland, 208
cholinergic innervation, 34
sympathetic innervation, 34
Sweating, 200, 202
Sydenham's chorea, 156
Sympathetic ganglia, 24f
norepinephrine cells in, 211–212
Sympathetic nervous system, 33–36. *See also* Autonomic nervous system
acetylcholine and, 208
clinical aspects of function, 35–36
control of circadian rhythms, 199
innervation of abdominal and pelvic viscera, 35
innervation of adrenal gland, 35
innervation of body wall, 34
innervation of eye, 35, 106
innervation of head and neck, 34–35
innervation of pineal, 202-203
innervation of thoracic viscera, 35
innervation of urinary bladder, 37
neurotransmitters of, 34
Sympathetic trunk, 34, 37f. *See also* Chain ganglia
cervical part of, 34
Synapse, 1, 2f, 19
Synaptic cleft, 2f, 19
Synaptic contact(s)
histogenesis of nervous system and, 14
neuron deprived of, 21
Synaptic delay, 19
Synaptic potential, 20. *See also* Excitatory postsynaptic potential(s); Inhibitory postsynaptic potential(s)
Synaptic vesicle(s), 2f, 19
Syncope, 102
Syntax, 190. *See also* Aphasia
Syphilis, 241
Syringomyelia, 74f, 75
System review, 235
Systemic lupus erythematosus, 39

Tactile agnosia, 190
Tactile discrimination, 51–59, 55f, 109. *See also* Stereognosis; Two-point discrimination
loss of, 58, 113, 115–117, 184
pathways of, 51–57
physiologic aspects of, 57–58
spinal cord lesions and, 73
testing of, 51
Tactile localization, 240
Taste, 90, 186. *See also* Special visceral afferent(s)
loss of, 107
Taste bud, 100, 202
Taste system, 99–100. *See also* Primary taste area
ascending taste (gustatory) tract, 91, 100, 202
Tear secretion. *See* Lacrimal gland
Tectopontine tract, 161
Tectorial membrane, 120f, 121
Tectospinal tract, 64, 65, 66f, 67, 89f, 90, 90f-92f, 94, 161
auditory reflexes and, 125
motor activity and, 63–64
Tectum, of midbrain, 82, 93, 212f. *See also* Inferior colliculus; Superior colliculus; Tectospinal tract
Teeth, pain sensation from, 109
Tegmentum
of medulla, 79
of midbrain, 93
of pons, 90
Tela choroidea, 77–78, 177
Telencephalic limbic system, 193–197, 194f
Telencephalon, 198

Temperature sensation, 41–50, 109
loss of, 113, 115–117
pathways for, 42–47
spinal cord lesions and, 73
spinal cord tumor and, 76
syringomyelia and, 75
testing of, 240
Temporal bone, 121
Temporal lobe, 4, 148f, 149f
amygdala and, 195
auditory cortex of, 122, 123f, 124. *See also* Auditory cortex; Primary auditory cortex
eye movements and, 171f, 172–173
herniation of, 105, 241
heteromodal association areas of. *See* Temporoparietal association area. *See also* Heteromodal association area(s).
hippocampus and, 194f, 195
visual field defect with lesions of, 165
Temporal lobe epilepsy, 195
Temporal pattern, of sound, 122
Temporal pole, 5f, 7f, 162f, 177, 189, 193, 195, 205f
Temporalis muscle, 107, 109
Temporoparietal association area, 173, 185, 187–188, 195. *See also* Heteromodal association areas
lesions of, 187–188
Tendon(s), 28–29. *See also* Golgi tendon organ(s)
Tensor tympani muscle, 107, 125
Tensor veli palatini muscle, 107
Tentorium cerebelli, 6f, 95, 105, 135, 230, 241
Terminal ganglia, of parasympathetic nervous system, 36, 99. *See also* Ciliary ganglion; Otic ganglion; Pterygopalatine ganglion; Submandibular ganglion
Testosterone, 201
Thalamic fasciculus, 151, 152f
Thalamic nuclei, 133, 180–182. *See also* Thalamus
destruction of, 47
intralaminar, 87
pain and, 47
sensory, 122
with subcortical and diffuse cortical connections, 181–182
Thalamic reticular nucleus. *See* Reticular nucleus, of thalamus
Thalamic syndrome. *See* Central pain
Thalamocortical connection(s), 54, 127, 143, 174, 178, 179f, 180f, 206
to layer IV of cerebral cortex, 175
topographic pattern of, 179f, 180–182
Thalamocortical neuron(s)
basal ganglia disinhibition of, 156–157
basal ganglia inhibition by indirect loop, 153, 153f
Thalamus, 80f, 94, 142–143, 143f, 148f, 150f, 174, 177–178, 179f, 180f, 209f, 212f, 216f, 217f. *See also* Anterior nuclear group; Intralaminar nuclei; Lateral nuclear group; Medial thalamic nuclei; Reticular nucleus; Ventral nuclear group
amygdala and, 196
blood supply to, 224f, 226
functions of, 178
hippocampal formation and, 195
influence of substantia nigra and globus pallidus on, 151, 152f
internal capsule and, 180–181, 180f
isocortex and, 175
lesions of, 49, 58
pain and, 46–47
Thermal sensation. *See* Temperature sensation
Thermal test. *See* Caloric test
Thermoregulation, 198, 200–201
Theta activity, 242
Thiamine. *See* Vitamin B1
Third ventricle, 5f, 6f, 80f, 143f, 177, 202, 227, 228f
Thoracic branch, of vagus nerve, 102
Thoracic spinal cord, 7, 10f
Thoracic spinal nerve(s), 7
lateral cutaneous rami of, 44f
Thoracic spine, bullet lodged in, 68, 76
Thoracic splanchnic nerve(s), 35. *See also* Splanchnic nerve
innervation of abdominal vicera, 35
innervation of adrenal gland, 35
Thoracic viscera
sympathetic innervation of, 35
vagal system and, 100
Thoracolumbar outflow, of sympathetic system, 33
Threshold stimulus, 19, 20
Thrombosis, 221, 223
of anterior spinal artery, 75–76, 76f
Thyroid-stimulating hormone, 201
Thyrotropin-releasing hormone, 218
Tic, 157
Tic douloureux, 110
Tickling sensation, 51
Tinnitus, 124, 133
Tissue plasminogen activator, 67, 96, 118, 192
Titubation, 144
Tongue. *See also* Taste *entries*
atrophy of, 97, 103, 113
facial nerve and, 106–107
motor innervation of, 89, 97
paralysis of, 103, 112
sensory innervation of
general sensation, 101, 109
taste, 101
Tonotopic organization, 122, 124, 185
Topographic organization. *See also* Homunculus; Retinotopic organization; Somatotopic organization; Tonotopic organization
of basal ganglia loops, 150–151
of cortical input to striatum, 150
of raphe projections, 213
Touch, 51–59, 56f
light. *See* Light touch
localization of, 185
pathways of, 42, 51–57
sensation of, 41–42. *See also* Tactile discrimination
spinal cord lesions and, 58–59, 59f, 73
Touch-pressure sensation, 41–42
Tourette's syndrome, 157

Toxin(s)
effect on synaptic transmission, 20
neuromuscular junction and, 21
Trabeculae, 7
Trachea
cough reflex and, 103
sensory innervation from cranial nerve X, 100
Tracheotomy, 99
Tract, 3
Tractotomy, of spinothalamic tract, 48
Tractus solitarius. *See* Solitary tract
Trail ending, 28f, 29–30. *See also* Gamma motoneuron
Transverse cervical nerve, 43f, 44f
Transverse pontine fiber(s), 141
Transverse temporal gyri, 122, 123f, 185. *See also* Auditory cortex; Auditory association area
Trapezius muscle, 97, 238
Trapezoid body, 91, 91f, 123f, 124
nuclei of, 122, 124
Tremor, 145, 146, 155, 156, 240
in cerebellar dysfunction, 145–146
of Parkinson's disease, 156
Triceps reflex, 240
Trigeminal ganglion, 45f, 46, 89, 109, 217f
Trigeminal nerve. *See* Cranial nerve V
Trigeminal neuralgia. *See* Tic douloureux
Trigeminal pathways
to cerebellum, 137, 141
to cerebral cortex, 45f, 46–47, 108f, 109–110
lesions of, 49, 110
to reticular formation, 46–47
Trigeminothalamic tract(s), 45f, 46–47, 92f–94f, 184
dorsal trigeminothalamic tract, 109
lesions of, 49
ventral trigeminothalamic tract, 109
Trigger zone, 110
Trochlear nerve. *See* Cranial nerve IV
Trochlear nucleus, 64, 84, 84f, 93f, 94, 105, 131, 170
Trophic factor(s)
CNS synapses and, 21
in development of nervous system, 14
neuromuscular junction and, 21, 69–70
Trophic hormone(s), 201
Tryptophan, 210, 213
Tuber cinereum, 197
Tuberal region, of hypothalamus, 197, 199. *See also* Lateral tuberal nuclei
Tuberohypophyseal projection(s), 210
Tuberoinfundibular projection(s), 210
Tuberomammillary nucleus, 199
Tumor
brain, 69, 125, 229–230, 234, 241
brain stem, 112, 230
cerebellar, 230
clivus, 103
pineal gland, 118
pituitary, 165–166
spinal cord, 69, 76
Tuning curve, 122
Tuning fork test(s), 124–125
Tunnel vision, 165, 224
Two-point discrimination, 51, 184
testing of, 58, 240
Tympanic branch, of glossopharyngeal nerve, 101
Tympanic membrane, 119, 120f, 124
Tyrosine, 210
Tyrosine hydroxylase, 210

Ulnar nerve, 43f, 44f
Uncinate fasciculus, 130
Uncus, 7f, 195, 196f, 205f, 240. *See also* Herniation, of temporal lobe
Unimodal association area(s), 175, 177, 178f
auditory, 185
somatosensory, 184–185
visual, 185–186
Unit potential(s), 20
Unmyelinated fiber(s), 1–3, 25
conduction velocity of, 18, 25t
Upper motoneuron(s), 61
Upper motoneuron lesion(s), 70–72, 75
Uremia, 229
Urethra, external sphincter of, 37, 37f
Urinary bladder
lesions that affect function of, 38, 73
motor innervation of, 36–37, 37f
proprioceptors in wall of, 37
Urinary tract. *See* Genitourinary tract
Urination, voluntary control of, 38. *See also* Micturition
incontinence, 38, 230
Utricle, 120f, 127–128, 130

Vagal system, 98–103, 98f. *See also* Cranial nerve VII; Cranial nerve IX; Cranial nerve X; Cranial nerve XI; Nervus intermedius
cell columns of origin, 98–99
external course and distribution of nerves of, 101–102
general visceral sensory portion of, 100–101
innervation of branchial muscles, 99
innervation of viscera, 99
reflexes of, 102–103
somatic sensory innervation of auricle and external auditory meatus, 101
taste functions of, 99–100
Vagal trigone, 79, 80f
Vagus nerve. *See* Cranial nerve X
Varicella virus, 50
Vasoactive intestinal peptide, 46, 215
Vasodilatation, Horner's syndrome and, 35
Vasogenic edema, 229
Vasopressin, 20, 199–200, 218
Vasopressin receptor(s), 218
Vasospasm, of digital arteries, 39
Venous sinus. *See* Dural venous sinus
Ventral acoustic stria, 122, 123f
Ventral amygdaloid pathway, 194f, 196–197, 199
Ventral anterior thalamic nucleus, 151, 152f, 154, 179f, 188
Ventral cochlear nucleus, 122
Ventral corticospinal tract, 11f, 62f, 63, 66, 66f, 74f, 81f
Ventral funiculus, 9, 10f

Ventral horn(s), 9, 10f, 24f
cell columns of, 11f
lesions of, 75
Ventral lateral thalamic nucleus, 133, 141f, 142, 143, 151, 151f, 152f, 179f, 186
caudal portion of, 182
oralis portion of, 184
Ventral median fissure, 9, 10f, 78f
Ventral mesencephalic tegmentum, 139
Ventral nuclear group of thalamus, 177, 180
Ventral pallidum, 149, 149t, 154, 203
Ventral posterolateral nucleus (VPL), 45f, 46, 47, 49, 54, 55f, 133, 179f, 184, 186
Ventral posteromedial nucleus (VPM), 45f, 47, 49, 100, 108f, 109, 179f, 184
parvocellular division of, 186
Ventral root(s), 7, 10f, 24f
lesions of, 70f, 73
pain and, 42
Ventral spinocerebellar tract, 11f, 52, 53f, 54, 88f-90f, 140f, 141
Ventral striatum, 149, 149f, 149t, 152, 154, 181, 189, 197, 216f, 217f, 218
Ventral tegmental area (VTA), 87, 149, 149t, 154, 203, 211, 211f, 216f
Ventral tegmental decussation, 64, 71f, 94, 94f
Ventral trigeminothalamic tract, 109
Ventral white commissure, 10f, 42, 45f, 46, 62f, 63, 75
Ventricle(s), 6–7. *See also* Cerebral aqueduct; Fourth ventricle, Lateral ventricles, Third ventricle
cerebrospinal fluid circulation in, 227
choroid plexuses in, 227, 230
Ventrobasal complex, 46
Ventrolateral sulcus, 9, 10f, 78, 79f
Ventromedial brain stem system, 67
Ventromedial nucleus, of the hypothalamus, 198f, 199, 201–202, 216f
Verbal paraphasia, 192
Vergence eye movements, 169, 173, 184
Vermis, 91f, 129f, 135, 144, 162f, 171f, 172
Vertebra(ae), 8f
Vertebral artery, 95, 95f, 221, 222f, 225f
dissection from injury, 113
occlusion of, 113
Vertebral column, 7
Vertical diplopia, 105
Vertical nystagmus, 133
Vertical saccade(s), 170
Vertigo, 95, 128, 132–133
Vesical plexus, 37
Vesical reflex, 37–38
Vesicle(s), of developing brain, 12–13
Vestibular cortex, 184, 186-187
Vestibular ganglion (of Scarpa), 128, 129, 129f
Vestibular hair cell(s), 127, 128
Vestibular nuclei, 67, 80f, 84f, 85f, 89, 90f, 91f, 92, 130, 137, 140, 140f, 142, 172. *See also* Descending (inferior) vestibular nucleus; Medial vestibular nucleus; Lateral vestibular nucleus; Superior vestibular nucleus
damage to, 113, 132
Vestibular system, 127–133. *See also* Vestibulospinal tract
cortex, 184, 186–187
functions of, 127
clinical testing of, 132
inner ear, 127–128
sensory aspects of stimulation, 133
vestibular nerve, 89, 129–130, 129f, 140. *See also* Cranial nerve VIII
Vestibule, of inner ear, 120f, 121
Vestibulocerebellar connection(s), 130
Vestibulocochlear nerve. *See* Cranial nerve VIII
Vestibulo-ocular system, 91, 131–133, 169, 172–173
clinical tests of function, 132–133
organization of, 172
reflexes of, 131–132, 169
testing and identifying abnormalities in, 172–173
Vestibulospinal tract, 65, 74f, 130–131
decerebrate rigidity and, 131
lesions of, 70
medial longitudinal fasciculus and, 65
motor activity and, 65
Vestibulothalamocortical pathway, 130, 133, 179f
Vibration sense, 51–52
loss of, 58, 113, 115–117, 146
spinal cord lesions and, 73
testing of, 58, 240
Virchow-Robin space, 228
Visceral afferent fiber(s), 4, 47, 85–86, 90, 100. *See also* General visceral afferent fiber(s); Special visceral afferent fiber(s)
Visceral fiber(s), 23
Visceral motor fiber(s). *See* General visceral efferent fiber(s); Special visceral efferent fiber(s)
Visceral motor neuron(s), 4, 33
Visceral pain, 47–48
Visceral reflex(es), 24f, 100
Visceral sensory column, of brain stem, 98–99
Visceral sensory pathways, 100, 202
Vision, 158–166, 185–186. *See also* Eye(s)
Visual acuity, 158, 165
decreased, 167, 172, 173
testing of, 172, 236, 238
Visual agnosia, 189–190
Visual association area, 163, 175, 179f, 185–186. *See also* Peristriate cortex
Visual cortex, 161, 162f, 163, 170f, 171f, 172, 179f
lesions of, 165
near-point reaction and, 168
receptive field characteristics of, 163–164
Visual evoked potential(s), 243
Visual field, 159f, 162f, 185
testing of, 238
Visual field defect(s), 159f, 185
altitudinal pattern, 165
lesions causing, 165
testing for, 164–165
Visual pathway(s), 158, 159f, 161–163
information processing in, 163–164

lesions of, 164–165
magnocellular stream, 164
parvocellular stream, 164
Visual perception, 163
Visual pigment, 158
Visually guided saccade(s), 163
Vitamin B_1 deficiency, 146
Vitamin B_{12} deficiency, 69
Vocalization. *See* Speech
Volitional saccade(s), 169
Volitional visually guided saccade(s), 169
Voltage-gated channel(s), 16, 20
Voltage-sensitive channel(s). *See* Voltage-gated channel(s)
Volume conduction, 242
Voluntary muscle fiber, 2f. *See also* Skeletal muscle(s); Somatic muscle fiber(s)
Vomiting, 230
reflex, 103
Von Frey hairs, 51
VPL. *See* Ventral posterolateral nucleus
VPM. *See* Ventral posteromedial nucleus
VTA. *See* Ventral tegmental area

Wakefulness, 87–88, 154, 209
Walking, 54, 155. *See also* Locomotion
Wallenberg's syndrome, 112f, 113–114
Wallerian degeneration, 68
Water balance, 199, 200
Wax, in ear, 125
Weber test, 124–125, 238
Weber's syndrome, 111, 116–118, 117f
Weigert method, 88
Wernicke's aphasia. *See* Fluent aphasia
Wernicke's area, 185, 187, 191, 191f
lesions of, 192
Wernicke-Korsakoff disease, 146
White matter, 3
spinal cord, 9
White ramus(i) communicans(tes), 24f, 34
Wolverines. *See* Go Blue
Writing test, 237
Wryneck, 157

X-cell(s), 164
X-ray study, conventional, 244

Y-cell(s), 164
Yoked pairs of extraocular muscles, 172

Zinc metabolism, 206
Zona incerta, 148f, 151, 152f